The RATIONALITY of IRRATIONALITY

Schizophrenia, Criminal Insanity and Neurosis

The Fallen Empires of Psychoanalysis,
Medical Models & Cognitive-Behavioral Theories

The RATIONALITY of IRRATIONALITY

Schizophrenia, Criminal Insanity and Neurosis

The Fallen Empires of Psychoanalysis, Medical Models & Cognitive-Behavioral Theories

Yacov Rofé & Yochay Rofé

Bar-Ilan University, Israel

World Scientific

NEW JERSEY • LONDON • SINGAPORE • BEIJING • SHANGHAI • HONG KONG • TAIPEI • CHENNAI • TOKYO

Published by

World Scientific Publishing Co. Pte. Ltd.
5 Toh Tuck Link, Singapore 596224
USA office: 27 Warren Street, Suite 401-402, Hackensack, NJ 07601
UK office: 57 Shelton Street, Covent Garden, London WC2H 9HE

British Library Cataloguing-in-Publication Data
A catalogue record for this book is available from the British Library.

THE RATIONALITY OF IRRATIONALITY
Schizophrenia, Criminal Insanity and Neurosis

ISBN 978-981-120-888-1

For any available supplementary material, please visit
https://www.worldscientific.com/worldscibooks/10.1142/11514#t=suppl

Typeset by Stallion Press
Email: enquiries@stallionpress.com

Contents

Acknowledgements

It is unusual to find an eminent scholar willing to support a theory that contradicts the conclusions of much of the scientific research conducted over the past century regarding the underlying causes of mad behaviors. I therefore owe a deep debt of gratitude to Professor Robert Aumann, laureate of the 2005 Nobel Prize in economics, for his courageous support of Psycho-Bizarreness Theory.

In addition, I deeply appreciate the support of Professor Kalman J. Kaplan of the Department of Psychiatry at the University of Illinois College of Medicine. He has published numerous studies in various areas of psychopathology, schizophrenia, and suicide. Dr. Kaplan's rejection of the deterministic disease-models of modern psychopathology is consistent with Psycho-Bizarreness Theory's claim that madness is a decision which individuals make in accordance with their evaluation of the current reality demands, rather than a condition that has been inflicted upon them.

I would also like to express my appreciation to three distinguished psychologists who endorsed this book and expressed their support for Psycho-Bizarreness Theory. Professor Daniel Algom of Tel-Aviv University; Professor Yuval Wolf, former Dean of the Faculty of Social Sciences at Bar-Ilan University; and Professor Aharon Tziner, former Dean of the Faculty of Behavioral Sciences at Netanya Academic College, Israel.

Special thanks go to Professor Leonard Weller, former Dean of the Faculty of Social Sciences at Bar-Ilan University, for his thoughtful comments on my work.

I would like to extend my heartfelt gratitude to Professor Joseph Deutsch, Dean of the Faculty of Social Sciences, and to Mr. Shmuel Amrani, Head of Administration, Faculty of Social Sciences, Bar-Ilan University, for recommending my work to the Moshe Schnitzer Foundation for Research on the Israeli Economy and Society at Bar-Ilan University.

Yochay Rofé, co-author of this book and of two articles, discussing conversion disorder (Rofé & Rofé, 2013) and fear and phobia (Rofé & Rofé, 2015) from the perspective of the new theory. He was introduced to the theory when he attended my course on psychopathology at Bar-Ilan, while studying for his a master's degree public health (MPH). His experience as an assistant lecturer at Bar-Ilan University and as a medical student at Tel-Aviv University qualified him as a scientist and researcher with the means and tools to develop the theory's insights — against prevailing opinion within the scientific community. I am blessed to have such a talented son.

Finally, I wish to express my deepest love and appreciation to my eldest son Yoav, whose suggestions greatly improved the new theory; to my beloved daughter Esti, an exceptionally talented musician; and to the light of my life, my dear wife, Sara, for her encouragement and support.

Preface

This book has six fundamental objectives which are essential for a new genuine understanding of the development and treatment of psychological disorders.

The first objective is to demonstrate the belief that schizophrenia is a brain disease, like Parkinson's disease, Alzheimer's disease and multiple sclerosis — an idea which has been universally accepted for more than a century — is completely wrong. Unfortunately, this theory, which in recent years has expanded to include nearly all types of behavioral disorders, has motivated the development of appalling treatments, such as lobotomy, electroconvulsive therapy and shock insulin therapy. Even today's antipsychotic drugs, widely considered a boon of modern medicine, come with an array of serious harmful effects, including cardiovascular disease, Alzheimer's disease and even death when administered over extended periods of time, as is typical with schizophrenic patients. What's more, the brain-disease theory continues to prevail despite significant empirical data refuting its validity. Examples of such data include the significant percentage of schizophrenic patients who display no brain abnormalities; the failure to identify neurological defect specific to schizophrenia; and the many patients who recover from this disorder without pharmacological intervention.

While each of the above data should have been enough to overthrow the disease concept of schizophrenia, this theory continues to prevail because of: 1) the significant correlations between schizophrenia and genetic defects or brain impairments; 2) the inability of traditional psychological theories to explain this data, which led to sustained hopes that the biological mechanisms of schizophrenia will be discovered in the near future. Accordingly, in an effort to eradicate this pseudo-scientific belief, this book presents a new theory of psychopathology that both explains these correlational studies in psychological terms and resolves the many fundamental problems that have plagued the disease model of schizophrenia.

The second objective of this book is to show that that despite the complete failure of psychoanalysis, Freud made an invaluable contribution to psychopathology in his exceptional clinical intuition that all mad behaviors share a similar etiology. Medical models have seemingly succeeded disproving this assumption by attributing schizophrenia to genetic defects and neurological impairments, based on the above correlational studies. Additional challenges to psychoanalysis were presented by research which refuted Freud's notion of symptom substitution and by cognitive-behavior theories whose therapeutic methods proved to be more effective than psychoanalysis for behavioral disorders, such as obsessive-compulsive disorder (OCD), conversion disorder, panic disorder and agoraphobia. Numerous studies refuting the existence of repression, which constitutes the most important concept of psychoanalysis, served to invalidate this theory completely. Nevertheless, these data do not necessarily refute Freud's underlying idea that all mad behaviors share a common etiology. In fact, this idea constitutes the core assumption of the new theory presented in this book and the key to the understanding mad behaviors. But while Freud attributed the cause of madness to childhood traumas, this new theory makes the revolutionary claim, supported by a significant amount of research and clinical data, that madness is a direct result of stress (which itself may be the consequence of environmental, psychological or neurological factors).

The third objective of this book concerns the axiomatic assumption, common to all psychopathological theories, that behavioral disorders are controlled by irrational mechanisms. The theory presented in this book views this assumption as the root of the bitter dispute among theories of psychopathology, which have remained unchanged since the beginning of the previous century. Accordingly, this book aims to demonstrate that a breakthrough in resolving this theoretical deadlock can be obtained only by abandoning this assumption in favor of its antithesis: madness is a rational coping mechanism which individuals intuitively choose when confronted with intolerable levels of stress.

Another fundamental principle of the new theory, which is necessary for the understanding of behavioral disorders, is that mad behaviors are akin to an economic product which individuals may "purchase": patients choose a specific madness from a virtual market of potential disorders in accordance with their unique psychological needs, when they intuitively feel that it will enable them to overcome their stress. The main goal of this "purchase" is repression, defined as a deliberate distraction from a given stressor, as suggested by Freud in his original version of this concept. However, while Freud and his followers argued that repression causes madness, the new theory makes the opposite claim: patients intuitively choose a specific madness in order to block the accessibility of stress-related thoughts. Hence, contrary to psychoanalytic doctrine, the new theory states that madness causes repression, rather than vice versa.

The specific mad behavior must also increase patients' control over the stressor and/or provides some social privileges, such as sympathy or monitory rewards. Moreover, like consumer decision-making processes, the choice of a specific symptom is determined by the availability of this behavior in the individual's memory store, which in turn is affected by various channels of information (e.g., mass media, family, peer group and suggestions). Another principle that affects this choice is cost-benefit considerations: The specific mad behavior will only be adopted if the individual intuitively feels that it can effectively reduce his or her emotional distress.

The fourth objective of this book is to provide operational criteria that will enable the diagnosis bizarre behaviors or madness, which Freud categorized as neurosis and psychosis. In its first two editions, the Diagnostic Statistical Manual of Mental Disorders (DSM), the world's most prominent diagnostic system, excluded psychoses from the list of psychological disorders. This decision was made following a large number of studies suggesting that psychoses are actually brain diseases, rather than psychological disorders. Later, with the scientific deterioration of psychoanalysis, the DSM-III and succeeding editions chose to remove neurosis as well, denying that the behavioral disorders classified in this category (e.g., panic disorder, agoraphobia, OCD, anorexia nervosa and dissociative-identity disorder) share common characteristics. In doing so, the DSM completely removed madness as a legitimate scientific category.

While a growing number of investigators have harshly criticized the DSM, none have addressed the DSM's assertion that neuroses lacks common characteristics which separate them from other deviant behaviors. The new theory challenges this claim by providing five major and two secondary criteria, which enable us to classify both neuroses and psychoses into one diagnostic category, as originally suggested by Freud.

The fifth objective of this book is to show that the new theory is able to integrate within its theoretical framework all therapeutic methods pertaining to schizophrenia and neuroses, including psychoanalytic, cognitive-behavioral, religious, placebo and drug therapies. This achievement, which none of the traditional theories could obtain despite significant efforts, became possible largely because of the new theory's re-conception of unawareness. According to this model, patients become unaware of the conscious adoption and maintenance of their mad behaviors through a set of cognitive processes that lead patients to believe that such behaviors are beyond their conscious control. This new conception of unawareness resolves several fundamental controversies in psychopathology relating to conversion disorder, dissociative-identity disorder, panic disorder and agoraphobia.

The sixth and final objective of this book is to redefine the diagnosis and etiology of criminal insanity, as well as, the liability for punishment. Currently, there exist no objective measure for the diagnosis of criminal insanity, and a diagnosis is generally determined by the subjective evaluation of psychiatrists. Furthermore, theories of psychopathology, including both psychoanalysis and medical models, view such people as suffering from either mental illness or brain disease and thus exonerate them from, at the very least, conscious responsibility for their criminal acts. The new theory presented in this book applies the same criteria used for the diagnosis of madness to the diagnosis of criminal insanity. It argues that these individuals commit their criminal acts deliberately for selfish purposes, such as the inflation of their self–esteem and fame, enabling them to relieve their emotional distress. Accordingly, they ought to be held fully responsible for their actions by the justice system.

In conclusion, it would seem that none of the traditional theories are able to account for the development of psychological disorders or for the mechanisms controlling therapeutic changes. Moreover, they are incapable of integrating the relevant research and clinical data within a single theoretical framework. Unfortunately, despite the tremendous amounts of resources expended over the last century by the scientific community in the effort to understand the mystery of psychological disorders, the result has been a failure. The theory proposed in this book outlines a path for psychopathology that promises to finally open the door to a new, comprehensive understanding of these disorders.

Introduction

The Need for a New Theory of Psychopathology

The Scientific Collapse of Psychoanalysis

Despite extensive research throughout the last century, the underlying causes of schizophrenia and other types of bizarre behaviors remain a mystery. These behaviors appear senseless, disrupt the individual's daily life, and moreover, leave patients ignorant of the underlying causes of their dramatic behavioral change. The range of manifested behaviors is baffling as well. Two cases reviewed in this book involve the schizophrenic patients Theodore John Kaczynski and John F. Nash. Kaczynski, also known as the Unabomber, was a professor of mathematics at the University of California, Berkeley (Graysmith, 1996), and Nash was a Nobel Prize winning economist (Nasar, 1998). While the former became a serial killer, the latter displayed behaviors, which, though extremely bizarre, were not violent. What caused these two remarkably intelligent individuals, both supposedly suffering from the same illness, to display such dramatically disruptive and seemingly senseless behaviors, each in a radically different way?

This mystery is not restricted to schizophrenia. William Ellery Leonard (1927), for example, a poet, writer, and professor at the University of Wisconsin, experienced an intense panic attack upon seeing a freight train from a distance and subsequently displayed agoraphobic symptoms, preventing him from leaving his home. Why did a freight train suddenly cause Leonard such an extreme level of anxiety? Why did this panic attack subsequently evolve into agoraphobia? Is there any common denominator between Leonard's behavior and those of Kaczynski and Nash?

Other cases of madness reviewed in this book include **filicidal mothers**, who claim to have heard voices instructing them to kill their children (Valenca, Mendlowicz, Nascimento, & Nardi (2011); patients with **dissociative identity disorder** (DID), previously termed multiple personality disorder, some of whom commit burglary, kidnapping, murder, or rape (e.g., Behnke, 1997; Dinwiddie, North, & Yutzy, 1993; James, 1998; Nakic & Thomas, 2012; Perr, 1991; Saks & Behanke, 1997; Steinberg, Garver, Moeller et al., 1993); and patients suffering from **obsessive neurosis**, which causes them to experience extremely hostile obsessive thoughts, such as those of one mother who confesses, "I'm having terrible thoughts about stabbing my children (crying). That's terrible – isn't it? I've been having thoughts of hurting others too... I love my kids. How could I have these horrible thoughts of hurting them?" (McAndrew, 1989, p. 312, 316). Like schizophrenia, these behaviors come across as senseless, severely disruptive, and the seemingly contrary to the individual's conscious intentions.

Until now, psychoanalysis was the only theory that made the explanation of bizarre behaviors the focus of its inquiry (see Emmelkamp, 1982; Searle, 1992; Shevrin & Dickman, 1980; Woody, 2003). The inability of patients to explain the underlying causes of their dramatic, behavioral changes and their failure to exercise control over these behaviors led Sigmund Freud to believe that these psychological disorders must be controlled by irrational mechanisms, which are beyond the conscious mind. As noted by Shevrin and Dickman (1980), "the clinical phenomena that led to the assumption of unconscious processes often takes the form of a patient describing a bothersome condition that the patient can neither account for nor control" (p. 422). Similarly, Woody (2003) noted that "the unconscious is invoked to explain behavior that is remarkable or portentous and inscrutable: actions and thoughts that seem otherwise inexplicable — bizarre behavior ... " (p. 190). Likewise, Emmelkamp (1982) noted, in reference to several examples of bizarre behavioral deviations, "although there is little empirical support for the psychoanalytic point of view … one cannot help but be impressed by some of the clinical observations [of bizarre behaviors] … made by psychoanalysts, especially by Freud and Fenichel" (p. 181).

Freud classified moderate levels of bizarre behaviors in which there was no indication of detachment from reality, such as panic disorder, obsessive-compulsive disorder (OCD), conversion disorder, dissociative-identity disorder (DID), and anorexia nervosa, as **neurosis**. In contrast, extreme levels of bizarre behaviors, where patients displayed severe distortion of reality, manifested by hallucinations, delusions, and disorganized speech, as is typically observed in schizophrenia, were categorized as **psychosis**. The senseless nature of these behaviors led Freud, and the entire scientific community in this field, to believe they were controlled by irrational mechanisms. Furthermore, since there were no extant factors that could justify the radical change in patients' behaviors, they were attributed by Freud and his followers to repressed childhood traumas or psychological conflicts, which under certain stressful conditions trigger the unconscious to take over and disrupt the individual's daily functioning.

However, two major problems challenge the validity of the psychoanalytic theory. One problem concerns the inability of psychoanalysis to account for the significant relationship between schizophrenia — the most extreme level of bizarre behaviors — and genetic/neurological flaws (e.g., Mistry, Harrison, Smith et al., 2018; Neelam, Garg, & Marshall, 2011; Sakamoto, & Crowley, 2018). As noted by Willick (2002),

> there is perhaps no better example of a psychoanalytic theory that has turned out to be incorrect than the once prevalent theory regarding the etiology of schizophrenia. This theory, or perhaps I should say conviction, about the cause of schizophrenia had three components. It was believed, first, that the damage to the ego and its functioning took place primarily

> in the first one or two years of life; second, that the major cause was to be found in profoundly inadequate caretaking; and, third, that in most cases there was no fundamental organic process responsible for the illness (p. 28).

The second problem relates to numerous studies that refute the existence of repression, the "cornerstone on which the whole structure of psychoanalysis rests" (Freud, 1914, p. 16). Contrary to Freud's concept of repression, numerous studies have found that people tend to remember their traumatic experiences (see reviews by McNally, Clancy, & Barrett, 2004; Piper, Lillevik, & Kritzer, 2008). Even so, advocates of psychoanalysis have claimed that repression does exist, as some studies have reported that trauma does indeed impair memory (e.g., Brown, Scheflin, & Whitfield, 1999; Cheit, 1998; Chu, Frey, Ganzel, & Matthews, 1999). Similar to religious sect, proponents refused to abandon Freud's theory despite the fact that careful examination of studies, seemingly supporting Freudian repression, have revealed serious methodological problems (e.g., see McNally, Clancy, & Barrett, 2004; Piper, Pope, & Borowiecki, 2000).

In an attempt to reconcile this theoretical dispute, Erdelyi (2006) claimed that Freud defined repression as a conscious and deliberate forgetting, a statement based on a significant number of studies. However, researchers have harshly criticized this conceptualization of repression. McNally (2006), for example, noted that by restricting repression to deliberate forgetting, Erdelyi "deprives it of its distinctive psychoanalytic character … Freud did not earn his reputation as a bold and original thinker by blandly affirming that people sometimes try not to think about unpleasant things" (p. 526; see also Bonanno, 2006; Crews, 2006; Kihlstrom, 2006; Macmillan, 2006).

In 2008, Rofé attempted to resolve the theoretical conflicts and further debunk Freud's theory by showing that studies not only refuted Freud's claim that people tend to forget trauma, but also questioned four additional components of Freudian repression that are necessary for the validation of this concept. These include (1) the existence of an autonomous unconscious entity, which supposedly preserves the repressed traumas for an indefinite period of time and controls the manifestation of the resulting bizarre behaviors; (2) the assumption that repression has a pathogenic effect upon the individual's physiological and psychological systems as it prevents a discharge of harmful tension and causes an inaccurate perception of reality; (3) the suggestion that repressed childhood trauma is the cause of neurotic disorders; and (4) the claim that the lifting of repression is a necessary condition for a genuine recovery. A thorough review of the literature reveals that none of the Freudian components of repression elicit empirical support. Accordingly, Rofé (2008) concluded that "the Freudian notion of repression cannot be used as a scientific psychological concept, as its empirical status precludes this possibility" (p. 76). These findings indicate that Freud's theory failed not only in explaining schizophrenia but neuroses as well. Thus, as noted by Bornstein (2001), "psychoanalysis remains a paradox — one of the 20th century's great intellectual achievements and at the same time one of its most resounding scientific failures" (p. 17). Similarly, Kihlsrom (2015), one of the leading cognitive investigators, arrived to conclusion that "from a scientific point of view, classical Freudian psychoanalysis is dead as both a theory of the mind and a mode of therapy."

The poor scientific state of psychoanalysis, along with a lack of better psychological explanations, has reinforced the conviction that bizarre behavioral disorders must be the consequence of brain impairments. Accordingly, advocates of medical models decried the possibility that an alternative psychological theory would be able to explain bizarre behaviors using one set of theoretical concepts. As noted by Wakefield (1999),

> a parsimonious theory of all such breakdowns is highly unlikely. Previous claims to have formulated general

> theories of the etiology of all mental disorders — from the sexual theory of the neuroses to irrational ideas to operant conditioning — have consistently proven unsatisfactory and degenerated into ideologies masked as scientific theories (p. 969).

Inadequacy of Medical Models

When one examines the history of the belief that mental disorders are the consequence of brain disease, as Harrington (2019) has recently done, it is astonishing to find that numerous researchers still refuse to abandon this belief in the face of repeated failures to demonstrate its validity. Despite lacking direct data to support their position, advocates of medical models in the 1980's (e.g., Andreasen, 1985) took advantage of developments in neuroscience, genetics, and psychopharmacology, along with the inability of traditional psychological theories to explain these findings, in order "to overthrow the Freudian and to bring back the brain as the primary object of psychiatric research, diagnosis, and treatment. It was a simple explanatory story, one with clear heroes and villains, and above all a satisfactory a happy ending" (Harrington, 2019, p. xiv). The ultimate scientific collapse of psychoanalysis, along with neurological impairments observed among patients suffering behavioral disorders, and the supposed efficacy of psychiatric drugs, was seen as robust evidence of the neurological origin of such disorders.

However, this book aims to demonstrate that the belief that schizophrenia and other types of bizarre behaviors, such as those listed above, are a brain disease is misguided. Moreover, though there is little question regarding the scientific failure of psychoanalysis, Freud's basic assumption that bizarre behaviors share the same diagnostic criteria and etiology is in fact a contribution and prerequisite for the understanding of bizarre behaviors. This idea strongly contradicts medical models' view that behavioral disorders are neurological diseases, as it is medically impossible that a variety of diseases with completely different symptoms will share the same etiology. Medical models partly succeeded in dismantling Freud's theoretical assumption on this matter, at the beginning of the last century, when they led the scientific community to believe that schizophrenia is a brain disease. Their second, far-reaching pseudo-victory, which has altogether buried Freud's contribution in this matter, has occurred in more recent years with their growing political power in the American Psychiatric Association, following the scientific deterioration of psychoanalysis. Advocates of these models have utilized this opportunity to eradicate Freud's diagnostic category of neuroses from the Diagnostic Statistical Manual (DSM), the most influential diagnostic reference in the world. The DSM's task force arrived at the conclusion that "there is no group of conditions which together comprise 'neurosis'" (American Psychiatric Association, 1976, p. 11; see also Bayer & Spitzer, 1985), without objectively examining the scientific validity of this claim. Moreover, although the DSM's task force claimed to be theoretically neutral, in reality, medical models implicitly determined its categories (e.g., Burstow, 2005; Follette & Houts, 1996; Pilecki, Clegg, & McKay, 2011). As a result, the DSM has become, in fact, a medical book, where psychological disorders are categorized as neurological diseases (see Grinker, 2010; Warelow & Holmes, 2011), as opposed to the DSM-I (American Psychiatric Association, 1952) and DSM-II (American Psychiatric Association, 1968) which were based on Freud's diagnostic categories. Not only has researchers undermined the scientific credibility of the DSM, but the American Psychiatric Association has been accused for behaving

> very much like a corporation seeking profit and influence rather than a scientific organization charged with the crucially important task of defining mental disorders. Some have argued that the motivations of the APA are not scientific but primarily financial...Rather than engaging with the scholarly criticisms of the DSM-5 and mounting a credible defense of their scientific

> work, the APA worked to suppress critical discussion... This led Gary Greenberg to compare the APA to "bumbling Kremlin bureaucrats" — and to question whether a private guild with close ties to the pharmaceutical industry should be entrusted by the public to create the diagnostic manual used by all helping professions (Lacasse, 2014, p. 5).

This book aims to demonstrate that the idea that behavioral disorders are brain diseases lacks scientific validity, not only regarding neuroses, but regarding schizophrenia as well. The reason psychoanalysis lost the battle against medical models was not because Freud's idea of bizarreness was wrong. Rather, this was the result of other issues, such as the lack of empirical support for the notion that these disorders are the consequence of childhood repressed trauma and the inability of psychoanalysis to explain the neurological data, which seemingly support the disease conception of behavioral disorders. The lack of an adequate psychological theory that could validate Freud's vision, enabled medical models not only to maintain their century-old misleading belief that schizophrenia is a brain disease, but expand this conviction to neuroses as well. The following five areas of research demonstrate the problematic state of this theory and thc urgent need for an alternative theoretical approach. Not only are all these data able to disprove the idea of brain disease, but each of them is sufficient on their own to invalidate this theory.

1. Lack of Evidence of a Specific Brain Abnormality: Despite intensive research, the disease model of schizophrenia still lacks empirical validation. Williams (2012) notes, in his book Rethinking Madness, that proponents of the disease model hypothesis have been forced to admit that no clear evidence has been found of a biochemical imbalance that is consistently associated with schizophrenia. Similarly, Burley and his colleagues (2015) note that, while many neurological variables are "seen in many schizophrenic individuals, there is no one neurological marker seen consistently across patients" (p. 32; see also Harrington, 2019; Whitker, 2015; Pies, 2011).

2. Schizophrenia in the Absence of Brain Abnormality: The majority of those diagnosed with schizophrenia show no neuro-pathological or biochemical abnormalities. Moreover, the same bio-physiological abnormalities found in some patients diagnosed with schizophrenia can be found in individuals who do not suffer from the disorder (see also Boyle, 2002; Siebert, 2000). As noted by Williams (2012), in his extensive review of the literature, "the majority of patients diagnosed with schizophrenia do not show brain abnormalities at all...while a number of healthy subjects do" (p. 26; see also Whitaker, 2010). Furthermore, findings refute the myth that schizophrenic symptoms are the consequence of progressive brain impairments, as originally assumed by Kraepelin (see review by Zipursky, Reilly & Murray, 2013). In fact, adverse neuro-anatomical changes do not necessarily precede the development of schizophrenia, but may occur over the course of this disorder (e.g., Guo, Palaniyappan, Liddle et al., 2016). These changes may be the result of adverse effects of antipsychotic drugs, substance abuse, low physical activity and stress (e.g., Fusar-Poli, Smieskova, Kempton et al., 2013; Keedy, Reilly, Bishop, Weiden et al., 2015; Torres, Portera-Olivera, Borgwardt et al., 2013; Williams, 2012; Zipursky et al., 2013), and not necessarily the effect of genetic factors.

3. Inability to Explain Heterogeneity of Symptoms: Medical models are unable to explain how the same disease can cause extreme differences in symptomatology within a specific behavioral disorder. This claim is valid not only for schizophrenia, but also for neurotic disorders, which neurologists now attribute to neurological impairments. For example, in recent years, advocates of these models have attributed the cause of conversion disorder, in which individuals display physical disabilities (e.g., paralysis, blindness, psychogenic movements and epilepsy) in the absence of neurological defect, to abnormal neurological activity (e.g., Stone, LaFrance, Brown et al., 2011). However, medical models are not only unable to explain how the large variability of symptoms occurs, they cannot even explain how neurological defects could cause these symptoms.

4. Recovery Through Psychotherapy: Many schizophrenic patients completely recover from their "neurological disease" purely through psychological intervention (see Bradshaw, 1998; Karon, 2008; Mackler, 2014; Siebert, 2000; Whitaker, 2010; Williams, 2012). Given the irreversibility of neurological damage, it is difficult to see how these results are compatible with the idea of brain disease. As noted by Siebert (1999) "psychotherapy and milieu therapy, without medications, have led even the most severely disrupted individuals with schizophrenia to full recovery and beyond. Many people diagnosed with schizophrenia have recovered on their own without any treatment, something never accomplished by a person with Parkinson's Alzheimer's, or multiple sclerosis" (p. 179). Similarly, Siebert (2000), notes in reference to the rapid spontaneous recovery of a young women diagnosed with paranoid schizophrenia, that "this incident and questions raised about psychiatric practices suggest that something is seriously wrong with psychiatry" (p. 34). Similar claims can be applied to neurotic disorders, such as conversion disorder, which as stated above neurologists have ascribed to brain abnormality. It is difficult to see how medical models can explain how psychological and religious therapy often result in full recovery from this disorder (see a review by Rofé & Rofé, 2013).

5. Drugs Hinder Recovery: Studies reviewed by Whitaker (2010) reveal that while nearly two thirds of schizophrenic patients in undeveloped countries (e.g., Agra, India, Nigeria, and Columbia) had good outcomes, and slightly more than one-third had become chronically ill, in wealthier countries only 37% of patients had good outcome and 59% became chronically ill. While only 16% of patients in the poor countries regularly took antipsychotics, 61% did so in the developed countries. In Agra and India, where the recovery rate was highest, only 3% used medication, whereas patients in Moscow displayed the lowest recovery rates but the highest usage of medications. Williams (2012), concluded in summarizing relevant findings that "the long-term use of antipsychotics increases the likelihood of the development of a chronic psychotic condition and significantly reduces the likelihood of recovery, as well as carrying the high likelihood of causing other serious physical, cognitive, and emotional impairments" (p. 58, see also Whitaker, 2015).

Medical models, and in fact all traditional theories of psychopathology including psychoanalysis, are unable to explain several fundamental issues associated with neurosis. These include

1) *The dramatic increase in the prevalence both of eating disorders* (e.g., Lucas, Beard, O'Fallon, & Kurland, 1991; Mitchell & Eckert, 1987; Willi, Giacometti, & Limacher, 1990), and of *Dissociative Identity Disorder (DID)* (e.g., Lilienfeld Kirsch, Sarbin, Lynn et al., 1999; Mai, 1995; Merskey, 1995; North, Ryall, Ricci, & Wetzel, 1993) in recent years;

2) *The fact that these increases have been restricted to Western societies and that Westernization through mass media affected the increase rates of these disorders in non-Western countries* (e.g., Bhadrinath, 1990; Keel & Klump, 2003; King, 1993; Pate, Pumariega, Hester, & Garner, 1992);

3) *Data indicating that nearly all neurotic disorders are more prevalent among females, as opposed to schizophrenia, which is more prevalent among males* (see review by Rofé, 2000, and studies reviewed in this book). Although gender differences are found in a variety of physiological diseases, this explanation is not sufficient as long as advocates of medical models present no direct evidence demonstrating that these differences are linked to gender-based neurological differences (e.g., see Keynejad, Carson, David, & Nicholson, 2017).

It is also worthwhile to recall the following remarks of Thomam Insel, director of the National Institute of Mental Health (NIMH), in 2013

> Thirty years after the biological psychiatrists declared victory, all of psychiatry's diagnostic categories were still

> based, not on any biological markers of disease, but merely 'on consensus about clusters of clinical symptoms'. In the rest of medicine... this would be 'equivalent to creating diagnostic systems based on the nature of chest pain or quality of fever' (Harrington, 2019, p. xvi; see also Frances, 2013).

The New Theory of Madness

Although the medical model of schizophrenia is confronted with serious difficulties, this theoretical position prevails mainly because no better explanation has been suggested. Accordingly, the main objective of this book is to suggest a new theory, Psycho-Bizarreness Theory, also known as The Intuitive Rational-Choice Theory of Madness, which can resolve the above problems, while taking into consideration those data which seemingly support the disease model of schizophrenia. It is important to emphasize that although the focus of the new theory is to demonstrate the inadequacy of medical models, it challenges the validity of all theories of psychopathology, including the conditioning (Bouton, Mineka, & Barlow, 2001; Mineka & Oehlberg, 2008) and cognitive (Clark, 1986, 1988) theories of panic disorder and agoraphobia, which are the dominant explanations of these disorders.

As will be specified in the discussion section of Part III, cognitive-behavioral theories suffer from various shortcomings, such as their inability to explain the extremely resistance to extinction of panic disorder despite many years of exposure to the feared stimuli, the fact that agoraphobia may developed in the absence of any anxiety-provoking event, the rarity of these disorders among children despite the fact that children are more prone to develop fears and phobias than adults, and the higher prevalence of these disorders among women than men. Furthermore, both theories are unable to explain bizarre phobia toward innocent stimuli, such as chocolate and train, which severely disrupt the daily functioning of those who suffer from these phobias. Another fundamental problem that challenges the validity of the conditioning-cognitive theories of panic disorder and agoraphobia is their inability to integrate each other's findings within their own theoretical framework (see review by Rofé & Rofé, 2015).

Overall, this book aims to show that the poor scientific state of traditional theories has come about mainly because of their common axiomatic assumption that behavioral disorders reflect mental or physical illnesses that stem from irrational processes or neurological impairments. In contrast, Psycho-Bizarreness Theory views these behaviors as economic products which individuals may choose to consume when they are confronted with extreme levels of stress. It makes no distinction between schizophrenia and other types of bizarre behaviors; and most importantly, promotes the antithesis of the traditional axiomatic assumption, i.e., that these behaviors are rational coping mechanisms which in fact improve the individual's quality of life. This radical theoretical assumption enables the new theory to integrate research and clinical data pertaining to the development and treatment of these disorders from all schools of thoughts, into one coherent theoretical system.

The Structure of This Book

This book consists of four parts, which discuss various aspects of Psycho-Bizarreness Theory. **Part I** presents the major concepts of Psycho-Bizarreness Theory. This includes the diagnostic criteria of mad behaviors, a new definition of repression, and principles that guide individuals to choose a specific mad behavior. It demonstrates that schizophrenia is a response to an intolerable level of stress and that the same theoretical concepts are applicable to criminal insanity and neurosis. It also shows the damaging effects of both antipsychotics and antidepressants, and the fact that psychotherapy can result in a complete recovery from schizophrenia. Although the latter issue mostly relates to Part III, which discusses therapy, it is discussed in Part I because supposed efficacy of drug treatment is part of the medical models' campaign to validate their theoretical position that schizophrenia is a brain disease.

Part II presents the complexity of self-deceptive processes by which patients become unaware of their involvement in the adoption and maintenance of mad behaviors. The new model of unawareness resolves several fundamental issues that are unaccounted for by rival theories. One such issue concerns the seemingly paradoxical coexistence of both unawareness of the underlying causes of mad behaviors and evidence indicating that patients have some conscious control over these behaviors. Another example is the lack of a satisfactory explanation for why some patients acknowledge their "illness," while others, such as those suffering from schizophrenia, anorexics, and OCD, deny that their behavior is deviant. In addition, the new model can resolve a number of fundamental theoretical conflicts, relating to conversion disorder, DID, panic disorder, and agoraphobia.

Part III discusses the mechanisms of therapeutic change from the standpoint of Psycho-Bizarreness Theory: What brings patients to abandon their maladaptive behaviors? This understanding enables the integration therapies pertaining to neuroses and schizophrenia, recommended by rival theories, into one coherent theoretical framework. Part III also suggests a new therapeutic intervention that may facilitate recovery. The essence of this intervention is to increase patients' awareness of the faulty coping mechanisms they are using and to help them develop more adequate coping behaviors.

Part IV is a general discussion that summarizes Psycho-Bizarreness Theory's main theoretical achievements and its practical implications.

This book is a scientific document that is based on a vast amount of research and clinical data, and is expected to make a revolutionary scientific impact in this field. Although the major target audience is professionals in mental health, it also addresses scholars who are interested in understanding the mysteries surrounding this field. The book has an important message for the justice system as well. The dominant conviction that serial killers like the Unabomber, DID patients, and filicidal mothers, who commit the most horrendous of crimes, may be "innocent due to insanity" must be abandoned. These behaviors, like madness in general, are goal-oriented deliberately adopted by people who have been confronted with intolerable level of stress. Accordingly, while their stressful conditions need to be taken into account, they should be punished similarly to sane criminals.

Part I

Psycho-Bizarreness Theory Versus Medical Models

Foundations of Psycho-Bizarreness Theory

Psycho-Bizarreness Theory (PBT) is not completely new. Earlier versions of this theory, along with significant research and clinical data, have been published in two books (Rofé, 1989, 2000). It has also received positive reviews in Psychiatric Services (Sarma & Garfield, 2001) and Contemporary Psychology (Lester, 2002). In recent articles PBT demonstrated its ability to integrate all therapeutic methods pertaining to neurosis into one theoretical framework (Rofé, 2010) and explains all data, including neurological findings, relevant to the development and treatment of conversion disorder (Rofé & Rofé, 2013). The new theory also resolves the theoretical confusion regarding the explanation of phobia by distinguishing between bizarre (e.g., agoraphobia and chocolate phobia) and non-bizarre phobia, such as dog phobia (Rofé & Rofé, 2015). In more recent article empirical diagnostic criteria were provided for distinguishing between bizarre behaviors, consisting of neuroses and psychoses, and non-bizarre behaviors, which challenge the decision to exclude neuroses from DSM (Rofé, 2016). The main concepts of this theory are presented below.

Diagnostic Criteria of Madness

As mentioned above, one of the major problems with Freud's theory is that it does not allow for empirical criteria that can effectively distinguish bizarre behaviors from non-bizarre behaviors (e.g., Bayer & Spizer, 1985; Millon, 1983, 1986). Accordingly, providing a clear, empirical definition of these criteria is a prerequisite for the acceptance of PBT's claim that schizophrenia is the most extreme form of madness which shares the same etiology as other types of mad behaviors. To this end, a significant amount of clinical and research evidence, which was overlooked by the DSM's task force when it made the decision to exclude neurosis from the DSM, as well as a recent study (Rofé, 2016), indicates that both neuroses and psychoses, are multidimensional concepts that share five major and two secondary criteria. Usually, all the five major criteria must be present for the classification of a given behavior to be categorized as bizarre. The secondary criteria are two characteristics that are not necessary to diagnose bizarre behavior, but may be important in some exceptional cases, as will be clarified below.

Major Criteria

Criterion 1: Mad behaviors intensively preoccupy the individual and severely disrupt their daily functioning. For example, obsessive-compulsive disorder (OCD) is a time-consuming disorder that occupies an individual for more than one hour a day, significantly interfering with his or her daily functioning (American Psychiatric Association, 2000; Rofé, 2000, pp. 98–115). Similarly, 49% of eating disorder patients spend more than 3 hours each day on their eating rituals and 16% spend over 8 hours (Sunday, Halmi, & Einhorn, 1995). Similar data can be observed with all forms of neuroses and psychoses. Mad behaviors also place a burden on the family, community, and society in general.

Criterion 2: The individual displays dramatic and spontaneous behavioral changes in the absence of a specific event that is uniquely linked with this shift and has been unquestionably proven as its cause. For example, a variety of **obsessive-compulsive rituals** (Rachman & Hodgson, 1980; Samuels et al., 2002) and **conversion symptoms** (e.g., see Blanchard & Hersen, 1976; Brady & Lind, 1961; Fukunishi et al., 2001; Griffiths & Ellis, 2007; Prüter, Kunert, & Hoff, 2001) occur in the absence of a unique factor or event (e.g., neurological, environmental, or social trigger) that is consistently associated with or definitively causes these dramatic behavioral changes. In some cases, the onset may be gradual, such as with **conversion disorder** (e.g., Akdemir & Ünal, 2006; American Psychiatric Association, 2000; Stone,

Warlow, & Sharpe, 2012; Wittkower, Rodger, Scott, & Semeonoff, 1941) and **anorexia nervosa**, which progressively deteriorate until reaching a dramatic point of radical change. However, there is no observable event that is exclusively associated with or can account for the progressive behavioral change.

Researchers often report findings that seem to indicate that a certain event is the cause of a given behavioral disorder. Such evidence, however, violates the criterion of spontaneous onset only if the event has been unequivocally proven as a sufficient condition for the development o f a specific disorder, or is exclusively associated with this disorder. To date, no such proof has been found for any of the neurotic or psychotic disorders. For example, although advocates of medical models have expressed no doubt that schizophrenia is a brain disease (e.g., see Wikllick, 2002), skeptics challenge the scientific basis of these models. As noted by Prendergast in reference to Williams' (2012) book *Rethinking Madness*, which challenges the disease explanation of schizophrenia, "after over 100 years and billions of dollars spent on research looking for schizophrenia and other related psychotic disorders in the brain, we still have not found any substantial evidence that these disorders are actually caused by a brain disease." Similarly, Robbins (2002) noted that

> despite research of an extent and duration, that has few if any parallel in medicine, no neurobiological defect or marker, or combination of markers, has yet been discovered that reliably distinguish schizophrenias from control subjects. (p. 311; see also Boyle, 2002; Moncrieff, 2014; Siebert, 1999)

Criterion 3: Bizarre behaviors are extremely rare, apparently due to the considerable social embarrassment and impediment of daily functioning generated by such behaviors. Based on relevant data regarding psychological disorders, the prevalence of these behaviors in the general population is usually lower than 3% (American Psychiatric Association, 2000).

Criterion 4: The individual is unaware of the underlying causes of the behavioral change. This criterion is based on a substantial amount of clinical data, which led Freud to attribute these behaviors to the unconscious mind.

Criterion 5: Bizarre behaviors are stigmatized as mental or physical illness and people often refer to them as simply as “|weird” or “unusual.” As noted by Carson, Butcher, and Coleman (1988) “almost by definition … abnormal behavior is behavior that is *unintelligible* to the vast majority of persons observing it” (p. 17). Similarly, Bandura (1969) states, “the designation of behavior as pathological thus involves social judgments … Consequently, the *appropriateness* of symbolic, affective, or social responses to given situations constitutes one major criterion in labeling ‘symptomatic’ behavior” (p. 3). Indeed, neurotic and psychotic disorders are perceived by the medical community as a form of mental illness (e.g., American Psychiatric Association, 2000).

Secondary Criteria

The two secondary criteria are stress and depression. These criteria can be used to exclude some exceptional deviant behaviors that seem to meet the five major criteria, but whose onset is not related to stress or depression. For example, while one may argue that autism meets the five major criteria, its onset is definitely not associated with stress or depression. Secondary criteria can also be used to avoid incorrect diagnoses when a behavior fulfills only four of the major criteria, such as in criminal cases, which the current diagnostic approach sometimes misidentifies as normal criminal behavior instead of criminal insanity.

Differential Diagnosis

PBT’s criteria enable us to distinguish between neuroses and psychoses. Although both meet all these criteria, in psychoses their effects are more pronounced in four of the five criteria. Therefore, in psychoses (1) the patient's attention is more intensively preoccupied; (2) there is a lower prevalence rate; (3) patients are not only unaware of the underlying causes of their behaviors but are usually unaware that their behaviors are deviant; and (4) patients are more socially stigmatized. Additionally, psychotic symptoms are qualitatively different from neurotic behaviors, as only psychotic patients display hallucinations, delusions, and disorganized speech. Non-Bizarre ***behaviors*** fulfill either none of PBT's five major criteria (e.g., dentist's phobia) or fewer than five (e.g., posttraumatic stress disorder [PTSD]).

To further examine PBT's diagnostic criteria, a new study was conducted (see Rofé, 2016). A total of 15 psychiatrists and 50 clinical psychologists completed a questionnaire in which they were asked to evaluate 12 randomly arranged deviant behaviors, on each of PBT's major criteria of bizarreness (e.g., to what extent does each of the deviant behaviors occupy people who suffer from them; to what extent is the individual unaware of the underlying causes of his/her behavioral change), on a scale of 1–7. The deviant behaviors consisted of neurotic and psychotic disorders (e.g., agoraphobia, OCD, conversion disorder, schizophrenia) and other forms of deviant behaviors (e.g., flight phobia and PTSD). Findings revealed that neurosis and psychosis are the only disorders that meet all five of the criteria, compared to specific phobias that met none. Psychosis scored significantly higher on all five of the criteria when compared to neurosis. PTSD only met the first criterion (the disorder intensively preoccupies the patients' attention).

Thus, PBT makes a sharp distinction between bizarre behaviors, that is, those behaviors that meet the five major criteria, such as schizophrenia, criminal insanity and neuroses, and non-bizarre behaviors, such as PTSD, depression, normal criminal behaviors, and simple phobias. PBT is limited to the explanation of bizarre behaviors; non-bizarre behaviors need to be explained by different theoretical concepts.

Numerous clinical examples reviewed in this book, particularly in Part I (see also Rofé, 2000), strongly support PBT's diagnostic criteria. This diagnostic approach is consistent with Freud's original classification, which dominated the first two editions of the *DSM* (American Psychiatric Association, 1952, 1968). PBT's diagnostic approach is more accurate than the *DSM's* anti-Freudian diagnostic approach, which was based on the consensus of one group of experts who were theoretically biased toward the medical model and may have been motivated by personal interests (e.g., Burstow, 2005; Follette & Houts, 1996; Pilecki, Clegg, & McKay, 2011). Most importantly, these diagnostic criteria are strongly linked with a theory that accounts for both the etiology of relevant behaviors and the processes by which they are developed, as will be demonstrated later on. As noted by Follette and Houts (1996) "without a theory categories proliferate, any atheoretical system will eventually fall of its own weight as will classification systems that are based on inadequate theory" (p. 1122; see also Grinker, 2010; Pilecki et al., 2011).

Etiology

PBT's basic assumption is that bizarre behaviors are a response to extreme levels of stress, which exceed the individual's coping abilities. Stress is defined as a situation that results in an inconvenient emotional state, regardless of whether its source is environmental, psychological, or neurological. These triggers includes stressful life-events, social rejection, low self-esteem, unacceptable impulses, and coping abilities deficits which may be result of brain impairments or inadequate social development. Historical traumas, such as child abuse or parental loss, are considered stressful if they exert negative emotional distress on the individual's current experiences.

When individuals are confronted with intolerable levels of stress their behavioral options in handling the situation are limited. They will often choose to remain emotionally distressed, adopt drastic measures, such as suicide, substance abuse and aggression, and/or search for help or therapy. However, PBT's unique contribution to the understanding of people's reactions to intolerable levels of stress is that a minority of these people will unconsciously choose a particular mad behavior because it effectively meets their specific coping demands, as will be clarified later. Extreme intolerable emotional distress, particularly depression, must precede in order for individuals to consider the employment of mad behaviors. This is consistent with the fact that depression characterizes all types of neuroses (see review by Rofé, 2000, 2010) as well as psychoses (e.g., Ramírez, Arranz, Sanchez, Centeno, & San, 2006, Rofé, 2000; Whitehead, Moss, Cardno, & Lewis, 2003). Thus, unlike traditional theories of psychopathology, which view *anxiety* as the core of psychiatric disorders (e.g., Eysenck, 1976; Eysenck & Rachman, 1965; Freud, 1936/1963; 1926/1964), PBT considers *depression* to be the underlying motivational cause of madness. Even when patients display symptoms of anxiety, such as agoraphobia, panic disorder and OCD (which are traditionally viewed as anxiety disorders — *DSM-IV*, American Psychiatric Association, 1994), it is depression, rather than anxiety, which motivates the adoption and maintenance of these behaviors.

The idea that madness is a coping mechanism aimed primarily at alleviating an extremely unbearable level of depression is consistent with Guntrip's (1969) claim that "the psychoneuroses are, basically, defenses against internal bad-object situations which would otherwise set up depressive … states" (p. 23). Similarly, Zigler and Glick (1984) noted that "the psychic pain of dysphoric mood leads the depressive to employ coping mechanisms, which themselves may be maladaptive" (pp. 55–56). Accordingly, from their standpoint, paranoia and mania are "employed by individuals to ward off a breakthrough into consciousness of depressive thought and its accompanying painful affective concomitants" (p. 57).

Stress alone may not be sufficient to produce the extreme emotional distress needed in order to motivate people to consider the adoption of madness. Several additional factors affect the individual's response to a current stressor. These include ***genetic predisposition to depression and anxiety*** (e.g., see review by Bozorgmehr et al., 2018; Mistry, Harrison, Smith, Escott-Price, & Zammit, 2018; Routledge et al., 2017; Tennant, 2002), **lack of social support** (e.g., Martin & Brantley, 2004; Romanov, Varjonen, Krio, & Koskenvuo, 2003; Uchino et al., 2018), **poor coping abilities** (e.g., Kant, D'Zurilla, & Maydeu-Olivares, 1997), and **childhood trauma** (e.g., Bremner, Southwick, Johnson, Yehuda, & Charney, 1993; Yama, Tovey, & Fogas, 1993).

Repression

As with the concept of bizarreness and the notion that these behaviors have a common etiology, PBT preserve Freud's idea that repression is the key to understanding these behaviors, provided that this concept is radically changed in accordance with clinical and research data. As will be specified throughout this book, numerous case studies demonstrate that blocking the accessibility of stress-related thoughts is a major psychological need of schizophrenic, criminally insane, and neurotic patients. This evidence is consistent with Freud's clinical observations regarding the necessity of repression for the understanding of behavioral disorders. As noted by Freud (1914), in his vigorous attempt to defend repression

> If anyone should seek to regard the theory of repression and of resistance as assumptions instead of as results following from psychoanalysis, I shall oppose him most emphatically … the doctrine of repression is the outcome of psycho-analytic work, a theoretical inference legitimately drawn from innumerable observations. (p. 298)

However, while it would be a mistake to overlook Freud's clinical observations, it is equally anti-scientific to overlook the abundance of studies that refute the existence of Freudian repression as do psychoanalytic advocates (e.g., Boag, 2012, 2015). Therefore, PBT suggests abandoning the psychoanalytic concept of repression, as specified above, which differs from Freud's original idea (see review by Rofé, 2008). Repression needs to be restricted to the essence of this concept, defined by Freud (1915) as "turning something away and keeping it at a distance from the conscious" (p. 147). What's more, the unconscious was not a critical theme in Freud's original conception of repression. As noted by Erdelyi and Goldberg (1979) "in his very earliest writings (e.g., Freud, 1894/1962) repression was treated as a potentially conscious mechanism … at least at times, repression is a "conscious, deliberate act" (p. 365; see also Erdelyi, 2006). This statement is consistent with laboratory studies, which show that repression is nothing more than conscious distraction (see reviews by Holmes, 1974, 1990). Accordingly, *PBT defines repression as a coping mechanism by which the individual blocks the accessibility of stress-related thoughts through deliberate distractive means. Thus, while this new definition of repression preserves Freud's basic notion, which, as will be demonstrated, plays a vital role in understanding mad behaviors, it is not subject to the critique of studies which refute the existence of the psychoanalytic doctrine of repression* (e.g., McNally, Clancy, & Barrett, 2004; Piper, Lillevk, & Kritzer, 2008; Rofé, 2008).

However, in order for repression to facilitate our understanding of madness, two additional modifications of the Freudian concept must be made. First, according to psychoanalysis, repression is pathogenic as it exerts negative effects on the individual's daily adjustment and may cause psychophysiological illnesses and/or a large variety of behavioral disorders (e.g., Alexander, 1950; Dollard & Miller, 1950; Eagle, 2000; Fenichel, 1946; Freud, 1915a, 1926, 1936). In contrast, PBT's repression is beneficial to adjustment, as it blocks the accessibility of stress-related thoughts and encouraging positive thinking, and thereby relieving the individual's emotional distress. This claim is consistent with a significant amount of research showing that among the nonclinical population, repressive-avoidance strategies of threatening stimuli have no pathogenic impact and may even have positive emotional and behavioral effects (see review by Rofé, 2008). Second, in sharp contrast with psychoanalysis, *in PBT repression is the consequence rather than the cause of madness*. In other words, when facing stress that exceeds the individual's coping abilities, some people will *deliberately choose mad behaviors that heavily occupy their attention to the extent that they become unaware of their stressors*. The major benefit of this behavioral resolution is distraction: the patient's attention becomes so heavily preoccupied by the mad behavior that it can no longer access stress-related thoughts.

While bizarre behaviors can generate unawareness of the stressor, this coping strategy would have little distractive value if patients remained aware of their conscious involvement in the adoption of these behaviors. Accordingly, as will be discussed in Part II, PBT claims that the choice of a specific symptom is intuitive and made with little or no conscious awareness. The individual may intuitively feel that a certain unusual behavior, proposed by current or past experiences, is the most efficient possible reaction for relieving his or her intolerable emotional distress. Consequently, some people will spontaneously adopt such a behavior, resulting in immediate emotional relief, largely due to its high distractive value. Although the decision to implement the intuitive/unconscious choice is conscious, patients become unaware of the Knowledge of Self-Involvement (KSI) or the True Reason (TR) for acting bizarrely through a variety of cognitive processes that cause the forgetting of this information. Subsequently, patients develop a self-deceptive belief that attributes the cause of their symptoms to factors beyond their conscious control, and thus stabilizes the unawareness of KSI/TR (see Part II).

Choice of Symptoms

PBT claims that the selection of a specific madness is similar to the purchasing of a product. The choice of a specific mad behavior is determined by the same three principles that guide a consumer's decision-making process (e.g., see Wänke & Friese, 2005). The major principle that affects the choice of a specific madness is **controllability**: the specific mad behavior must not only block the accessibility of stress-related thoughts but also increase the patient's ability to exercise control over the stressor and\or provide social rewards. For example, in times of war, soldiers are likely to adopt conversion disorders, such as paralysis, blindness, or epilepsy, rather than anorexia nervosa. As noted by Dohrenwend and Dohrenwend (1969) regarding psychiatric symptoms developed by soldiers during World War II, "the patient's symptoms became his means to escape from further combat, and, not surprisingly, few recovered to the point where they could be returned to the front" (pp. 114–115). Similarly, as will be demonstrated later, people who blame themselves for their failures in coping with life's demands, and thereby suffer from low self-esteem, are likely to choose a mad behavior, such as schizophrenia, that can artificially inflate their self-esteem, rather than other types of madness.

The second guiding principle is **availability**. Similar to the consumer who chooses a product based on various channels of information available to him, the choice of a suitable mad behavior is affected by various factors that increase the individual's awareness of this behavior, such as the media, personal experiences, family, and peers (see Rofé, 2000). For example, clinical evidence suggests that subjects may utilize their current or past injuries or illnesses to develop a neurotic disorder that suits their coping needs, for instance conversion disorder (Rofé, 2000; Rofé & Rofé, 2013). Similarly, studies to be reviewed later demonstrate that mass media has played a significant role in the dramatic increase of eating disorders and dissociative-identity disorder (DID).

The third principle is net **cost-benefit analysis**, which states that a mad behavior will be chosen only if the individual intuitively feels that it can reduce his or her intolerable suffer. For example, as will be specified later, this principle can explain gender differences in the prevalence of neurotic disorders: men are less likely to adopt these disorders (e.g., agoraphobia and conversion disorder), both because of the higher social embarrassment and because they increase the risk of unemployment, which is more costly for men than women. Another example to be elaborated upon in Part III, are studies indicating that increasing the cost of the symptom (e.g., withdrawal of attention, monetary rewards and hospital privileges), motivates patients to abandon their deviant behavior (see also Rofé, 2010; Rofé & Rofé, 2013). However, the benefit patients derive from the bizarre behavior in combatting depression is so great that patients may be reluctant to abandon this behavior even when this may risk their life, as will be specified later when discussing the case study of the Unabomber.

Rationality Versus Irrationality

PBT's claim that madness is a rational behavior is to some extent consistent with both Freud's psychoanalytic theory and with Scottish existential psychiatrist, Robert Laing's (1964) approach to schizophrenia. As noted by Herbert Simon (1978), the late cognitive psychologist and Nobel Prize-winning economist

> It is perhaps … surprising to discover how pervasive assumptions of rationality are in psychoanalytic theory — confirming the suspicion that there is indeed method in madness … Almost all explanations of pathological behavior in the psychoanalytic literature … explain the patient's illness in terms of the functions it performs for him. (p. 3)

Similarly, Laing noted that

> the experience and behavior that gets labeled schizophrenic is a special sort of strategy that a person invents in order to live in an unlivable situation … the person has come to be placed

> in an untenable position. He cannot make a move … without being beset by contradictory pressures both internally, from himself, and externally, from those around him. He is, as it were, in a position of checkmate. (p. 187)

However, although Freud acknowledged that madness serves important psychological functions, primarily in reducing the patient's level of anxiety, he explicitly viewed bizarre behaviors as irrational. This is so mainly because these behaviors are attributed to childhood events, which are no longer relevant to current reality demands. Freud's conception of irrationality is most prominent in regard to schizophrenia, in which the Ego (i.e., the cognitive rational system that navigates the individual's responses to reality) ceases to function. Although Laing's suggestion is more congruent with PBT's idea of rationality, he provided no explanation as to how schizophrenic symptoms improve the patient's quality of life. Most importantly, he provided no comprehensive explanation of the cardinal issues surrounding schizophrenia, such as the cognitive mechanisms that control the patient's behaviors and the manner by which the heterogeneity of the symptoms occurs. The same critique is applicable to Williams (2012), who, similar to Laing, claims that schizophrenia is a rational behavior.

PBT's unique contribution in this matter is that it views not only schizophrenia, but all types of deviant behaviors that fulfill the aforementioned criteria of madness, including criminal insanity and neuroses, as rational behaviors. Moreover, PBT resolves fundamental issues in this area, such as the psychological functions of madness, and the variability of symptoms within and among different disorders. It is therefore succeeds in integrating a huge number of clinical and research data from seemingly incompatible schools of thoughts into one theoretical system.

It may be argued that the high cost that individuals pay for their mad behaviors is incompatible with rationality, as they seem to work against their best interests. For example, the Unabomber's high risk of arrest for the murders he committed and the expected death penalty, make his behavior seem completely irrational. However, studies from the field of economics indicate that when experiencing emotional distress, the choice of a specific product is determined by the individual's immediate need to relieve tension, rather than by long-term considerations (Shiv & Fedorikhin, 1999, 2002). Thus, given the extreme emotional distress to which neurotics and psychotics are exposed, mad behaviors are rational because they serve patients' immediate psychological needs relieving their emotional distress through the repressive and controllable values of these behaviors. Moreover, rationality is not defined in terms of an optimum solution, but rather a decision made within the boundaries determined by information available to individuals at the decision-making stage, together with psychophysiological and environmental constraints (e.g., March, 1978; Simon, 1955, 1956). Robert Aumann (2016), the Nobel Prize-winning economist, noted in a letter of support for this book, that PBT

> fits in very well with the concept of rationality as understood in economics, where a person's behavior is considered 'rational' if under his circumstances, it advances his goals. In turn, this is well rooted in evolutionary theory; under the doctrine of 'survival of fittest,' the behavior of organisms has evolved in order to serve the organism's interest. Thus, Rofe's theory, revolutionary as it sounds, fits well into the frameworks of economics, game theory and evolution.

It seems that the reason for the contradictory attitudes between psychologists and economists regarding the nature of the human being is largely due to the seemingly senseless behaviors of mad people, which psychology, especially psychoanalysis, interpret as though they are controlled by irrational mechanisms. Thus, while succeeding in validating the thesis that mad behaviors are fundamentally rational PBT will also help settle the philosophical question of whether the human being is a rational or irrational creature.

Schizophrenia, Criminal Insanity and Neuroses: Brain Diseases or Rational-Coping Mechanisms?

As specified below, schizophrenic patients have two types of deviant behaviors. One type refers to bizarre behaviors, such as hallucinations, delusions and disorganized speech, which medical models have termed positive symptoms. The second type relates to sever personality deficits, such as severe lack of social skills and cognitive impairments, which medical models have termed negative symptoms. Medical models labeled these behaviors "symptoms" because of the significant correlation between schizophrenia and genetic mutations and brain abnormalities, interpreted as reflection of a brain disease.

PBT claims that this interpretation is completely wrong. This belief appeared to be the most plausible explanation of schizophrenia in the absence of a theory which could provide an alternative explanation for this correlation. This new theory denies the validity of this interpretation by claiming that schizophrenia, and so other types of bizarre behaviors, is purely the result of stress. This intolerable emotional state may be the result of severe personality deficits, caused by brain impairments, or purely the consequence of environmental or psychological factors. The positive symptoms are rational coping mechanisms which individuals may intuitively adopt when they are subjected to an intolerable level of stress.

From this new standpoint, the numerous studies which examined brain abnormalities made no direct contribution to the understanding of schizophrenia. They merely help pinpoint one of the major sources of stress that often motivates individuals to adopt the schizophrenic coping mechanism, mistakenly labeled by medical models as "positive symptoms". The new theory claims that the only research method which can to determine, at this stage of investigation, which of the above two alternative theories is correct, is to fist examine cases of schizophrenia with no evidence of brain abnormalities. Conclusions derived from these cases can then be generalized to include cases with brain abnormalities.

Before specifying the relevant data, which constitutes the primary purpose of Part-I, nine goals that an ideal theory of schizophrenia should meet, will be specified. These goals, which cover nearly all the problems that challenge the validity of traditional psychopathological theories, will then be used as a tool to examine the theoretical merits of PBT versus medical models. This evaluation, however, must wait for the end of this book, after all the aspects of the new theory have been fully discussed and considered. Part-I examines the validity of PBT versus medical models by formulating a number of hypotheses, which are derived from six of the nine theoretical goals. If case studies and data reviewed in Part-I confirm these hypotheses, they would provide sufficient support to PBT, thereby disproving the medical conception of schizophrenia. The other three goals relate to issues of unawareness and therapy which are covered in Part-II and III.

Misinterpretation of Neurological Impairments

The belief that schizophrenia is a brain disease, originally promoted by Emil Kraepelin (1856–1926; see Ebert & Bar, 2010; Falkai et al., 2015), became universally accepted mainly because of the significant correlation between schizophrenia and neurological impairments, which are usually the result of genetic flaws (e.g., Keshavan, Diwadkar, Montrose, Rajarethinam et al., 2005; Nuechterlein, Subotnik, Ventura, Green et al., 2012; Reichenberg & Harvey, 2007; Schiffman, Maeda,

Hayashi, Michelsen et al., 2006; Tandon, Keshavan, & Nasrallah, 2008), and sometimes of obstetric complications (e.g., Kunugi, 2003). However, as noted by Williams (2012), this hypothesis "has relied heavily upon this mistaking of correlation with causation, particularly maintaining the assumption that correlations between schizophrenia and brain anomalies (when and if they are found) imply that these brain anomalies must be the primary causative agent of such experiences" (p. 33). Moreover, as stated above, despite extensive research efforts, there is no significant evidence that these disorders are actually caused by a brain disease (e.g., Boyle, 2002; Siebert, 1999, 2000; Zipursky et al., 2013). Nor can medical models explain the large heterogeneity of schizophrenic symptoms, which is unlike that of any other neurological disease. It is also difficult to see how these models account for the fact that many schizophrenic patients fully recover without medication, which never occurs with other types of brain disease (see Siebert, 1999, 2000).

In light of these serious difficulties, it is puzzling that this belief became "so reasonable and credible… how is the presentation of 'schizophrenia as a brain disease' managed in such a way that the absence of direct evidence will not be noticed or not seem important?" (Boyle, 2002, p. 9). The only reasonable answer seems to be the absence of a more plausible explanation. Although Freud and his followers understandably defied this conceptualization (e.g., see Karon, 2008; Robbins, 2002; Silver, 2008; Szalek, 2015), their efforts failed, mainly because of psychoanalysis' inability to address genetic-neurological data (e.g., Willick, 2002).

PBT acknowledges the correlational studies, but disagrees with the interpretation of this data. While medical models claim that neurological impairments directly cause schizophrenia, as in Parkinson's and Alzheimer's diseases, according to PBT these impairments only cause an intolerable level of stress (e.g., see Wisner, Chiappelli, Savransky et al., 2019), which then motivates the individual to adopt the pathological coping mechanisms characteristic of schizophrenia. From this standpoint, while stress may be the consequence of environmental events, unacceptable impulses, and/or poor coping skills, as will be elaborated on later, it may also be the result of neurological impairments (see review by Zipursky et al., 2013). A vast number of studies reviewed in this book, indicate that schizophrenic patients with neurological impairments typically have severe attention deficits, low cognitive abilities, and poor social skills. Consequently, they are likely to experience acute social isolation and poor adjustment over the course of childhood, adolescence, and adulthood (Gureje, Aderibigbe, Olley, & Bamidele, 1994; Levitt, Shenton, McCarley, Faux, & Ludwig, 1994).

Such frustrating life experiences, which may also be the result of environmental events and/or other psychological factors even among individuals without brain abnormalities, are likely to generate a profound sense of incompetence, in which the self is perceived as the core reason for the patient's unhappy life experiences. While a common reactions among such individuals include substance abuse, addictions and suicide (e.g., Balhara & Verma, 2012; Bilge, Handan, Rumeysa, & Alp, 2015), some unconsciously prefer to develop schizophrenia because it provides two powerful psychological means to alleviate their intolerable levels of depression (1) repression: the bizarre behaviors block the accessibility of stress-related thoughts; (2) controllability: the specific schizophrenic behaviors enable the patient to inflate their self-esteem and/or attribute the cause for their miserable life-conditions to external sources.

PBT resolves the problem of the extreme heterogeneity in schizophrenic symptomatology by using the three principles of choice of symptoms, specified above. Another prominent advantage of this theoretical position is that it can explain cases with no evidence of brain impairments. This sheds light on findings that show that schizophrenia may develop in the absence of brain abnormality (e.g., see Williams, 2012).

The idea that schizophrenia is a rational-coping mechanism, rather than a brain disease, suggests that the major therapeutic intervention should be stress management, rather than pharmaceutical interventions. From this perspective, the barbaric treatments of schizophrenia, such as prefrontal lobotomies (e.g., De Mille, 1962; Hakola, Puranen, Repo, & Tiihonen, 1993) and insulin shock (e.g., Doroshow, 2006; Jones, 2000), were criminal acts against helpless people. To a large extent, this claim is also applicable to antipsychotic therapy, which is currently the major treatment approach for schizophrenia, as it may cause disastrous outcomes for the individual's cognitive and physiological systems, as will be elaborated on later.

Negative and Positive Symptoms

In their attempt to reinforce the idea that schizophrenia is a brain disease, medical models distinguish between two types of symptoms (1) negative symptoms, which refer to personality deficits, such as impaired attention, poor social skills, apathy, poverty of speech, poor rapport, and difficulty with abstract thinking; and (2) positive symptoms, which refer to schizophrenic-specific bizarre behaviors, such as hallucinations, delusions, and disorganized speech (e.g., see *DSM-5*, 2013; Buchanan, 2007; Moller, 1995; Skodlar, Henriksen, Sass, Nelson, & Parnas, 2013). PBT claims that these terms are misleading as they are not symptoms in the same sense as symptoms of physical illness. The negative symptoms are personality traits that usually characterize schizophrenics who have neurological impairments. They are the very cause of patients' stressful situations, which then motivate the adoption of schizophrenia. The positive symptoms are mad behaviors, which patients deliberately adopt in response to their intolerable levels of stress — which are the consequence of their inability to cope mainly as a result of the negative symptoms. This theoretical position may explain the fact that the "negative symptoms" do not respond to drug treatment, as will be elaborated upon later. PBT's theoretical position is also consistent with findings showing that disrupting patients' coping mechanism by increasing their awareness that they suffer from illness, aggravates their level of depression and the risk of suicide (e.g., Acosta, Aguilar, Cejas & Gracia, 2013; Balhara & Verma, 2012; Crumlish, Whitty, Kamali, Clarke, Browne et al., 2005; Ekinci, Ugurlu, Albayrak, Albayrak, Arslan et al., 2012; Lysaker et al., 2007; Melle & Barrett, 2012; Murri, Amore, Calcagno, Respino et al., 2016; Kao & Liu, 2011).

Inadequate Research Methods

Medical models focused their research efforts on investigating brain abnormalities because they believed that schizophrenia is a brain disease. However, research focused on the brain would not be adequate to advance the understanding of this disorder if, as claimed by PBT, schizophrenia is a psychological disorder that develops in response to stress. At best, these studies may help us understand the neurological cause of certain personality structures, which tend to place the individual at risk of developing schizophrenia due to severe deficiencies in coping skills.

Another research problem that challenges the validity of medical models concerns schizophrenics with no evidence of brain impairments. Traditionally, medical models have first examined cases in which there are brain impairments and then generalize the conclusions derived from these studies to cases with no evidence of brain impairments (e.g., Amador & Paul-Odouard, 2000; Capps, 2011; Nasar, 1998). Researchers took for granted that all schizophrenics necessarily suffer from brain impairments, even when there was no evidence to support of this claim. PBT claims that this research method has resulted in misleading conclusions and that the order of investigation should be reversed. Cases with no evidence of brain impairments should be studied first and then it can be determined whether the conclusions from these cases can promote the understanding of cases in which there are brain abnormalities.

Accordingly, PBT recommends the use of case study, as originally employed by Freud and his followers, rather than correlational studies, as the primary research method of schizophrenia and other types of madness. Case studies with no evidence of neurological impairments appear to provide the best means of examining PBT's main ideas. This methodology enables us to clarify whether (1) schizophrenia has greater similarity to other bizarre behaviors, such as criminal insanity and neuroses, than to brain diseases, such as Parkinson's and Alzheimer's disease; (2) stress is the underlying motivational cause of this disorder; (3) the major function of bizarre behaviors is repression, namely to block the accessibility of stress-related thoughts; (4) the choice of specific symptoms is determined by the individual's need to exercise control over the stressor, the availability of suitable means, and cost-benefit analysis.

"Case studies are considered most appropriate as tools in the critical, early phases of a new … theory, when key variables and their relationships are being explored" (Gibbert, Ruigrok, & Wicki, 2008, p. 1). Similarly, as noted by Flyvbjerg (2006), in order to understand a complex issue in-depth, case-study research is necessary (see also Bowers & Favolden, 1996; Brewin & Andrews, 1997; Zaidah, 2007). One may argue that case studies are not an acceptable scientific method for testing hypotheses. However, Flyvbjerg (2006) noted, following Karl Popper, that the method of case studies is "one of the most rigorous tests to which scientific proposition can be subjected." (p. 47)

Thus, while all research data must be taken into consideration, including correlational studies between schizophrenia and genetic defects or neurological impairments, case study must be the major research tool for understanding the underlying causes of schizophrenia. This method can be used to clarify the true interpretation of correlational studies, that is, whether neurological impairments directly cause schizophrenia, or just cause severe deficits of coping mechanisms, which leads to intolerable levels of stress and the adoption of this disorder. Therefore, the method of case study is very useful when examining PBT's major concepts.

Theoretical Goals

Another method to examine the validity of PBT is to compare this theory with rival approaches on nine cardinal issues that an ideal theory of psychopathology is expected to resolve. As will be demonstrated throughout this book, while PBT is able to solve all these issues, rival theories lack the ability to properly address any of them. Furthermore, resolving these problems enables one to obtain the most ambitious goal of an ideal theory of psychopathology: integrating relevant but seemingly incompatible data from all schools of thought, including psychoanalysis, behavior-cognitive theory, and medical models, into one theoretical framework.

1. **Diagnostic Criteria:** If schizophrenia were indeed a neurological disease, rather than a psychological disorder, it would be expected that, after so many years of research, medical models would have found neurochemical diagnostic measures for this disorder. At the very least, there should not be more common diagnostic characteristics between schizophrenia, criminal insanity, and neurotic disorders than there are between schizophrenia and neurological diseases, such as Parkinson's and Alzheimer's diseases and multiple sclerosis. However, unlike PBT's diagnostic measures which are common to all types of mad behaviors and are able to differentiate these behaviors from other deviant behaviors, medical models have failed to identify neurological diagnostic criteria, as will be demonstrated in Part I.

2. **Etiology:** If stress alone were able to account for cases of schizophrenia with no evidence of neurological impairments or genetic flaws, this would seriously damage the credibility of the disease conception of this disorder. This would have an even stronger effect if the same concept could also be applied to schizophrenic patients with brain impairments. An even greater theoretical challenge would be

to demonstrate that stress sits at the root of other types of bizarre behaviors, such as criminal insanity and neuroses.

3. **Heterogeneity of Symptoms:** As stated earlier, schizophrenic symptoms are extremely diverse. Although this poses difficulties for medical models, it does not challenge their validity, as there is no available theory that can explain these differences either. Advocates of medical models would claim that the complexity of the brain has hindered their ability to resolve this problem, as they have claimed regarding other challenging issues (e.g., see Wakefield, 1999). Therefore, if PBT were able to explain these differences, it would seriously challenge the validity of medical models, especially if the same concepts can also be applied to explain the heterogeneity of other bizarre behaviors.

4. **Psychological Functions of Madness:** From the point of view of medical models, none of the bizarre symptoms, and certainly not those of schizophrenics, have any psychological value, much in the same way as symptoms of brain diseases such as Alzheimer's and Parkinson's disease, which lack psychological value. In contrast, from the standpoint of PBT, mad behaviors are goal-directed behaviors, which serve the patients' needs of repression and controllability.

5. **Choice of Symptoms:** According to PBT, patients intuitively choose their mad behaviors. Similar to consumers' decision-making processes, the choice of a specific mad behavior is determined by the patient's controllability demands, his or her available cognitive experiences, and cost-benefit considerations.

6. **Sociocultural Effects:** Additional problems that challenge the validity of medical models concern the effects of sociocultural factors on the prevalence of mad behaviors. These include the dramatic increase of eating disorders and DID in Western countries, their rarity in non-Western society, the high prevalence of OCD among religious groups, and gender differences, that is, the fact that nearly all neuroses

are more prevalent among females, as opposed to schizophrenia, which is more prevalent among males. As will be demonstrated in Part I, only PBT can account for these sociocultural variations.

7. **Awareness–Unawareness:** Clinical data indicate that although patients are unaware of the underlying causes of their bizarre behaviors, they are consciously involved in the display of these behaviors. For example, the Unabomber was unaware of the causes of his criminal acts and yet he took active precautions not to be arrested, which motivated some researchers to claim that he consciously planned these behaviors and deny that he suffered from schizophrenia (e.g., see Magid, 2000). Similarly, subjects with hysterical seizures have the ability to prevent injury, tongue biting, and post seizure confusion, when falling to the ground (e.g., Blanchard & Hersen, 1976; Nicol, 1969). In the same manner, those with hysterical paralysis fail to display the symptoms of immobility when distracted (e.g., Cassady et al., 2005; Kihlstrom, 1994, p. 382; Merskey, 1995) or weakened during sleep (e.g., Laurema, 1993). Likewise, kleptomaniacs are seemingly unable to resist their bizarre impulse to steal, yet avoid stealing when immediate arrest is probable (*DSM-IV*, American Psychiatric Association, 1994). It is difficult to see how existing theories can resolve these seemingly contradictory facts. An ideal theory of psychopathology would be expected to suggest an alternative explanation for the Freudian unconscious, which undermines the role of the conscious in the development and treatment of mad behaviors.

8. **Resolutions of Theoretical Conflicts:** The scientific credibility of a theory is partly determined by its ability to resolve theoretical conflicts in its field of investigation. In this respect, PBT makes three important theoretical contributions, as will be specified in the "discussion" section of Part II. One theoretical conflict concerns the etiology of conversion disorder. While according to psychoanalysis, this is a psychological disorder, in which a psychological trauma

is unconsciously converted into a false illness, neurologists claim that it is the result of abnormal neurological functioning (e.g., Stone et al., 2011; see also the *DSM-5*, American Psychological Association, 2013). The second dispute relates to the trauma model of DID, which views this disorder as a coping mechanism by people who were subjected to childhood trauma (e.g., see Bremner, 2008; Gleaves, 1996), as opposed to the socio-cognitive theory, which claims that it is a role enactment (e.g., see Boysen & VanBergen, 2014.) The third area is the controversy regarding panic disorder and agoraphobia, which behaviorists, cognitivists, and advocates of medical models attribute to conditioning, irrational thinking and brain abnormalities, respectively. This last problem becomes more complicated as none of these theorists can explain bizarre phobias, such as train phobia, chocolate phobia, and rat germ phobia, which meet PBT's criteria of bizarreness (see review by Rofé & Rofé, 2015). Not only does PBT resolve these theoretical conflicts, it also integrates research and clinical data pertaining to these disorders into one theoretical framework.

9. **Therapy:** Theories of psychopathology (e.g., psychoanalysis, behavior–cognitive theories, and medical models) have each developed therapeutic techniques for the treatment of mad behaviors. However, despite extensive research efforts no theory has succeeded in integrating these therapeutic methods into a single theoretical framework (see review by Feixas & Botella, 2004; Lampropoulos, 2000, 2001). As will be demonstrated partly in Part I and more extensively in Part III, PBT is the only theory that can achieve this ambitious theoretical goal, which includes the explanation of curative effects of psychological methods on schizophrenia. Additional evidence that weakens medical models is a group of studies reviewed in Part I demonstrating the limited efficacy of drug treatments and their disastrous effects on both the physiological and cognitive systems of schizophrenic patients.

Hypotheses: An Empirical Examination of PBT

Part I aims to examine the validity of a number of specific hypotheses derived from the theoretical goals mentioned above, chiefly through case studies.

1. Schizophrenia criminal insanity and neuroses meet five of PBT major criteria of bizarreness. Sometimes a deviant behavior may fulfill only four of the five criteria. In these cases, the behavior should be diagnosed as bizarre if it meets PBT's two secondary criteria as well.
2. All mad behaviors are a response to stress, regardless of whether the source of the stress is environmental (e.g., family conflicts or military stress), psychological (e.g., unacceptable impulses and low self-esteem), or neurological that causes poor coping abilities.
3. Although there may be other causes, schizophrenia, and criminal-insanity, usually develop when individuals experience a profound sense of incompetence that severely damages their self-esteem, resulting in self-loathing. This hypothesis is consistent with "an accumulating amount of empirical studies [testifying] that the self is disturbed in schizophrenia spectrum disorders but is not in other disorders (Henriksen & Parnas, 2016, P. 1; see also Skodlar & Henriksen, 2019). In most cases, this painful psychological state is associated with severe deficiencies in social skills which results in an extreme state of social isolation. As noted by Saks (2007) "[one] of the worst aspects of schizophrenia is the profound isolation — the constant awareness that you're different, some sort of alien, not really human" (p. 193). While researchers limit this stressful experiences to schizophrenia, PBT extends it to criminal insanity as well. However, in contrast to both schizophrenia and criminal insanity, neuroses

tend to develop in response to environmental stress or unacceptable impulses.

4. The major psychological function of bizarre behavior is repression. This means that the schizophrenic behaviors, such as delusions, hallucinations, and disorganized speech, intensively preoccupy the individual's attention, and thus block the accessibility of stress-related thoughts.
5. Schizophrenic patients are reluctant to acknowledge that they suffer from illness, both because it sabotages the distractive value of the symptom and because it damages their attempt to inflate their self-esteem or attribute the cause for their "illness" to external sources. Accordingly, increasing patients' awareness of their "illnesses" may increase their level of depression as well as the likelihood of suicide.
6. The choice of a specific bizarre behavior is determined by PBT's three principles: the symptom must reinforce the individual's need of controllability in reducing the stressor; its choice is affected by the patient's available conscious and unconscious experiences; and it is adopted only if it benefits the individual by alleviating his or her emotional distress.
7. The prevalence of bizarre behaviors among different social groups is affected by the individual's available experiences and cost-benefit analysis.

Case Studies Without Evidence of Brain Impairments

This section addresses case studies of schizophrenia and criminal insanity with no evidence of neurological impairments or genetic flaws. Most cases have received publicity in both the media and research literature. As will be demonstrated, these cases meet PBT's diagnostic criteria of bizarre behaviors and are explainable by the same set of theoretical concepts suggested by this theory. Cases of schizophrenia and criminal insanity were mixed in order to demonstrate that, often, these types of behaviors share the same etiology, despite significant differences in their symptomatology: both are confronted with stresses that severely damage their self-esteem. While both have the same psychological functions of repression and enhancement of one's sense of competence, they differ in their choices due to differences in the availability of their personal experiences, which increase the saliency of specific types of bizarre behaviors, and cost-benefit considerations.

1. **The Unabomber — The Schizophrenic Serial Killer:** This case refers to Theodore John Kaczynski, also known as the Unabomber, who was a professor of mathematics at the University of California, Berkeley. In 1971, at the age of 29, he resigned from the university, moved to a remote cabin with no electricity or running water and began living as hermit. Between 1978 and 1995, Kaczynski mailed bombs to various locations, including universities and airlines, killing 3 and injuring 23. Kaczynski sent a letter to the New York Times on April 24, 1995, promising to desist from the bombings he claimed were necessary to direct attention to the erosion of human freedom caused by modern technologies. The Unabomber was diagnosed with paranoid schizophrenia, and although he had the option to plead insanity, and thus escape the death penalty, he vehemently resisted this option. Instead, he unsuccessfully tried to fire his court-appointed lawyers when they did not adhere to his seemingly irrational request (Graysmith, 1996).

Amador and Paul-Odouard (2000), based on evidence that schizophrenics typically deny their illness, as well as studies indicating that poor insight is linked to frontal lobe dysfunction, arrived at the conclusion that the Unabomber must have suffered from brain damage. Not only is there no direct evidence to support this claim, but the authors also overlooked psychological factors mentioned by other researchers as possible causes for the Unabomber's behavior. These include (1) severe lack of social competence caused by inadequate socialization; (2) inability to communicate with females, which according to his confession caused "acute sexual starvation";

and (3) a deep sense of inferiority and severe levels of depression (e.g., Leeper, Carwile, & Huber, 2002; Magid, 2009; Zuk & Zuk, 2000). Furthermore, denial is not limited to schizophrenia, but is also seen in neurotic disorders, such as anorexia nervosa (Bruch, 1978; Gottheil, Backup, & Cornelison, 1969; Vandereycken, 2006a), and certain forms OCD (e.g., compulsive cleaners, see Foa, 1979; Kozak & Foa, 1994; Rachman & Hodgson, 1980). However, as with the Unabomber, no evidence has been presented that indicates these patients suffer from a brain disease. Moreover, as will be discussed later, the phenomenon of denial can be explained by rational, simpler concepts.

Another fundamental problem that is inexplicable by medical models concerns the heterogeneity of schizophrenic symptoms. Even if they had been able to corroborate the presence of neurological impairments, Amador and Paul-Odouard still should have been required to explain which specific impairment had caused the Unabomber's delusion concerning the corruption of industrial society and his criminal insanity. It seems unlikely that such complicated behaviors could have been caused by neurological impairments, which led Magid (2009) to claim that Kaczynski's transformation into the Unabomber resulted from "conscious choices" rather than from a brain disorder.

> Kaczynski extensively planned, prepared, and pondered before engaging in specific attacks, suggesting heightened culpability. His crime was the product of careful deliberation, not uncontrollable impulse or delusion (p. 20).

However, while it is difficult to dismiss evidence suggesting that Kaczynski's criminal behavior was fully intentional, it is equally difficult to accept Magid's claim that these actions were normal criminal behavior. The Unabomber's criminal behavior appears senseless because it lacks incentives that motivate normal criminal behaviors, such as monetary, sexual rewards, and revenge. Conscious deliberate behavior also characterizes other bizarre criminal incidents, such as that of Charles Cullen (Yorker et al., 2006), a case which will be discussed in more detail later. These behaviors seem senseless, and therefore require a different explanation from that of common criminal acts.

PBT's theoretical contribution in this respect is that it is capable of resolving the above problems and applying the same set of concepts for explaining a variety of bizarre behaviors. The Unabomber is one of a series of case studies that confirm PBT's theoretical position. **First,** unlike medical models, which lack objective diagnostic classification, **PBT's diagnostic criteria** enable us to diagnose the Unabomber as a mad person. Thus, in accordance with the first hypothesis above, the Unabomber's delusion and criminal behaviors intensively preoccupied his attention and severely disrupted his daily functioning (criterion 1); his radical behavioral change occurred in the absence of a specific observable event that is uniquely associated with and can account for this effect (criterion 2); he was unaware of both the underlying causes of his behavior and that his behavior was abnormal (criterion 3); his delusion and criminal behaviors are extremely rare (criterion 4); his behaviors were stigmatized as crazy or as a reflection of illness by the psychiatric diagnostic system (criteria 5).

Second, this case also confirms PBT's second hypothesis that mad behaviors develop in response to stress. The Unabomber was extremely lonely, a condition mainly the result of poor social skills. Dr. Sally C. Johnson, who diagnosed him with paranoid schizophrenia, cited "an almost total absence of interpersonal relationships" (Sally, 1998, p. 47). Although he gained impressive academic success, he was miserable and depressed. Due to his notable deficit in social skills, he could not maintain functioning relationships with women or satisfy his intense sexual desires, leaving him in a constant state of frustration. While genetic factors may be involved in affecting personality tendencies (e.g., Horwitz, Luong, & Charles,

2008; Kandler, Gottschling, & Spinath, 2016; Lukaszewski & Roney, 2013), it seems that the major variable behind the development of the Unabomber's handicapped personality was his social environment as a child. His mother fixated on the advancement of his intellectual abilities and neglected to promote the development of his social skills. Kaczynski and his brother were not seen outside playing with other children, as their mother kept them inside and encouraged them to study (Leeper et al., 2002). "His parents focused on developing his intellectual and academic abilities at the expense of normal childhood ... By age eight or nine, it was apparent that Kaczynski was not socially accepted by other children of his age. Moreover, his family relocated several times, only compounding the problem" (Magid, 2009, p. 7). Often, schools compensate for parents' mistakes in this respect by providing social environment in which students can develop adequate social skills. However, Kaczynski missed these opportunities because his school allowed him to skip the sixth and eleventh grades without taking into consideration the severe negative impact this would have on his social development. Thus, he was deprived of normal social experiences and instead learned with much older students who had no interest in him. This isolation intensified when he enrolled at Harvard University at the young age of 16. He experienced a deep sense of inferiority and severe levels of depression (e.g., Leeper et al., 2002; Magid, 2009; Zuk & Zuk, 2000).

Hence, he lacked basic social competence, and as revealed by both research (e.g., Uhrlass, Schofield, Coles, & Gibb, 2009; Williams & Galliher, 2006; Zaitsoff, Fehon, & Grilo, 2009), and case studies (e.g., Derossett, 2013; Rodger, 2014), deficient social skills can severely damage a person's self-esteem, lead to depression, and often precede the onset of psychosis and suicide.

Third, in accordance with PBT, the Unabomber's schizophrenic symptoms served two major psychological functions. His continuous engagement in building homemade bombs and planning his next "mission," along with taking precautions not to be caught, served as a **powerful repressive tool**. These bizarre behaviors also enhanced Kaczynski's controllability over his sense of incompetence by boosting his self-esteem. His grandiose delusion that he could change industrial society and modern civilization **provided him with imaginary control** over the society he felt had rejected him (see Magid, 2009, p. 8). As noted by Zuk and Zuk (2000) the Unabomber felt he had a messianic mission to share with the world.

> It seems reasonable that he assumed the message was one that was legitimate, somewhat messianic, one that would have the support and endorsement of a deity. If it was necessary to threaten the destruction of individuals in pursuit of his messianic mission, he probably felt he had an entitlement. If in the course of his effort to inform the world he would be captured and perhaps put to death for murder, he was prepared because his demise would promote a presumed wish to become a martyr. (p. 334)

Hence, in terms of cost-benefit, the Unabomber's schizophrenic symptoms were a beneficial coping mechanism, which reduced his unbearable levels of depression and reduced his risk of suicide. The Unabomber also enjoyed celebrity status and thrived on the attention he received in the media, as is typically observed with serial killers (Haggerty, 2009).

His refusal to confess that he suffered from mental illness, despite the risk of receiving the death penalty, reflects the high benefit that the symptoms yielded. It seems probable that the Unabomber's denial of his "illness" was due to the high emotional toll he would have suffered had he confessed that he was mentally ill, as proposed by his lawyers. This confession would mean not only abandoning his coping mechanism and reexposing himself to the original unbearable stress, but also an additional blow to his self-esteem, which might have pushed him to suicide. Amador and Paul-Odouard's (2000) claim that the Unabomber's denial was irrational and stemmed from brain disease might have been accepted as the most reasonable explanation in the absence of PBT; with the new explanation, however, this behavior appears entirely rational.

As specified earlier, similar to consumer's decision processes, the choice of a specific bizarre behavior is affected by the individual's available experiences. One experience that motivated the Unabomber to develop his specific delusion regarding the corruption of industrial society was his familiarity with the French philosopher Jacques Ellul. The Unabomber was so captivated by Ellul's ideas that he read his book, *The Technological Society*, **six** times. He became convinced that continued scientific and technical progress would inevitably result in the extinction of the individual's liberty and threaten people's wellbeing. The second experience, apparently was influenced by Ellul's attitude toward modernity, was his decision to move to a secluded cabin and become self-sufficient, thereby distancing himself from the modern society that had rejected him. He soon realized he could not live in a fully self-sufficient manner because industrial development had destroyed the land around him. But "the ultimate catalyst which drove him to begin his campaign of bombings was when he went out for a walk to one of his favorite wild spots, only to find that it had been destroyed and replaced with a road." As noted by the Unabomber:

> That summer there were too many people around my cabin so I decided I needed some peace. I went back to the plateau and when I got there I found they had put a road right through the middle of it ... You just can't imagine how upset I was. It was from that point on I decided that, rather than trying to acquire further wilderness skills, I would work on getting back at the system. Revenge (see Kaczynski, 1999)

Another significant experience that might have contributed to his specific choice was witnessing numerous riots and protests, such as the People's Park Riot of May 1969, an extremely violent event at which police officers shot students (Carley, 2013). A further factor that affected the Unabomber's choice of mad behavior is the availability of weapons in the United States.

It should be noted that PBT does not preclude the possibility that the Unabomber did have some brain abnormality which contributed to his deficit of social skills and or affected his violent behavior. However, this does not refute PBT's fundamental claim that an extreme level of stress was the direct cause of his schizophrenic behavior and that his madness was goal-directed behavior, rather than the consequence of brain disease.

2. **John Nash — A Masterpiece of Craziness:** There is, perhaps, no better example to illustrate PBT's claim that schizophrenia is a rational behavior than the case study of Nobel Laureate, John Nash (see Biography by Nasar, 1998). Not only were Nash's schizophrenic symptoms goal-directed behaviors as they alleviated his emotional distress through their repression and controllability values, as is typical of all bizarre/mad behaviors, but they were also exceptionally sophisticated behaviors, especially because of their symbolic meanings, as will be illustrated below.

Similar to the Unabomber, Nash's schizophrenia meets **PBT's five criteria of madness**. The symptoms occupied his attention and severely affected his daily activities (criterion 1); the onset of his bizarre behaviors was not linked to a specific event that could account by itself for the dramatic change in his behavior (criterion 2); he was unaware of the underlying cause of his behavior (criterion 3); his schizophrenic behaviors were extremely rare (criterion 4); his behaviors were stigmatized as the reflection of an illness (criterion 5).

Furthermore, etiologically, Nash's schizophrenic symptoms can be seen as a response to extreme levels of stress. Before reviewing the specific stressors that preceded his mental breakdown, it is important to note that, like the Unabomber, Nash had poor social skills, which constituted a major source of stress. Nasar (1998), who provided the most detailed and remarkable account of Nash's biography, noted "his contemporaries, on the whole, found him immediately strange. They described him as 'aloof,' 'haughty,' 'without affect,' 'detached,' 'spooky,' 'isolated,' and 'queer.' Nash mingled rather than mixed with his peers … " (p. 13). "The boys made him the butt of various pranks" (p. 43). His sister, Martha, wrote

> Johnny was always different. [My parents] knew he was different…. Mother insisted I do things for him, that I include him in my friendships … but I wasn't too keen on showing off my somewhat odd brother. (Nasar, 1998, p. 32)

His fellow students made similar notes:

> He was a country boy unsophisticated even by our standards … He behaved oddly, playing a single chord on the piano over and over, leaving an ice cream cone melting on top of his castoff clothing in the lounge, walking on his roommate's sleeping body to turn off the light. (Nasar, 1998, p. 42)

> Nash was out of the ordinary … If he was in a room with twenty people, and they were talking, if you asked an observer who struck you as odd it would have been Nash. (Nasar, 1998, p. 73)

Nash's inadequate social skills are also illustrated by the fact that three faculty members at Princeton University voiced strong opposition to offering him an assistant professorship due to his social manners. One professor felt that he simply would not be able to tolerate Nash, "whom he regarded as aggressive, abrasive and arrogant, in such a small department" (Nasar, 1998, p. 132).

While it seems likely that years of social rejection left him with feelings of inferiority and negatively affected his self-esteem, they were probably not substantial enough to motivate the adoption of deviant behaviors, as seen with the Unabomber and other cases to be reviewed below. This may have been the case particularly because of the positive experiences he had with the two women in his life, which helped to boost his self-esteem. For Nash, "who had never even known a woman other than his mother and sister" (Nasar, 1998, p. 174), his secret liaison with Eleanor [his mistress] was not only a pleasant sexual experience, but also a highly ego enhancing affair. His wife, Alicia, "a beautiful young physics student who adored him" (Nasar, 1998, p. 15), and of whom he was proud, surely raised his confidence as well.

Nevertheless, the prolonged period of social rejection weakened Nash's ability to tolerate stress. As claimed by Nasar (1998), schizophrenia may not be the result of a single stressor but rather the consequence of the cumulative effects of a number of stressors. While stress plays a vital role in the development of schizophrenia, it does not necessarily mean a single dramatic event precipitates this disorder. As noted by Nasar (1998) "certain events are definite stressors, but it's not famine or war. It's idiosyncratic. It's things that get to the soul and self-identity and expectations of oneself … Rather than a single trauma, a string of events from childhood through young adulthood produces strains that mount like straws on the proverbial camel's back" (p. 188). Three specific personal stressors dramatically aggravated Nash's emotional distress, which motivated him to adopt schizophrenia as a coping mechanism.

The first stressor concerned Nash's extremely ambitious personality, which was influenced by his strong feelings of inferiority resulting from years of social rejection. As noted by Nasar (1998), although "he was told that he had a brilliant future in mathematics … for a teenager who had endured a lifetime of rejection by peers, the warm praise of such professors … was too little … Nash craved a more universal form of recognition … " (p. 44). "Nash was interested that everyone would recognize how smart he was, not because he needed this admiration, but anybody who didn't recognize it wasn't on top of things … He seized opportunities to boast his accomplishments" (p. 67). However, Nash's self-esteem further deteriorated when his need for superiority was denied in the course of two important events.

Nash hoped to get a position at Princeton University but thanks to his personality he was rejected by the members of the mathematics faculty. "The thought must have occurred to Nash that he was being rejected less on the basis of his work than on the basis of his personality. It was an even greater blow [to his self-esteem] because the same faculty made it clear that John Milnor, only a junior by this time, would one day become part of the Princeton faculty" (p. 132). Similarly, his expectation of receiving a promotion and tenure at MIT was not fulfilled, because faculty members felt he was a poor teacher and an even worse colleague. MIT promised to reconsider his promotion once his new article was published. "Nash, however, was furious" (p. 224).

Additionally, Nash was extremely disappointed when he did not receive the Fields Medal, the mathematics' equivalent of the Nobel Prize, or the less prestigious Bôcher Prize. Perhaps the best indication of his disappointment in himself regarding his academic achievements can be observed in his statement, "what, thirty already, and still no prize, no offer from Harvard, no tenure even? And you thought you were such a great mathematician? A genius? Ha, ha, ha!" (p. 229).

The second stressor was his bisexual tendencies. Capps (2003, 2004, 2005) has thoroughly reviewed evidence indicating that Nash had homosexual desires. Based on Erikson and Freud's theories, Capps suggests that Nash's paranoid delusions were mainly the result of acute identity confusion and his efforts to repress his homosexual desires after his marriage to Alicia. It seems that these desires aggravated his negative self-loathing particularly due to his "merciless superego" (Nash's own term, Nasar, 1998, p. 317) and his guilt, which was "directly connected, but not limited, to his feelings about homosexuality" (Nasar, 1998, p. 327). Nash imagined himself as "a religious figure of great, but secret importance" (Nasar, 1998, p. 275) destined to replace the Pope (see Capps, 2004). It seems that this delusion was associated with Nash's desire to gain a "gay liberation" and compensate for his unbearable guilt. As noted by Capps (2004) with regard to Nash's homosexual desires, Nash was seeking "some sort of vindication as a man who had suffered far too much at the hands of his "merciless superego" (p. 211). The "gay liberation" was so important to Nash that it was one of the main topics of conversation with his son, John Stier, after their reconciliation. Even during "very dark hours he clung to a vision of liberation — which later became, more concretely, a wish for sexual liberation" (Nasar, 1998, p. 328).

The third stressor, perhaps even worse than the previous two, concerned his wife's pregnancy and the death of his father. Nash's breakdown and his hospitalization occurred when Alicia was giving birth to their son, John Charles. It seems unlikely that his wife's pregnancy and the birth of his child constituted stressful events, as Nash felt proud when his mistress, Eleanor, had announced her pregnancy 5 years earlier (Nasar, 1998, pp. 175, 235). Moreover, he reminded Alicia when she had suggested waiting a few years before having children, "that the whole purpose of marriage, in his view, was to produce children" (p. 235). Therefore, it seems the expected birth precipitated Nash's mental breakdown for other reasons. **First**, the birth reminded him of the trauma associated with his first son's birth and his parent's subsequent discovery of his mistress and son. The shock to his parents was enormous. His father contacted him via a long-distance call, an unusual occurrence as they communicated exclusively by letters, and told him sternly "don't come home … Go right to Boston and make this right. Marry the girl" (Nasar, 1998, p. 208). Soon afterward, his father suffered a massive heart attack and died. The death shocked Nash, and the possibility that he had hastened his father's death disturbed him greatly. His mother accused Eleanor of causing her husband's death, and "it is quite possible that she said something similar to her son, or implied as much" (Nasar, 1998, p. 209). "What is almost certainly the case is that Nash blamed himself" (Capps, 2005, p. 367). **Second**, Capps (2003) notes that the expected birth was traumatic because it "confronted him with a crisis of commitment … The archaic voice of his father, saying perhaps, 'You are not man enough to assume responsibility for the consequences of your actions'" (p. 378).

It seems likely that these accumulating stressors increased Nash's self-loathing, because he perceived himself as fully responsible for his inability to cope, and thus motivated the adoption of his schizophrenic disorder. It may well be that genetic predisposition gave rise to certain components of Nash's personality, such as his poor social skills, and that this factor aggravated his emotional distress. However, these effects do not negate PBT's claim that Nash's delusions and hallucinations were rational coping mechanisms that effectively reduced his emotional distress. The major psychological function of his mad behaviors was repression: these behaviors intensively preoccupied his mind so that unbearable stressful thoughts became inaccessible. Thus, contrary to psychoanalytic conception that Nash's paranoid delusions were the "effect of the repression of homoerotic desires" (Capps, 2005, P. 371), Nash's delusions and hallucinations were, from PBT's standpoint, repressive tools that blocked the accessibility of stress-related thoughts, including homosexual desires.

While it is beyond the scope of this book to analyze all of Nash's delusions, which are discussed by both Nasar (1998) and Capps (2003, 2004, 2005), a number of examples can sufficiently illustrate the psychological functions of his mad behaviors. These examples also demonstrate the symbolic and complex meanings of Nash's symptoms and the sophisticated way these meanings were encoded in his mind, thereby undermining the theory of brain disease. One example is when Nash entered the common room of Hartfley Rodgers at MIT, while pointing to the story on the front page of the *New York Times*, and announced that

> Abstract powers from outer space, or perhaps it was foreign governments, were communicating with him through the

> New York Times. The messages, which were meant only for him, were encrypted and required close analysis. Others couldn't decode the messages. He was being allowed to share the secrets of the world. (Nasar, 1998, pp. 241–242)

Although this delusion appears insane and irrational, it is, in fact, exceptionally clever, both in its symbolic meanings and in its psychological repression and controllability functions. The abstract powers represent his "merciless super-ego," which generated stressful thoughts, intense feelings of guilt and severe damage to his self-esteem, is consistent with the psychoanalytic suggestion that in some cases "the patient's problems result from the extremely severe superego" (Szalek, 2015, p. 115). The extreme emotional distress which these thoughts produced drove him into repressing them using his schizophrenic behaviors. These thoughts were encrypted and labeled as "the secrets of the world" to further distance himself from accessing them. Nash encrypted his emotionally-charged thoughts the same way a mathematician would encode his knowledge. This delusion inflated Nash's self-esteem as the "abstract powers" or "foreign government" had shared the secrets of the world" only with him.

Often, his schizophrenic symptoms were insufficient in blocking the accessibility of his stress-related thoughts. Nash noted, despite the "horror of hospital and illness, these ideas keep coming into my head and I can't prevent it" (p. Nasar, 1998, p. 258). Therefore, he utilized his exceptional creative abilities to invent various tricks that served as additional barriers to prevent him from accessing his "secrets" — the stress-related thoughts. One example of such a distractive activity was Nash's decision to focus on Alicia's secrets in an attempt to further distance himself from his own repressed stressors. "He behaved as if she knew some secret but wouldn't share it with him" (Nasar, 1998, p. 248). Nash became so persistent with the delusion that "he threatened to hit her" if she did not tell him (p. 249). As noted by Capps (2003), Alicia suspected that Nash's inquiries into her secrets "were an act designed to deflect attention from himself" (p. 367), and to further repress his anxiety-provoking thoughts. He made Alicia part of the conspiracy plot against him, in an attempt to externalize the underlying causes of his psychological difficulties.

Nash was so distressed by his thoughts and his constant battle to repress them that he felt as though his head was "a bloated windbag, with voices which dispute within" (Nasar, 1998, p. 328). He invested a vast amount of time and energy in forming a fictional world government (e.g., sending letters to all the embassies in Washington, Nasar, 1998, p. 244), seeing himself as the leader of a great movement for world peace, and referring to himself as "the prince of peace" (p. 255) or "a religious figure of great, but secret importance" (Nasar, 1998, p. 275). While these delusions aimed to inflate Nash's self-esteem and constituted effective repressive measures, they also bore symbolic meanings. "The prince of peace" may have symbolized his wish to establish peace within his psyche by resolving his unbearable psychological conflicts. Similarly, it is possible that he adopted a position of religious importance because he believed he could change the laws forbidding bisexual behaviors if he were to possess religious authority.

The dual symbolic meaning of Nash's delusions are also illustrated by Nash's rejection of a prestigious offer from the University of Chicago to be a head of the mathematics department, stating that he was expected to become "Emperor of Antarctica." This statement represents his failure to gain the world's respect: although the position of Emperor is respected, serving as "Emperor of Antarctica," a barren and empty place, is not the most impressive role he could have created for himself, indicating that he did not believe himself worthy of more. In addition, Nash told a student that he was on the cover of *Life* magazine but that his photograph had been disguised to make him look like Pope John XXIII. He mentioned two signs proving the photograph was of him and not of the Pope (1) unlike Nash, John was not the Pope's given name, but rather a name that he had chosen for himself; (2) the number 23 was Nash's favorite prime number. While this delusion boosted his self-esteem allowing both for comparison between himself and the leader of the Catholic world and the belief that his photograph had been publicized by a well-known magazine, it also reflects Nash's negative perception of himself in that the magazine had to "disguise" his real face because of his disgraceful behaviors.

In analyzing Nash's delusional perception of himself as the Pope, Capps (2003) claims that this delusion "reflected primitive feelings of guilt and rage" over his function as "papa" and his failure "to live up to his obligations as a father to Eleanor's son" (p. 383). However, while delusions may contain negative messages, as was prominent in Nash's case, one of the function of these cognitions is to increase the schizophrenic's self-esteem. As demonstrated in the previous case, enhancing self-esteem was one of the central functions of the Unabomber's schizophrenic symptoms. This claim is also consistent with studies showing that motivating patients to abandon their positive symptoms (i.e., hallucinations and delusions) by increasing their awareness that they suffer from illness, leads to depression, low self-esteem, hopelessness, and suicidal behavior (e.g., Acosta et al., 2013; Balhara & Verma, 2012; Crumlish et al., 2005; Ekinci et al., 2012; Kao & Liu, 2011; Konsztowicz & Lepage, 2019; Lysaker et al., 2007; Melle & Barrett, 2012). Accordingly, Nash's positive symptoms were so important to him because of their repressive and controllability values that he felt that "taking away his delusions and hallucinations would be taking away his genius, his most treasured gift" (Weiden, 2002).

Nash's contradictory messages were also demonstrated by his ongoing delusion that "he was the left foot of God and that God was walking on the earth" (Nasar, 1998, p. 258). While there seems to be no higher ranked position than closeness to God, this delusion also implies that he did not perceive himself as important enough to serve as God's right foot, which indirectly refers to the perception of himself as a failure. Nash's psychological methods to reduce his intolerable level of depression not only included repression and grandiose delusions, but also delusions that aimed to project his failures and immoral behaviors on external factors. For example, in one of his letters, Nash wrote that "his career was being ruined by aliens from outer space" (Nasar, 1998, p. 243). Similarly, Nash accused one of the mathematics graduate students at MIT of searching through his trash to steal his ideas (p. 243). All this evidence indicates that schizophrenic bizarre behaviors are goal-directed behaviors that serve the patients' best interests.

Another delusion worth discussing is Nash's belief that he could renounce his American citizenship and replace it with a universal identity card, "one that declared him to be a citizen of the world" (Nasar, 1998, p. 271). Later, he also wished to obtain official refugee status. When his efforts failed, he disposed of his American passport, so that "in his own mind, Nash was now stateless … " (Nasar, 1998, p. 276). He was so decisive in his efforts to dissociate himself from his old identity that he refused to return to the United States even after Swiss authorities issued a deportation order and forced him to leave Geneva. His strong desire to disconnect himself from the United States was part of his repressive efforts to detach himself from anything that reminded him of his irreversible past. This may also account for the fact that in a conference he insisted on giving his lecture in what he called "Pidgin French," even though most of the speakers delivered their talks in English. Nash's self-loathing was so painful that he attempted to escape from himself by establishing a new identity completely detached from any memory of past experiences. This is consistent with Nasar's (1998) statement that Nash was:

> motivated as much by antagonism to his former existence as by an urge for self-expression, Nash particularly desired to supersede the old laws that governed his existence, and, quite literally, to substitute his own laws, and to escape, once and for all, from the jurisdiction under which he had once lived. (p. 271)

Nash's case is also unique due to the relatively large number of symptoms. While this can be interpreted as additional indication of his exceptional creative ability, it seems there were psychological reasons for this unusual abundance. Unlike the Unabomber and other cases to be discussed below (e.g., Charles Cullen), Nash did not develop schizophrenic symptoms that could intensively preoccupy his attention for a prolonged period. As specified above, the Unabomber's mad behaviors demanded a vast amount of cognitive and behavioral activity that effectively insulated his attention from the infiltration of stress-related thoughts. In contrast, most of Nash's delusions and hallucinations did not require intensive behavioral effort or cognitive activity, and certainly not for a prolonged period. Moreover, since his symptoms were symbolically associated with his stressors, they could not serve as strong preventative barriers. As a result, he had to produce more symptoms that, taken together, could intensively occupy his attention. However, they eventually became insufficient, which may explain his desperate efforts to acquire refugee status and escape from his original environment that reminded him of his stressors. The inadequacy of Nash's schizophrenic symptoms to block the accessibility of stress-related thoughts is consistent with experimental findings which show that patients who experience auditory hallucinations have more intrusive thoughts and are more distressed by them than control subjects without hallucinations (Morrison & Baker, 2000).

Nash's refusal to take medications was interpreted by researchers as a sign of his irrationality. For example, in an article titled "Why Did John Nash Stop His Medications" Weiden (2002) noted, "Nash would have to be persuaded that his voices and strong beliefs (delusions) were harmful to his intelligence, and those medications, by reducing his preoccupations, would help his concentration and intellect" (p. 390). Not only did Weiden fail to realize the important psychological functions of Nash's schizophrenic symptoms, but recent studies also indicate how fortunate Nash was that he stubbornly refused medications. An increasing number of studies, to be reviewed toward the end of Part I, reveal that antipsychotics increase the risk for metabolic syndrome, cardiovascular disease, excessive mortality, and significant cognitive damages.

Similar to the Unabomber, Nash's choice of symptoms was affected by the principle of availability. One of Nash's most prominent and unique symptoms was associated with numerology (e.g., see Nasar, 1998, p. 281), likely because "Nash was the greatest numerologist the world has ever seen" (Nasar, 1998, p. 335). Similarly, the fact that mathematics constituted the major focuses of his life may explain why "Nash's delusions and hallucinations often involved mathematics, numbers, and other mathematicians …" (Riplee, 2012). Another example of availability concerns his delusion regarding establishing a world government along with his persistent efforts to renounce his American citizenship and replace it with a universal identity card. Nasar noted in this regard that

> ideas of world government, and the related concept of world citizenship, were at their heyday during Nash's Princeton graduate-school days and permeated the 1950's science fiction that Nash devoured as a student … Princeton was the center of that movement, largely because of … Albert Einstein and John von Neumann … However, the one-worlder who fired Nash's imagination was a loner like himself, the Abbie Hoffman of the one-world movement. In 1948, Garry Davis, a leather-jacketed World War II bomber pilot, Broadway actor … had walked into the American embassy in Paris, turned in his U.S. passport, and renounced his American citizenship. He then tried to get the United Nations to declare him "the first citizen of the world." (pp. 270–271)

Nash's delusions were often associated with religious themes, and one was directly associated with the biblical story of Jacob and Esau (Nasar, 1998, p. 327). The availability of these ideas was due to his Sunday Bible classes (Nasar, 1998, p. 33), and to his upbringing in a traditional religious family.

In no other known case have schizophrenic symptoms reached as high a level of sophistication in their symbolic meanings, originality, and number of creative bizarre behaviors, as in the case of Nash. Although Nash's symptoms appear bizarre, careful examination reveals that they comprise a masterpiece of metaphors for his psychological condition, a masterpiece that only a genius such as Nash could invent. Some examples of these unique metaphors are (1) Nash's perception of himself as Emperor of Antarctica, which represented both his aspiration to be famous and his feelings of failure; (2) his belief that he was the left foot of God, symbolizing his recognition of his extraordinary abilities along with his deep sense of failure to implement his potential talents; (3) his claim that extraterrestrials were sending him messages, referring to the anxiety-provoking thoughts elicited by his merciless super-ego; (4) his conviction that the photograph of Pope John on the cover of Life magazine was actually a disguised photo of him, which again refers to his disappointment in himself for failing to earn recognition; (5) his reference to himself as "the prince of peace," which reflects his wish to settle his psychological conflicts and thus live in peace; (6) The title of "Absolute Zero," on his notebook, alluding to his perception of himself as a total failure. It is difficult to see how suggestions of brain impairments, such as Capps' (2011) claim that Nash's schizophrenic symptoms were the consequence of poor communication between the two hemispheres, or other rival theories can explain these extraordinary metaphors.

3. **Charles Cullen — The Angel of Death:** Cullen was a hospital nurse, who confessed to murdering as many as 40 patients over 16 years by injecting them with overdoses of various medications, such as insulin. Experts claim that he was responsible for the deaths of 400 patients (Graeber, 2013). Cullen had a long history of difficult circumstances. He attempted suicide multiple times, beginning from

as early an age as 9, felt lonely, experienced teasing, divorced his wife, and suffered from severe levels of depression (Graeber, 2013). In an interview with CBS' "60 Minutes," Cullen noted, regarding his suicide attempts, "I tried to kill myself throughout my life because I never really liked being who I was. I didn't feel I was worthy of anything" (Kroft, 2013). While repression, that is, blocking the accessibility of stress-related thoughts, played an important function in reducing his emotional distress, it seems that the major factor that caused him to choose this particular type of madness was controllability: the inflation of his self-esteem. While officially he was just another hospital nurse, in practice, his new position as a murderer, making life and death decisions, made him God-like. Furthermore, some of Cullen's attempts to kill his patients granted him the opportunity to increase his professional status in the hospital. As noted by Graeber (2013) "Cullen was the first to respond to the screaming 'code blue' and start resuscitating a failing patient. Because he had administered the cocktail of drugs that sent the victim into trouble, Cullen seemed almost magically prescient when he knew what drugs to administer to undo the damage and save the day." Thus, in terms of cost-benefit analysis, Cullen's seemingly senseless behavior was quite beneficial. It enabled him to reduce his intolerable level of depression so that he was no longer suicidal. By killing others he succeeded in saving his own life.

PBT's principle of availability may account for the reason why Cullen chose his specific bizarre criminal behavior. He utilized his profession and workplace to develop a unique pathological coping mechanism that served his repression and controllability needs with relatively low cost. As a nurse, Cullen was able to conceal his serial killings for many years particularly because he used medications normally employed to save people's lives. Drugs like digoxin, commonly used to help regulate heart rhythm, can become deadly when employed in large enough doses and injected into a patient's IV port. It was especially lethal to patients with a history of heart problems. Insulin was another drug Cullen frequently used, sending patients into spiraling diabetic comas and generally stressing their already fragile systems. The role of one's profession or workplace in choosing a specific bizarre behavior is seen in other cases, including those of Mordechai Vanunu, the Israeli nuclear spy, to be discussed below, and Andreas Lubitz, the 27-year-old copilot of German wings Flight 9525, who intentionally crashed into the French Alps on March 24, 2015 (Huggler, 2015), as will be discussed later.

Additionally, Cullen had a history of violent behavior prior to his serial killings. His wife filed two domestic-violence complaints against him and requested a restraining order. Furthermore, in March 1993, Cullen broke into the home of a coworker, whom he had once dated, while she and her young son slept, but left without waking them. Afterward, he began contacting the coworker frequently, leaving her numerous messages, and following her at work and around town until the woman filed a police report. He was arrested and then tried to commit suicide. Cullen pleaded guilty to trespassing and received 1-year probation. Thus, the choice of murder as his coping mechanism was driven by his specialized work in administering drugs and was compounded by his strong aggressive tendencies.

Charles Cullen's case meets all five of PBT's diagnostic criteria:

a. The murders intensively preoccupied his attention and severely disrupted his daily life, as he had to take precautions not to be arrested.
b. The dramatic change in his behavior could not be explained by any observable event beyond his conscious control.
c. He was unaware of the underlying causes of his own criminal behaviors and was therefore unable to explain the reasoning behind his actions. When asked about the reasons for his criminal acts, he first said he thought he was helping people by ending their suffering. However, Cullen told a different story when reminded of the fact that some were not close to death or suffering from great pain. He said there was "no justification" and that he "felt overwhelmed at that time." When pressed by

the interviewer from "60 Minutes," for an explanation for the families of his victims, he said "it felt like I needed to do something and I did. And that's not an answer to anything."

d. His criminal behavior was extremely rare.

e. His behavior was diagnosed as a reflection of madness (see Graeber, 2013).

4. **Mordechai Vanunu — *The Nuclear Spy*:**

a. **Background:** In 1986, Vanunu leaked classified information regarding Israel's nuclear capabilities and was subsequently sentenced to 18 years in prison (see biographical account by Toscano, 1990). Although Vanunu claimed that his actions were ideologically motivated, gaining the sympathy of various notable people around the world, including Nobel Laureates and the American astronomer — Carl Sagan (Toscano, 1990, p. 291), evidence reviewed below suggests that the underlying cause of his unusual criminal act was an extreme level of stress. This case is important because it indicates that the current diagnostic system lacks objective criteria for distinguishing between normal and criminal insanity, and may result in the miscarriage of justice.

Several months before the incident, Vanunu was fired from his low ranking position at the Israeli nuclear center, following eight and a half years of employment. This experience must have been particularly frustrating in light of his earlier failure to graduate Tel-Aviv University with a physics degree. Although he held a bachelor's degree in Greek philosophy and was studying for a master's degree, his career options were scarce. He also experienced chronic social alienation due to his extremely poor social skills (see Toscano, 1990, pp. 37, 55). As a part-time student at Ben-Gurion University in Beer-Shiva, he failed to establish meaningful relationships with fellow Jewish students. On the religiously divided campus, "Arabs soon became the only friends Vanunu could find" (Toscano, 1990, p. 37). Vanunu also had difficulty forming relationships with women, and he admitted to still being a virgin (Toscano, 1990, p. 67). The Israeli Supreme Court (1990) noted, with respect to his personality, that Vanunu was "an introverted person, egocentric and lonely, his personality structure is complex and problematic and from his life it seems that he did not find his place in the Israeli state and society" (p. 272). Vanunu's disappointment with himself is reflected in a diary he kept. In August 1982 he wrote

> what have I achieved until now? … Why am I not relaxed and settled, satisfied with something or enjoying something? I have never been ready to take responsibility for myself … Once I thought if you aren't ready, commit suicide and be released from the job given to you, from miseries you see in life. Release the world and your surroundings from your despairing and depressing personality. I am a failure in life. I don't want contact with anyone in society. What will be in the future? … What is my path in life? What am I doing with myself in this world? (Toscano, 1990, p. 29)

Similarly, the Israeli Supreme Court (1990) noted that Vanunu made tremendous efforts to earn a more respectable position in society than did his parents and other family members. "Unfortunately, he did not succeed, he did not create a family of his own, and at quite an advanced age he was still wandering along the paths of life. His routine work as a factory technician [at the nuclear center], with no hope — perhaps no chance for promotion in this job … brought him to the conclusion that he had accomplished nothing in his life." (Supreme Court, 1990, p. 272).

Subsequent to his dismissal from the nuclear center, Vanunu visited a number of Eastern European and Asian countries before finally arriving in Sydney, where he settled. In less than 2 months he converted to Christianity and changed his name to John. This was a very significant behavioral change, raised as an Orthodox Jew, Vanunu must have been aware that Jewish religious law treats a convert as if he were dead. This spontaneous and hasty religious conversion seems very unusual and appears to be motivated by emotional, rather than by intellectual, reasons. As noted by Toscano (1990), before his conversion, Vanunu "never evidenced much interest in Christianity, certainly nothing strong enough to trigger such an important move in the space of a few months" (p. 75).

The impulsive and seemingly senseless nature of Vanunu's behavior is evident also in his obsession with the Israeli nuclear project. Upon meeting the daughter of British television reporter, after leaving Israel, he immediately "spilled the Dimona story to a stranger and asked whether she could arrange a meeting with her father" (p. 64). Although the desire for revenge, publicity, and recognition may have influenced Vanunu's behavior — as was claimed by the Israeli Supreme Court (1990) — these do not provide a satisfactory explanation for his immigration, his religious conversion, and his unusual criminal behavior. After losing their job, people will not normally take measures as extreme as committing treason. Similarly, financial motive cannot account for Vanunu's unusual behavior. As noted by Toscano (1990), the possibility of making money never crossed Vanunu's mind (p. 72). Indeed, as confirmed by the Israeli Supreme Court (1990), there is no evidence that Vanunu received any significant amount of money for his betrayal (p. 273).

Vanunu justified his actions on ideological grounds, saying, "in a democracy ... the people should decide the nuclear issue. He wanted to give Israelis the opportunity denied to them by their government" (Toscano, 1990. p. 120). However, Vanunu's pretension that he was motivated by concern for the Israeli public appears ludicrous in light of the fact that his actions "in the minds of many Israelis ... threatened the very existence of the Jewish state" (Toscano, 1990, p. 120). Furthermore, the Israeli Supreme Court, rejecting Vanunu's ideological explanation, noted that there are no indications in Vanunu's personal diary that his actions "stemmed from strong ideological motives" (p. 274).

b. **PBT's Explanation:** Vanunu's psychological condition was quite similar to that of the Unabomber. Both were socially incompetent, isolated, sexually deprived, and suffering from deep feelings of inferiority. Vanunu was actually in a worse psychological state than the Unabomber. Unlike the Unabomber, who achieved exceptional academic success and gained a very high position in his profession, Vanunu failed in every sphere of his life. It is also worthwhile to note that like Vanunu, the Unabomber became very angry and sought revenge, just before beginning his killing spree, once he discovered that wildland around his cabin was destroyed for the development of industrial projects.

Like the aforementioned case studies, Vanunu's behavior was motivated by an extreme level of stress that severely damaged his self-esteem. Much like the Unabomber's murderous anger, Vanunu's rage at his dismissal from the Israeli nuclear center was a trigger that elevated his emotional distress to an intolerable level and motivated his unusual behavior.

One major reason for his behavioral change was repression. His leaving Israel, his conversion to Christianity, and especially his preoccupation with the nuclear project, were aimed at effectively blocking the accessibility of stress-related thoughts. As noted by Toscano (1990), Vanunu "spent virtually all his free time at the church or with the parishioners" (p. 67). Similar to John Nash, who detached himself from his former identity — for example, by his stubborn refusal to return to the United States — Vanunu achieved the same goal by leaving Israel, detaching himself from his Jewish identity through conversion to Christianity and changing his name to John. His new identity within a completely different social environment enabled him to disassociate himself from his past and manage "a simple life doing simple work" (Toscano, 1990, p. 76; Vanunu was employed as a cab driver). The repressive function of his behavior is further reflected in his obsession with the Israeli nuclear project. He "reached a point where he could not rest or relax as a result of his quandary over an appropriate moral response to Israeli nuclear policy" (Toscano, 1990, p. 67).

However, the major reasons for choosing treason as a coping mechanism was not repression, as this need could be satisfied also by other means of bizarre behaviors. The two major causes of Vanunu's criminal behavior were the need to exercise control over his stressor and the availability of suitable means. Similar to the aforementioned case studies, Vanunu experienced a strong blow to his self-esteem. The treasonable act enabled him to boost his self-esteem, thereby reducing his intolerable level of depression and his risk of suicide.

Availability affected Vanunu's behavioral choice in two ways (1) he was involved in extreme left-wing politics and frequently protested against the government. As such, his radical betrayal can be compared to anorexics and OCD patients who exaggerate a socially normal behavior to an extreme level; (2) before he left Israel, Vanunu took photographs of the nuclear site. As noted by Toscano (1990), these "photographs preoccupied Vanunu from the moment the ferry steamed out of Haifa harbor" (p. 63). Hence, similar to Charles Cullen who utilized the hospital setting and its drugs to build his unique insane coping mechanism, Vanunu used his classified knowledge of the nuclear center to construct an effective coping mechanism that let him achieve the goal of overcoming his overwhelming emotional distress.

Diagnostically speaking, Vanunu's behavior can be classified as bizarre, as it fulfills at least six of PBT's seven diagnostic criteria. It certainly disrupted his daily functioning and intensively preoccupied his attention, as required by PBT's first criterion. It also meets PBT's second criterion, as his criminal activities cannot be attributed to normal incentives that usually motivate treason. Vanunu's inability to provide a tenable explanation for his behavior indicates that he was unaware of his own underlying motives and that he chose the strategy of denial to preserve his unawareness. This use of denial is similar to that of patients with anorexia nervosa and OCD (e.g., compulsive cleaning) who deny that they are suffering from a disorder. In this regard, Vanunu was not different from the Unabomber, who denied that he suffered from mental illness though doing so could entail a death penalty. Vanunu's behavior also meets the fourth criterion, seeing as was extremely rare, its perpetrator being described as having "committed the most heinous form of betrayal possible in Israel" (Toscano, 1990, p. 300). Regarding the fifth criterion, there is disagreement as to whether Vanunu's behavior was abnormal. Although most Israelis would have found his behavior aberrant, many others, especially outside Israel, regarded him as a hero. Nevertheless, it seems that Vanunu should be diagnosed as a criminal insane, rather than as a normal criminal, as he also fulfilled PBT's two secondary criteria of stress and depression.

It should be noted that in the absence of PBT, the court was not sufficiently aware that Vanunu was in an extremely stressful situation and that his unusual criminal behavior was aimed at combating his extreme level of depression and reducing the risk of suicide. Otherwise, his prison sentence might have been reduced to fewer than the 18 years decided. In this regard, it is worth mentioning that the former Israeli minister, Gonen Segev, who was convicted of spying for Iran for monetary rewards, was sentence to only eleven years in prison.

5. **L. Percy King — The Creative Paranoid Patient:** White (1964, pp. 76–84) described a case study of a paranoid schizophrenic, L. Percy King, who was hospitalized for 28 years. King attributed all his misfortunes and weaknesses, including his long hospitalization, compulsive masturbation, and homosexual desires, to a group of invisible pursuers who had been chasing him since he left his home state 30 years earlier. The patient ascribed occulated powers to this group, believing they controlled his mind and body. He described in detail their supernatural abilities, special controlling methods, terrifying immoral acts, and danger to other people. "These mind-reading pursuers can ruin or disgrace anyone. I do not believe anyone's life is safe with some of them around!" (White, 1964, p. 77). This case is similar to the aforementioned case studies in several fundamental respects.

a. **Diagnostic Criteria:** King meets PBT's five major diagnostic criteria. His psychotic symptoms intensively preoccupied his attention and severely disrupted his daily life (1); the dramatic change in his behavior could not be explained by any observable event that would necessarily cause this change (2); he was not aware of the underlying causes of his delusions nor the fact that his behavior was deviant (3); his schizophrenic symptoms were extremely rare (4); and both the medical professionals and the general public considered him to be mad (5).

b. **Stress:** Prior to his hospitalization, King was extremely depressed, suffered from self-inflicted wounds, and even tried to commit suicide. King experienced a deep sense of self-loathing stemming from extremely low self-esteem. White noted that King felt "strong self-contempt" because of

> his masturbation, his lack of manliness, his failure to prove his sexual adequacy … In King's case the threat to his inflated self-esteem was intolerable. All the contempt he was accustomed to direct upon others threatened to come showering back to him if he really possessed such a grave flaw in his manhood. (pp. 81–82)

While his low self-esteem was the source for the intolerable stress that motivated the adoption of his schizophrenic symptoms, King arrived at this state primarily because of his poor coping abilities, particularly his deficiency in social skills, which resulted in social isolation and a deep sense of incompetence. He described himself as odd, queer, shy, bashful, sedate, and so reserved that he was afraid to approach "young ladies to make dates for petting and necking parties" (p. 81). White notes that, given King's personality, which was highly pretentious, self-promoting, and contemptuous, acknowledgment of his character flaws was extremely painful.

No information is provided in this case study concerning other areas of King's life, such as family relationships and professional achievement, which may have been additional sources for King's sense of failure and incompetence. However, the available evidence indicates the direct cause for King's emotional state were psychological factors, rather than neurological impairments.

c. **Repression and Controllability**: King's stressful thoughts relating to his low self-esteem and lack of sufficient coping skills, refer to his experiences before he became psychotic. Accordingly, from PBT's theoretical standpoint, King's schizophrenic symptoms were goal-directed behaviors, aimed to fulfill two major psychological needs: repression and controllability. King's schizophrenic symptoms of hallucination and delusion gave him a powerful repressive tool, which effectively blocked the accessibility of stress-related thoughts. Most importantly, they enabled him to reduce his stressors by means of projection, that is, attributing the cause of his weaknesses to external sources. White noted on this that "by projection he protected his self-esteem from an unbearable blow" (p. 81). A second tactic, perhaps more powerful than projection, is the strategy of denial, in which the individual deliberately inflates his self-esteem by producing a fictional reality. While in the previous cases, the artificial intensification of self-esteem had some basis in reality or at least a symbolic meaning (as in the case of Nash) in King's case, this involved a complete detachment from reality. This is illustrated in King's statement regarding what would happen once people found out about his discovery of the invisible pursuers:

> his photo and write-up will be published in every important newspaper and magazine on earth ... he will receive so many tones of fan mail that the post office will have to employ extra mail trucks to handle it.... He and they would be invited to appear before the State Assembly, in special session, and will be invited to the State House ... ." (p. 83)

Although King's delusion was completely nonsensical, his bizarre behaviors were rationally based as this was the best means at his disposal to relieve his intolerable level of depression. Hallucinations and delusions of grandeur diminish the sense of incompetence, and, as noted by White, King became far less disordered and less distressed when he entered the hospital. This is consistent with other data indicating that delusions and hallucinations constitute effective barriers against depression (e.g., Hogarty, Goldberg, & Collaborative Study Group, 1973; Siris et al., 1984; Van Putten, Crumpton, & Yale 1976). Indeed, schizophrenics with active delusions appear less depressed and more content than those who have recovered and abandoned their delusions (e.g., Roberts, 1991). Also, low self-esteem is consistently associated with persecutory delusional ideation (e.g., Green et al., 2006). An additional benefit of King's psychotic symptoms was that they allowed him to discharge his sexual tension without experiencing guilt over his homosexual desires and masturbation.

Not enough information is given to determine the effect of the principle of availability on King's symptoms. Based on the provided data, it seems that two available experiences likely affected the development of his unique delusion: sexual sensations and strong feelings of guilt, resulting from his unacceptable sexual desires. It seems likely that King utilized these two experiences, along with his imaginative abilities, to create a delusion of pursuers who were endowed with "astounding, unheard of, utterly unbelievable occult powers" (White, 1964, p. 76), which enabled him to satisfy his sexual drives without guilt.

6. **Mr. X — Failure of Meeting the Mother/God's Expectations:** As demonstrated above, schizophrenia is usually associated with a severe deficiency in coping skills, which increases the likelihood of self-loathing or strong feelings of incompetence. However, occasionally, environmental stressors may motivate the adoption of the schizophrenic coping mechanism, provided that they induce intense feelings of self-loathing. One example demonstrating this possibility is that of a 31-year-old, married, university lecturer, diagnosed

as schizophrenic. Psychiatrists deemed him incurable after several years of unsuccessful medical treatment (Karon, 2008). The patient was not eating, not sleeping, and continually hallucinating. Electroconvulsive therapy (ECT) was strongly though pessimistically recommended. His wife stopped the ECT treatment and directed him to psychoanalytic therapy, which resulted in a dramatic change in his behavior. He began eating after 3 days and began working at an intellectually demanding job after 4 months. He remained in treatment for a total of 14 years, and over 20 years later, after the treatment was completed, the patient sent the therapist a note thanking him for "giving me my life back" (Karon, 2008; see also Silver, 2008).

Mr. X was a Jew who married a non-Jewish woman. "His mother literally told him, like the apocryphal Jewish mother stories that he did not have to worry about the wedding because she would not be there. She would commit suicide. Right up to the wedding, he was terrified that she would carry out her threat" (p. 15). Psychological evaluations revealed that Mr. X experienced "extreme feelings of inadequacy, guilt, and worthlessness" (p. 15), which were apparently due to feeling that he had failed to meet his parents' expectations. The schizophrenic symptoms developed right after he received his Ph.D. and took a job at a prestigious college.

Karon noted that Mr. X was "held together by the fantasy that if only he were good enough, then his parents would accept him." When this did not happen … "his defenses unraveled" (p. 14). Thus, it seems that the patient's self-esteem was extremely dependent upon his parents' approval, especially that of his mother, who for him, was like God. His mother's disappointment over his marriage to a non-Jewish woman damaged his self-esteem. However, he was able to continue functioning normally because of his belief that his mother would accept him as soon as he got his Ph.D. When this did not occur, he felt a profound sense of failure, which motivated him to adopt the schizophrenic coping pathology. Psychoanalytic therapy, to be discussed later, succeeded in curing the patient primarily by focusing on childhood events, which destroyed the mother's idealized image. Once the therapy succeeded in disconnecting the patient's self-worth from meeting his mother's expectations, he fully recovered. This case challenges the validity of medical models both because (1) it demonstrates that schizophrenia may be solely the result of environmental stress; and (2) full recovery was achieved by psychological means, as opposed to medical intervention, which had worsened the patient's condition.

7. **Miss. A. — Environmental-Shaming Stress:** Another case in which environmental stress may be sufficient in producing self-loathing and motivating the adoption of schizophrenia is the case study of Miss. A., a 45-year old woman who had been suffering from schizophrenia for more than twenty years. This patient is under the treatment of the first author of this book. Before developing schizophrenia, Miss. A was exceedingly intelligent, earning high academic scores on her high school exams and psychometric tests, and had good social ties. The onset of her schizophrenic symptoms occurred following a social shaming, which severely damaged her self-esteem. Her parents put her in mental hospitals for a short period, but were disappointed with the treatment and decided to take her home, as was the case with Mr. X.

Miss. A's case, like that of Mr. X., presents serious difficulties for those who might be tempted to attribute it to medical factors: there is no case of mental illness in her family, nor did the psychiatrists find any evidence of brain impairments. Moreover, unlike typical cases of schizophrenia, she had no history of adjustment difficulties and so was not at risk of developing deviant behaviors in a stressful environment. The cases of Miss. A. and Mr. X both demonstrate that individuals may develop schizophrenia if their environment sufficiently damages their self-image, even if they functioned normally up to that time. In accordance with PBT, the schizophrenic symptoms provided the patient with a powerful repressive tool. Additionally, the symptoms served her controllability needs as her delusions of being the Messiah and having the power to resurrect the dead enhanced her self-esteem and provided her full control over her parents.

8. **Molly — A Rapid Spontaneous Recovery:** This case refers to an eighteen-year-old woman diagnosed as an "acute paranoid schizophrenic (Siebert, 2000). Molly's parents brought her to the hospital and told the staff that Molly claimed God had talked to her and said she was going to give birth to the second Savior. During her stay she was very withdrawn and unwilling to participate in any ward activities. The nurses could not persuade her to comb her hair or put on makeup. The staff consensus was that she was so severely schizophrenic that she would probably spend the rest of her life in the ward.

Molly suffered several life-events that damaged her self-esteem and may have triggered the onset of her paranoid schizophrenia: She was an only child who had tried unsuccessfully to win her parents' love and praise. In an attempt to please her father, a musician, she joined the school orchestra; she was promoted to first chair in the clarinet section, but when she ran home from school to tell her father, his reaction was to smash her clarinet across the kitchen table and tell her, "You'll never amount to anything." Later, after graduation from high school, Molly entered nursing school. She was eager and excited for her first clinical assignment, but it turned into a shattering experience. She was harshly criticized by two patients; afterward she reported feeling "like the world fell in." Then Molly ran away from school, took a bus to another town to see her high school boyfriend, but he told her to go home, and that their relationship was over.

In a clinical interview, Siebert (2000) made the patient aware of her stressors by saying: "So your dad and mom didn't love you, the patients were critical and didn't like you, and your boyfriend just wanted to be friends. That made you feel very sad and lonely". Molly responded by saying "Yes, there didn't seem to be anyone in the whole world who cared for me at all." (p. 42). This interaction soon led Molly to recognize that her "crazy talk" with God was, in fact, a rational coping mechanism that enabled her to alleviate her intolerable stress (for the full interview see PBT's insight therapy in Part-III).

Two days later, upon meeting the "therapist", the patient said: "I've been thinking about what we talked about... I've been wondering. Do you think I imagined God's voice to make myself feel better?" Soon afterward, a dramatic change occurred in the patient behavior. She became a cheerful, talkative teenager, and spoke easily with her doctor, the nurses, and other patients. She started participating in patient activities, brushed and combed her hair, put on makeup, and asked for nicer looking dresses. Siebert reported that "the plans to commit her were dropped. A few days later, she was transferred to the open ward and she did so well that the doctors and nurses expected her to be discharged soon" (p. 42).

This case, like the above cases, not only challenge the validity of medical models of schizophrenia, but it fully consistent with PBT in terms of diagnostic criteria, etiology, goal-directed behavior, and therapy, as will be specified later in Part-III.

9–11. **Suicide-Criminal Insanity:** This section discusses three case studies: Adam Lanza, Elliot Rodger, and Andreas Lubitz, who each murdered innocent people and committed suicide. It aims to demonstrate that although these behaviors appear completely irrational, as their perpetrators seemingly reaped no benefit from them, they are no less rational than all the above cases of schizophrenia and criminal insanity. The same theoretical concepts used for the explanation of the above cases are applicable for the explanation of these three additional cases. Firstly, the underlying causes of these cases is an extreme level of stress and depression. Secondly, in all three cases the individual experienced self-loathing and the insane criminal behavior was aimed to inflate the individual's self-esteem. Thirdly, the choice of the bizarre criminal behavior was determined by PBT's three principles of choice of symptoms. Fourthly, all three cases meet PBT's diagnostic criteria of madness.

Adam Peter Lanza: This case refers to a 20-year-old man, who on December 14, 2012, fatally shot his mother, murdered 20 children and 6 adult staff members at the Sandy Hook Elementary School in

Newtown, CT, and then committed suicide (Derossett, 2013). Although Lanza was diagnosed with Asperger's syndrome at the age of 5 (e.g., Lysiak, 2013), it is hard to see how this diagnosis can account for his horrendous criminal behavior. As noted by Lysiak, "most in the medical community believe there is no linkage between autism and acts of violence ... Autism did not commit this horrible act" (pp. 212–213). Similarly, Derossett (2013) stated that "the aggression that Adam displayed during this rampage is not typical of someone who has autism" (p. 153). His autopsy did not reveal abnormality or tumors in his brain that might have triggered his behaviors (Derossett, 2013, p. 167). Similar to the above cases of schizophrenia, Lanza was highly intelligent and achieved exceptional academic success, but lacked social skills. A fellow classmate, who sat next to Lanza in their sophomore-year honors math class, said Lanza barely spoke a word all year but earned high marks. He was shy, introverted, and lacked any close friends (Derossett, 2013). Lanza's mother removed him from the Newtown public school system because she was unhappy with the school district's plans for her son. He did not have any social interaction at home, as his mother was reluctant to let others into her house. A group of neighbors with whom Lanza's mother played a weekly dice game said she always managed to avoid hosting the get-togethers, despite having been an active participant for over 15 years (Derossett, 2013). As noted by Lysiak (2013):

> Adam was nineteen, he had withdrawn almost completely and become a virtual shut-in, spending hours playing the first-person shooter game Call of Duty. In the months that preceded the shooting, Adam began to isolate himself in his bedroom, surrounded all day and night by violent images. (p. 211)

Elliot Rodger: This case refers to a 22-year-old man, who displayed similar insane criminal behavior to Adam Lanza and had a similar psychological profile. He murdered 6 people and wounded

14 others, on May 23, 2014, in Isla Vista, CA (Derossett, 2013). Like Lanza, Rodger (2014) was highly intelligent, as evidenced by his cleverly written manifesto, but lacked adequate social skills. He repeatedly mentioned his loneliness, and, particularly, his desperate and unsuccessful efforts to establish relationships with women. He described himself as shy, quiet, and incapable of making friends. Experiencing loneliness, social rejection and strong feelings of inferiority, Rodger began:

> To act weird and annoying to people just to get attention … people started to make fun of me, but I don't care … I was extremely unpopular, widely disliked, and viewed as the weirdest kid in the school … I never knew how to gain positive attention, only negative … I told everyone that I wanted to commit suicide … I sank into major depression. My feelings of inferiority were intensified … I realized how hopeless everything in my life was … The loneliness was torturing me so intensely … I sank into one of the worst depressions of my life … . (Rodger, 2014, pp. 41, 42, 54, 57, 93, 105)

Thus, like the aforementioned cases, Rodger was extremely depressed, lonely and suicidal.

The aggression and suicides of both Lanza and Rodger are consistent with numerous studies indicating that depression, particularly when accompanied with social isolation, is a risk factor for general aggression, intimate partner aggression, and self-aggression (e.g., see review by Dutton & Karakanta, 2013; Heinrich & Gullone, 2006). In addition, both sought retribution: Lanza took revenge on the school that had offended him (see Lysiak, 2013, p. 212), and Rodger acted in response to the social rejection he experienced, particularly by women.

> They treated me like an insignificant little mouse, but on the Day of Retribution, I would be a God to them. They will be

> the mice, and I will be the predator … All of the suffering, loneliness, rejection, and humiliation I had to experience . … (Rodger, 2014, p. 32)

Although revenge was an important motive in triggering Lanza and Rodger's criminal behaviors, it seems that this factor alone is insufficient in explaining their unusual criminal acts. It appears that like all aforementioned cases, Vanunu's in particular, the major factor behind these insane criminal behaviors was severe damage to their self-esteem. Therefore, it seems likely that they suffered from an intense level of self-loathing, as they could only blame themselves for their miserable life conditions. Like the other individuals involved in cases of bizarre behavior, both were apparently unaware of this motive. The question that remains to be clarified concerns the benefits that Lanza and Elliot could derive from their horrible criminal acts, taking into consideration that they may have known in advance that they would end their lives immediately afterward.

Lanza "researched mass shooting extensively, he had a 7 by 4-foot spreadsheet that had the names of shooters, the weapons they used, the number of killed or injured and more … Lanza researched more than 500 shootings in all" (Derossett, 2013, pp. 17–18). Neither depression nor the desire to take revenge can explain why Lanza invested so much time and energy researching previous acts of murder. It seems likely that Lanza searched for an unusual, cruel, and unique criminal act, committed by none before, because he wanted to immortalize himself, a goal that raised his self-esteem during the planning stage. As noted by Haggerty (2009) in his analytic article on the etiology of modern serial killers, while attention seeking is a major motivating factor for these behaviors, "fame also offers citizens the prospect of surviving beyond death" (p. 174). The motive of self-enhancement can also explain the fact that Rodger invested a significant amount of energy and time in writing his 140-page manifesto. In the absence of this motive, it is difficult to understand why an extremely depressed person who intended to commit suicide would invest so much energy in writing such a long, detailed manifesto. Rodger formulated a clear expression of this need in the following statement:

> I would be a God to them ... In order to completely abolish sex, women themselves would have to be abolished ... In order to carry this out, there must exist a new and powerful type of government, under the control of one divine ruler, such as myself. (Rodger, 2014, pp. 110, 136)

Thus, similar to the above cases, self-enhancement, even after death — was the major motive for the adoption of the crazy behavior of both Lanza and Rodger.

Andreas Lubitz: This case relates to 27-year-old copilot of Germanwings Flight 9525, who intentionally crashed into the French Alps on March 24, 2015 (Huggler, 2015a). Like the above cases, he was motivated by an extreme level of depression and a need to inflate his self-esteem, even if doing so entailed his death.

Lubitz grew up dreaming of flying and of one day becoming a pilot. Klaus Radker, the club's chairman, said: "it was his dream to fly from an early age and it was a dream he began to fulfill here, so when he went on to gain his commercial license and fly planes... he was very happy and proud" (Sawer, 2015a). Lubitz's descent into suicidal depression appears to have begun when he started experiencing blurred vision in December 2014 (Huggler, 2015a). His vision was already restricted to 30%, possibly because of a detached retina, and he was concerned about losing his eyesight (Gallagher & Hall, 2015). According to medical records, Lubitz was taking medication to combat his depression, anxiety disorders, and panic attacks. He was reportedly using a medication so strong that patients taking it are advised not to drive a car. During their search of Lubitz's apartment, detectives found a letter in a waste bin indicating that he had been declared unfit to work by a doctor (Glenn, 2015). Motivated by the fear that blindness would cause him to lose his pilot's license, he began conducting online research about methods of committing suicide before deciding to crash Flight 9525 (Huggler, 2015b).

An additional stressful event, which may have facilitated his suicidal act, was his breakup with his girlfriend. "Investigators believe his eyesight problems — coupled with a breakdown in his relationship with his long-term girlfriend — triggered the 'madness' that ended in mass murder" (Gallagher & Hall, 2015).

Thus, it is likely that as with the aforementioned cases, Lubitz experienced a profound sense of incompetence and a strong blow to his self-esteem, following the realization that he must give up his dream to be a pilot. While there is not much information about his childhood background, a neighbor whose brother was in the same year as Lubitz in high school related: "I didn't know him well, but to me he seemed a very private, perhaps a little bit withdrawn" (Sawer, 2015a). Accordingly, it is likely that he had similar type of personality as Lanza and Rodgers, with a deep sense of inferior feelings, which did not allow him to tolerate failures. This motivated him not only to commit suicide, and thus relieve his unbearable level of depression, but also to take additional actions to enhance his self-worth through an unusual criminal act. This may explain his extremely unusual and terrifying suicide, as reflected in his statement to his ex-girlfriend: "one day I will do something that will change the whole system, and then all will know my name and remember it" (The Irish Times, 2015, see also Gallagher & Hall, 2015).

An additional factor which affected the insane criminal behaviors of Lanza, Rodger, and Lubitz is the principle of availability. Lanza's choice was affected by the following factors (1) the availability of weapons in his home (Police also found a gun safe in one of the bedrooms of the house containing 1,400 more rounds of ammunition along with other firearms, such as a 45 caliber Henry rifle (Derossett, 2013); (2) his extensive training in shooting (his mother often took her sons to practice at shooting ranges, Derossett, 2013); and (3) his exposure to a variety of cases of mass killings in the media. He comprehensively studied the 2001 Norway shooting and the 2006 Amish school shooting in Nickel Mines, PA; (4) he spent a significant amount of time playing an aggressive video game, Call of Duty.

Availability is also evidenced in Rodger's (2014) criminal acts:

1. In line with studies demonstrating that aggression is directed toward the frustrating objects (e.g., see Berkowitz, 1993; see also Blair, 2010; and Marcus-Newhall, Pedersen, Carlson, & Miller, 2000), Rodger harbored extreme anger toward women to whom he attributed his chronic sexual deprivation (see Rodger, 2014). When Rodger saw a young couple behaving intimately in public, he noted:

   > I was absolutely livid with envious hatred … I wanted to do horrible things to that couple. I wanted to inflict pain on all young couples.… I was capable of killing them … I wanted to kill them slowly, to strip the skins off their flesh … The males deserve it for taking the females away from me, and the females deserve it for choosing those males instead of me. (p. 87)

2. Rodger (2014) was continuously exposed to video games containing high levels of aggression. One such game, with which he was intensively preoccupied from the age of 13 to the age of 19, was World of Warcraft (WoW). The following statements illustrate his addiction to this game:

   > I only saw school as something that took time away from WoW' … I planned to spend the whole time on WoW, leveling up my character and forgetting about my horrible school life … I fully indulged myself in my addiction

> to WoW ... I just couldn't handle the anguish in my life anymore, and I needed a break, no matter how unhealthy and time-consuming WoW would be for me ... The loneliness was torturing me so intensely that I even started up my WoW account and played constantly for the month of September .... (pp. 41, 42, 49, 71, 93)

Although Rodger's obsession with this game temporarily distracted him from his stress, it ultimately increased his aggressive thoughts, hostile attitude, and violent behavior (e.g., see meta-analysis study by Anderson et al., 2010; Huesmann, 2010). Additionally, Rodger was the son of British filmmaker, Peter Rodger, assistant director of The Hunger Games, a notably violent film. Rodgers had seen the film, which contains graphic scenes of teenagers killing one another for sport, with his father at the red-carpet premier. Furthermore, Rodger's grandfather was a famed British photojournalist who took photos of Jewish survivors and mass graves at the liberated concentration camps in the final weeks of World War II. Thus, Rodger was continuously exposed to violent scenes, which must have affected his decision to take aggressive measures in response to his intolerable emotional distress.

3. Rodger (2014) underwent firearm training (p. 109) and saved $5,000 to purchase various weapons for the "Day of Retribution" (pp. 116, 113). Easy access to weapons gave him greater opportunity to violently express his frustration, which would have been more difficult in countries where there is greater gun control.

Availability apparently affected Lubitz's criminal act as well. Much like Charles Cullen who used medications that were available at his workplace to commit murder, and Vanunu who took photographs of the nuclear site at his workplace, Lubitz utilized his position as a copilot to commit murder-suicide.

One may argue that the fact that all three murderers committed suicide is incompatible with PBT's cost-benefit principle. However, as noted previously, research indicates that when individuals are confronted with an extreme level of emotional distress, cost-benefit considerations are determined by the individual's immediate needs to relieve tension, rather than by long-term considerations (Shiv & Fedorikhin, 1999, 2002). While others may view suicide as an irrational decision, from the standpoint of the suicidal individual, it can be seen as a rational choice. This explanation is consistent with Lester's (1988, 1997) rational choice theory of suicide (see also Lester & Yang, 1996).

Lanza, Rodger, and Lubitz all — meet PBT's five criteria of madness. All were intensively preoccupied with their murderous and suicidal intentions, and this severely disrupted their daily life (criterion 1); there was no specific event exclusively associated with their unusual criminal acts that can explain these behaviors (criterion 2); although there is no way to determine whether they were aware of the underlying causes of their behaviors, it seems likely that the intensive preoccupation with the planning of criminal behavior made them unaware of these causes (criterion 3); their unusual criminal actions were extremely rare (criterion 4); their behaviors were clearly denounced as the actions of someone who was crazy or mad and were seen as a reflection of illness (criterion 5). Furthermore, all three cases meet PBT's two secondary criteria of stress and depression.

Schizophrenia With Genetic/Neurological Flaws

PBT claims that there are no fundamental differences between schizophrenia with and without brain impairments. Patients with either form suffer from severe stress and both types blame themselves for their inability to resolve their stressors. The main difference between the two has to do with the source of their self-loathing: in atypical schizophrenia, where there is no evidence of brain impairment, the inability to cope with life's basic demands stems from lack of social skills (as demonstrated in cases of the Unabomber, Percy King, and to some extent in the case of Nash), or from a stressful environment (as seen in the cases of Mr. X, Miss. A, and Molly). By contrast, in typical schizophrenia, patients suffer from neurological abnormalities (see Martin, Dzafic, Robinson, Reutens, & Mowry, 2016; Shenton, Dickey, Frumin, & Mccarley, 2001; Zipursky et al., 2013), which seems to be the major cause for the severe deficit in their coping abilities. Thus, as stated in the beginning of Part I, while advocates of medical models interpreted the significant correlations between schizophrenia and neurological/genetic flaws in terms of causality, PBT explains these correlations in terms of stress.

Indeed, prior to the development of their disorder, typical schizophrenics suffer from severe cognitive dysfunctions (e.g., Morgan et al., 2012; Nuechterlein et al., 2012; Reichenberg & Harvey, 2007), manifested as ***attention deficits*** (e.g., Cornblatt, Dworkin, Wolf, & Erlenmeyer-Kimling, 1996; Cornblatt, Obuchowski, Roberts, Pollack, & Erlenmeyer-Kimling, 1999; Freedman, Rock, Roberts, Cornblatt, & Erlenmeyer-Kimling, 1998; Oner & Munir, 2005; Reichenberg & Harvey, 2007), ***low IQ levels*** (e.g., Byrne, Hodges, Grant, Owens, & Johnstone, 1999; Cosway et al., 2000), and ***poor performance in intellectual and executive functioning*** (e.g., Byrne et al., 1999; Davidson et al., 1999; Ozan et al., 2010). Additionally, typical schizophrenic patients are often raised in ***pathogenic home environments***. Their parents tend to be hostile, critical, domineering, emotionally over-involved, deviant communicators, and frequently unmindful to the feelings and needs of others (Lukoff, Snyder, Ventura, & Nuechterlein, 1984; Olin & Mednick, 1996; Rund, 1994; Tienari et al., 1993; Velligan et al., 1996; Ver Eecke, 2003). As described by Coleman (1984), schizophrenics' parents are

> Deficient tutors: they create a family milieu inappropriate for training a child in cognitive abilities essential for categorizing experience, thinking coherently, and communicating meaningfully. Coupled with feelings of inadequacy and other damage to the child's emerging self-concept, this may help explain the later cognitive distortions, communication failures, difficulties in interpersonal relationships, and identity confusion that commonly occur in schizophrenia. (p. 378)

Inevitably, due to their severe cognitive deficits and pathogenic social environments, the typical schizophrenics feel incompetent in all areas of their lives. These cognitive and personality deficits may explain studies revealing that high-risk children, who have genetic vulnerability to schizophrenia, exhibit poor adjustment to the cognitive and social demands of school (Ayalon & Merom, 1985; Beckfield, 1985; Beisser, Glasser, & Grant, 1967; Cannon et al., 1997; Grubb & Watt, 1979; Lewine, Watt, & Fryer, 1978; Nagler & Glueck, 1985; Nagler & Mirsky, 1985; Olin & Mednick, 1996; Olin et al., 1998; Parnas & Jorgensen, 1989; Parnas, Schulsinger, Schulsinger, Mednick, & Teasdale, 1982; Rolf, 1972; Rolf & Garmezy, 1974; Schulsinger, 1976; Sohlberg & Yaniv, 1985; Spring & Coons, 1982; Watt, 1978; Watt & Lubensky, 1976; Watt, Grubb, & Erlenmeyer-Kimiling, 1982; Weintraub, Liebert, & Neale, 1975). These children also have disciplinary problems and distant relationships with their teachers. They are emotionally unstable, exhibit difficulties in controlling their impulses, and are prone to anger and depression.

Inadequate social skills: The most severe personality features of typical schizophrenics are observable from an early age. As with atypical schizophrenics, this seems to be the main reason for their profound sense of incompetence (e.g., Bellack, Morrison, Wixted, & Mueser, 1990; Cornblatt et al., 2012; Davidson et al., 1999; Dworkin, Lewis, Cornblatt, & Erlenmeyer-Kimling, 1994a,

1994b; Hans, Auerbach, Asarnow, Styr, & Marcus, 2000; Hans, Marcus, Henson, Auerbach, & Mirsky, 1992; Matheson et al., 2013; McClellan & McCurry, 1999; Munk-Jorgensen & Mortensen, 1992). While social environment plays an important role in the development of social deficiencies, the dominant factor seems to be neurological impairments. As noted by Cornblatt et al. (1996), schizophrenics' premorbid attention impairment predisposes them to poorer social competence, which in turn makes communication with others difficult, and inhibits their interactions with their peers.

Despite their shortcomings, in the vast majority of cases, the family and school systems do provide some level of social support and security, enabling premorbid individuals to cope with their stress. However, upon reaching adolescence and young adulthood, a stage characterized by the need to make appropriate adjustments toward independence (e.g., moving away from the family, choosing a vocation, and seeking a partner), high-risk individuals, who have genetic vulnerability to schizophrenia are likely to experience complete helplessness. Though most young people are reasonably optimistic and feel that they can exercise control over their future (Mussen, Conger, Kagan, & Huston, 1984), for the high-risk population the prospect of "the future" is more likely to induce feelings of despair, anxiety, and depression. Perhaps the most frustrating aspect for a high-risk adolescent is an inevitable intensification of social alienation at the very age when peer-group support is critical. Mussen et al. (1984) noted that emotionally unstable adolescents

> are likely to meet with rejection or indifference. In turn an awareness of not being accepted by peers and a lack of opportunity to participate in and learn from peer group activities further undermine self-confidence and increase a sense of social isolation. (p. 398)

Overall, typical schizophrenics display poor premorbid adjustment over the course of childhood, adolescence, and adulthood

(Gureje, Aderibigbe, Olley, & Bamidele, 1994; Hans et al., 2000; Levitt, Shenton, McCarley, Faux, & Ludwig, 1994).

Thus, PBT agrees with medical models that genetic predispositions can lead to severe brain impairments and that this often precedes the development of schizophrenia. A further point of agreement is that in many cases stressful life-events precede and may facilitate the onset of schizophrenia (see reviews by Lukoff et al., 1984; Phillips, Francey, Edwards, & McMurray, 2007; Teague, Drake, & Bartels, 1989; Walker & Diforio, 1997). However, PBT claims that these negative personality traits (e.g., poor social skills and attention deficits), termed in the literature as negative symptoms (e.g., see Buchanan, 2007; Moller, 1995; Skodlar et al., 2013), are equivalent to the stressors of atypical schizophrenics that cause their sense of incompetence. While these personality traits may be sufficient to produce the level of stress required to motivate the adoption of schizophrenia, this may also be facilitated by stressful life-events. In other words, this personality profile is the major cause of stressors that motivate these people to adopt the schizophrenic symptoms of delusions, hallucinations, or disorganized speech, which are referred to by the medical models as positive symptoms (e.g., see *DSM-5*, 2013).

In accordance with this claim, it seems reasonable that schizophrenia would be more common among people with intellectual disabilities than among the general population. Intellectual disability is linked with impairments in general abilities, adaptive functioning across social and practical domains, low self-esteem, depression, loneliness, and high risk for behavioral disorders, which is three to four times greater than among those with no intellectual disability (American Psychiatric Association, 2013; Crnic, Neece, McIntyre, Blacher, & Baker, 2017; Dagnan & Sandhu, 1999; Einfeld et al., 2006; Emerson, McCulloch, Graham, et al., 2010; Garaigordobil & Pérez, 2007; Gilmore, & Cuskelly, 2014; McGillivray & McCabe, 2007).

Accordingly, it is not surprising that schizophrenia is at least three times more prevalent among individuals with intellectual disabilities than among those without this disability (Greenwood, Husted, Bomba, Hodgkinson, & Bassett, 2004; Morgan, Leonard, Bourke, & Jablensky, 2008; Welch, Lawrie, Muir, & Johnstone, 2011). As would be expected, patients with intellectual disabilities display substantially greater negative symptoms, such as unchanging facial expression, inappropriate affect, speech deficiency, poor rapport, passive/apathetic social withdrawal, difficulty in abstract thinking and attention deficit) than those with an average IQ (Faraone, Ghirardi, Kuja-Halkola, Lichtenstein, & Larsson, 2017, Thapar, 2017; Welch et al., 2011), which is the core reason for their coping deficits. This means that individuals with intellectual disabilities are more likely to experience a deep sense of failure, social isolation, and self-loathing, which might motivate the adoption of the schizophrenic coping mechanism.

Sally: A case study of a patient named Sally (Meyer & Weaver, 2013, pp. 83–89), illustrates PBT's claim that genetic predisposition may results in deficit in coping skills, leads to self-loathing and motivates the adoption of schizophrenia. Sally had some genetic vulnerability to schizophrenia, as her maternal grandfather was known in the family as eccentric, and was seen by others as "crazy." Her parents had a troubled marriage and even separated for 10 months when Sally was 2 years old. Although they reunited, the marital conflicts continued. Sally was of above average intelligence, but her performance was only average or lower in most subjects. She had occasional friends but did not form any deep friendships. She was a quiet, mildly shy child and developed odd mannerisms, which "served to further distance her socially" (p. 84).

Upon graduation from high school, Sally moved to the dormitory at the nearby college she attended, where she developed her schizophrenic disorder. She started talking to herself, and her assigned roommate quickly moved to another room. The dorm counselor found Sally sitting in a chair, staring at the floor. She was unresponsive, and her limbs could be moved about as if she were plastic doll. Medical models would attribute Sally's schizophrenic symptoms to adverse neurochemical changes, which were supposedly triggered by environmental stress. In contrast, PBT claims that her symptoms were purely the result of an intolerable level of stress. Self-loathing, where she perceived herself as the core reason for her inability to cope, motivated her to adopt the schizophrenic symptoms.

The fact that Sally's schizophrenic breakdown coincided with a stressful social environment is consistent with a follow-up study that found that an improved social environment, such as a kibbutz where social interaction is highly valued (e.g., Sohlberg, 1986), facilitates the development of schizophrenia (Mirsky, Silberman, Latz, & Nagler, 1985). Not only do social interactions become more difficult and frustrating the more successful other peers are, but also the social comparisons, by which people determine their worth, become more harmful (see Wills' Downward social comparison theory, 1981).

Although Sally's schizophrenic symptoms were meaningless, they still were rational coping mechanism as they were goal-directed behaviors, fulfilling the same psychological functions as the aforementioned case studies. Her psycho-motor immobility intensively preoccupied her attention, blocked the accessibility of stress-related thoughts, and thus met Sally's need for repression. They served her controllability demands as well, as they immediately caused her frustrated roommates to leave her room and eventually distanced her from the stressful school environment. Not enough information is given regarding availability, but it may be that indifference, talking to oneself and psycho-motor immobility are spontaneous reactions by people with average cognitive development when no better means of distraction are available at their disposal.

Sally meets all five PBT's five madness criteria. While it is redundant to specify all the criteria, it should be mentioned that the patient's symptoms occurred in the absence of events that would necessarily cause the behavioral change. To counter this claim, rival approaches need to present suitable data that can explain the patient's specific symptoms and the timing that these behaviors occurred.

Jennifer Plowman: Jennifer was genetically predisposed to schizophrenia, as her biological mother was schizophrenic. The onset of her "positive symptoms" occurred during late adolescence, following several stressful events (see Schwartz, 2000, pp. 370–411). At age 13, Jennifer found out that she had been adopted. At this time, she also learned that, after giving birth to Jennifer at age 16, her biological mother had spent the next 10 years in and out of mental hospitals, and eventually died from an overdose of drugs with alcohol. Several years after learning this tragic news, Jennifer graduated from high school and began university, where she continued to do well in her studies. A few years later, her stepfather ran into financial problems and was forced to sell his business and their house. Sometime afterward, he died of a heart attack. Jennifer found a job as a file clerk but lost the job when she grew forgetful and sloppy in her work. Shortly afterward, she developed schizophrenic symptoms.

Jennifer's stepmother sent her to a hospital where she underwent a 3-day evaluation. Although Jennifer did not answer most of the questions on the mental status examination, she was not silent. She kept up a constant chatter in which she jumped from one topic to another. Her stepmother noted that Jennifer gave up showering, would laugh unexpectedly and would talk to herself when she was alone in her room. On one occasion when Jennifer was alone in her room, her stepmother heard her say, "stop laughing. I am not funny." Jennifer refused to leave the house and claimed that people could read her mind. The excerpt below, recorded during her intake interview, illustrates Jennifer's impaired informational processing:

> men need sex. I have sex 10,000 times. That window is in the room because you want patients to know the color of the world. I know the president. He lives in town … Where are the mikes and cameras hidden? Is this logomouth here to get me nervous? My father died last year, leer, jeer, tears on my pillow, pain in my heart over you, what can I do? There is

> nothing wrong with me, you know. I don't know why I am here. I'm fine. (Schwartz, 2000, p. 373)

Jennifer's disorganized speech can be seen as a deliberate coping mechanism aimed to alleviate her intolerable emotional distress. She was subjected to a series of stressors, which caused her to experience a deep sense of incompetence. The major source of her stressors, which are associated with a genetic predisposition to schizophrenia, was her negative personality traits, especially attention impairments and poor social skills. These stress-producing characteristics, together with several environmental stressors (learning about her biological mother and her medical history, the bankruptcy and death of her stepfather, and her dismissal from work), elevated her emotional distress to an intolerable level. The deliberate disruption of her perceptive and thinking processes, which did not require specific sophistication, enabled her to both block the accessibility and inhibit the production of thoughts relating to self-loathing, thereby alleviating her extreme level of depression.

Conclusions

Up to now, PBT has demonstrated its ability to integrate case studies of schizophrenia with no evidence of brain impairments and with those exhibiting genetic and brain defects in one theoretical framework. It also demonstrated that schizophrenia and criminal insanity share the same diagnostic criteria and have similar etiology. PBT has succeeded in showing that both schizophrenia and criminal insanity are rational coping mechanisms, and that the choice of a specific symptom resembles consumer's decision-making processes. The specific symptom is determined by the need to exercise control over the stressor, availability of suitable means and cost-benefit analysis. The advantages of PBT, compared to rival theories, and particularly medical models, are its ability to:

1. Integrate schizophrenic cases in which there is no evidence of genetic or neurochemical impairments with studies that have found genetic flaws and brain damage;
2. Account for this disorder's large variability in symptomatology;
3. Unify schizophrenia, criminal insanity under one theoretical framework.

In considering these advantages, it is important to remember that current explanations of schizophrenia are "still in controversy and remain unsatisfactory to researchers and clinicians. The central roadblock to progress in this field is the lack of a cohesive, integrated model that incorporates the known facts of the illness" (Keshavan, Nasrallah, & Tandon, 2011, p. 3).

Neurosis

As was mentioned in the introduction, Freud gained his substantial reputation thanks to his theoretical explanation of neurosis. Advocates of medical models utilized the weaknesses of psychoanalysis to remove this concept from the *DSM* and replace it with a list of diseases (e.g., see Grinker, 2010; Lacasse, 2014; Pilecki et al., 2011; Warelow & Holmes, 2011) to which they applied their misguided theoretical positions (e.g., see Andreasen, 1985; Wakefield, 1999). As demonstrated above, this was a wrong decision, as neuroses do indeed share similar diagnostic criteria, which distinguish them other deviant behaviors. The following section aims to strengthen both this clinical observation and Freud's insightful clinical intuition that all bizarre behaviors share the same etiology. The following section aims to demonstrate that Freud's clinical intuition that all bizarre behaviors share the same diagnostic criteria and etiology was correct. Similar to schizophrenia and criminal insanity, neurotic disorders meet PBT's criteria of madness, they are intentionally adopted when stress becomes intolerable, the major motivating cause is repression, and the specific symptom is determined by the principles of controllability, availability, and cost-benefit analysis. However, unlike schizophrenia and criminal insanity, the underlying cause of these behaviors is not usually self-loathing. Instead, neuroses are adopted when an individual is interested in forcing certain environmental changes or when he or she seeks to exercise control over anxiety-provoking impulses.

Research Findings

Numerous studies have confirmed the significant relationship between current stressful life-events and neurotic disorders. Examples include ***agoraphobia and panic disorder*** (e.g., Michelson, June, Vives, Testa, & Marchione, 1998; Milrod, Leon, & Shear, 2004; Scocco, Barbieri, & Frank, 2007; Venturello, Barzega, Maina, & Bogetto, 2002; Wardle, Hayward, Higgitt, Brewin, & Gray, 1997), **OCD** (e.g., de Silva & Marks, 1999; Gershuny, Baer, Radomsky, Wilson, & Jenike, 2003; Sasson et al., 2005), ***conversion disorder*** (see review by Rofé & Rofé, 2013), ***dissociative fugue*** (e.g., Glisky et al., 2004; Ishikura & Tashiro, 2002; Masserman, 1946), ***eating disorders*** (e.g., Beckman & Burns, 1990; Chesler, 1995; Okon, Greene, & Smith, 2003; Rabe-Jablonska, 2003), and **DID** (see review by Dalenberg et al., 2012).

Case Studies

In order to illustrate the effect of stress on the etiology of neuroses and to show that PBT's concepts are also applicable to neuroses, a number of case studies of neurotic disorders are presented below. These cases are divided into two major types of stressors: environmental stress and unacceptable impulses. In addition, this section will review studies that show how the choice of a specific symptom is affected by the individual's available experiences, such as medical conditions, family, peer group, and media exposure.

Environmental Stress

Leonard's Case Study of Train Phobia: This case is an autobiographical account of a professor at the University of Wisconsin, who suffered from agoraphobia. When he was 36-years old, Leonard experienced a sudden panic attack, while standing alone on a cliff overlooking a quiet lake — in the absence of any environmental factors that could justify the dramatic shift in his behavior

> Then on the tracks from behind … comes a freight train, blowing its whistle. Instantaneously diffused premonitions become acute panic. The cabin of that locomotive feels right over my head, as if about to engulf … My sub-consciousness knows what the torture is; and makes my voice shriek, as I rush back and forth on the bluffs: My God, won't that train go, my God, won't that train go away!' (Leonard, 1927, pp. 304–307).

The panic had such a dramatic impact on Leonard that when he was taken to his parents' home, he stated "Father and Mother, this looks like the end. I guess I am dying" (p. 308). Following this traumatic experience, Leonard was unable to go a short distance beyond his parents' home.

> In the morning, though feeling strangely weak in body, I start out on a little walk down the street. Within a hundred feet of the house I am compelled to rush back, in horror of being so far away … a hundred feet away … from home and security. I have never walked or ridden, alone or with others, as a normal man since that day. (p. 308)

Later, when the university authorities threatened to dismiss him due to his long absence, Leonard and his parents moved to an apartment across the street from the university (pp. 328–329). Leonard conducted a self-hypnosis 11 years after the onset of his symptoms, which enabled him to recall a childhood trauma at the age of two — he was almost run over by a passing train. Both Leonard, who had extensive knowledge of psychoanalytic theory, and advocates of psychoanalysis (e.g., Allport, 1929; Culler, 1930; Taylor & Culler, 1929, 1931; White & Watt, 1981), attributed these symptoms to repression of the train trauma. For example, White and Watt (1981) noted in reference to this case that

> not uncommonly a phobia assumes extreme proportions at some point in adult life after having been quiescent since early childhood. This requires the assumption that something has happened recently to increase the strength of the anxiety response so that it reaches a newly disruptive level. (p. 198)

However, it is difficult to accept this interpretation for the following reasons. First, a large number of studies show that people tend to remember, rather than forget, their childhood traumas (e.g., Piper et al., 2008; Rofé, 2008). Second, the train episode was recorded in a diary that Leonard's mother started keeping for him 3 days after the incident. She noted that Leonard had been "talking a great deal about it ever since" (p. 16), indicating that he remembered the event, rather than having repressed it. The fact that he rehearsed the traumatic event is inconsistent with the psychoanalytic assumption that repression is an involuntary, unconscious mechanism, which causes the immediate removal of the threatening experiences from the individual's conscious mind (e.g., Alexander, 1932; Cramer, 2001; Fenichel, 1946; Wilson & Dunn, 2004). Third, Leonard continued to travel by trains after the incident, so even if a fear had originally developed, it should have been extinguished through repeated exposure to locomotives. Leonard himself testified that he "developed no specialized fear of locomotives … on the contrary, trains became a childish passion" (p. 24). Fourth, even if Leonard was subconsciously affected by the train episode, he should have developed a train phobia, not agoraphobia. Fifth, a thorough review of controlled research shows no significant relationships between repressed traumas and specific neurotic symptoms (see review by Rofé, 2008).

Contrary to the psychoanalytic position, it seems that Leonard deliberately adopted the panic-agoraphobic symptoms as a coping mechanism, an idea that occurred to him intuitively upon seeing the freight train. The panic attack occurred at the age of 36, soon after his wife, the daughter of a highly respected family, committed suicide. The community regarded Leonard as being demanding and self-centered, and almost unanimously blamed him for her death. Leonard became extremely miserable and depressed, he was extensively preoccupied with the death of his wife, and it seems that the major function of his neurotic disorder was repression. Instead of being engaged in stress-related thoughts, such as self-criticism of his role in his wife's death, he chose to make himself the victim of a serious disease. The intensive preoccupation with his symptoms enabled him to block the accessibility of stress-related thoughts and relieve his intolerable level of depression. Additionally, the symptoms enabled him to distance himself from his ostracizing community, who blamed him for his wife's suicide, thereby avoiding potential rejection by colleagues at the university. Subsequently, when the university authorities threatened to fire him for his absence (p. 328) — when the controllability demands changed — he moved closer to the university to resume his teaching obligations, while maintaining his symptoms.

Another indication of Leonard's conscious involvement in the maintenance of his symptoms is the adjustment of his agoraphobic symptoms in accordance with his unique personal needs. Thus, although his agoraphobic symptoms did not allow him to travel far distances from the university, he did break this rule when it was essential for his adjustment needs. For example, Leonard was able to ride his bicycle and purchase merchandise downtown. He rationalized this violation of his "illness" by the deceptive excuse that he could control his phobia because "the speed of the bicycle magnified my beat … and even that, I had to make the purchases with dispatch" (p. 343; see also 346). Likewise, Leonard ventured to travel by train to meet his fiancée twice, stating that the train was like an "electric chair" for him (p. 347), in an attempt to maintain his self-deceptive belief of illness (see Part II).

Leonard's panic disorder was affected by the principle of availability as well. It seems likely that seeing the freight train brought to his mind the childhood train incident. Leonard's strong belief in psychoanalytic theory (see Leonard, 1927, pp. 323–324), caused him to intuitively choose to develop panic and agoraphobic symptoms because they suited his coping needs. He intentionally inflated his anxiety, which he was already experiencing due to stressful-life event, by focusing on the psychoanalytic idea that such anxiety was in fact the consequence of childhood trauma. While he chose the panic disorder mainly because it served his coping needs, he also chose it thanks to his strong belief in psychoanalytic theory. This allowed him to deceive himself into believing that the panic attack was forced upon him by the unconscious.

Regarding PBT's diagnostic criteria, Leonard's panic disorder fulfills both the five major and the two secondary criteria. The behavior intensively preoccupied his attention and disrupted his daily functioning (criterion 1); the radical change in his behavior cannot be associated with a specific factor that was exclusively linked to his symptoms (criterion 2); he was completely unaware of the underlying causes for the dramatic change in his behavior (criterion 3); his disorder was extremely rare (criterion 4); and Leonard himself stigmatized his behavior as a reflection of mental illness (criterion 5). Additionally, his symptoms fulfill PBT's secondary criteria, as they developed following a stressful life-event and Leonard experienced an extreme level of depression.

Brady and Lind's Case Study of Conversion Disorder: Conversion disorder is a neurotic disorder in which patients display deficits in motor or sensory function, such as paralysis or blindness, in the absence of neurological defects, which normally cause these symptoms. According to psychoanalysis, this disorder is the consequence of repressed trauma or conflict, which is unconsciously converted into physical symptoms (Breuer & Freud, 1895). This theoretical position has encountered serious problems, especially due to studies that refute the existence of Freudian repression (see a review by Rofé & Rofé, 2013). The understanding of this disorder has becoming more problematic in light of studies that suggest that this behavior is the consequence of neurological deficits (Van Beilen, Vogt, & Leenders, 2010), leading researchers to rename it as "*Functional Neurological Disorder*" (e.g., Keynejad et al., 2017; Stone et al., 2011; see also Reynolds, 2018). However, as stated in the introduction, the medical models' explanation is no sounder than psychoanalysis. PBT's theoretical position, which settles the disagreement between these two theoretical approaches, will be addressed toward the end of Part II. The case study presented below aims to demonstrate that, like the previous case, the underlying cause of conversion disorder is environmental stress. It also demonstrates that repression, as defined by PBT, is the central function of conversion disorder.

The case refers to a 40-year-old man who suddenly developed hysterical blindness (Brady & Lind, 1961). The patient was described as immature and irresponsible, he dropped out of school early and had trouble keeping even simple jobs. He depended greatly on his wife, whom he described as "often nervous and upset," and endured constant harassment from both his wife and her mother. Shortly after his marriage, at the age of 23, the patient was drafted into the army where he served for 3 years. While in the army, he developed an eye infection, which resulted in partial loss of vision in one eye. Consequently, he received a medical discharge and a small pension. Over the next 12 years, the patient held several simple jobs, none of which lasted more than a year, and he largely depended on aid from relatives and public assistance. During this period, he suffered a recurrence of his eye infection. He requested an increase in his pension, but was refused because his visual acuity had not decreased.

On one occasion, while grocery shopping with his wife and her mother, without any immediate precipitating event, the patient suddenly became completely blind in both eyes. This blindness occurred at a time when his wife and mother-in-law were being unusually demanding, requiring him to perform various chores under their supervision. It seems that the stress he was experiencing grew intolerable as his wife and mother-in-law grew more demanding and critical, and the preoccupation with his blindness enabled him to cope with the surrounding stressors. The patient's attention was further occupied with extensive medical examinations (which failed to find a physiological cause for his blindness), prolonged and unsuccessful psychiatric treatment, as well as learning to navigate life with his disability (e.g., attempting to learn Braille).

This case challenges the medical explanation of conversion disorder, as medical examinations failed to identify physiological cause for his specific symptom. Moreover, the case is consistent with Freud's concept of conversion disorder, since the preoccupation with the stressor is replaced with illness-related thoughts. In Freudian terms, the individual's psychological energy is converted into preoccupation with a fictitious physical ailment. Thus, the recommendation of medical model advocates to change the name of conversion disorder (e.g., Ding & Kanaan, 2016; Keynejad et al., 2017; Stone et al., 2011), though supported to some extent by the *DSM-5* (American Psychiatric Association, 2013), should be rejected.

The hysteric blindness also met the patient's controllability need by successfully halting the constant demands and criticism of his wife and mother-in-law. The patient chose this specific behavior because of its availability via his eye infections, exaggerating them to the point of blindness. This case strengthens PBT's claim that bizarre behaviors are goal-directed behaviors and that a specific symptom is chosen in accordance with the individual's controllability demands and available experiences.

This case also reinforces the usefulness of PBT's diagnostic criteria of madness. The symptoms heavily occupied the patient's attention and severely disrupted his daily functioning, which meets the first criteria. The sudden onset of his symptom occurred in the absence of any event that was exclusively linked with and could account for this behavioral change (criterion 2); the patient was unaware of the cause of his blindness (criterion 3); his disorder was extremely rare (criterion 4); and his blindness was stigmatized as a reflection of mental illness (criterion 5).

Brandt and Mackenzie's (1987) Case Study of OCD: This case refers to a 26-year-old woman who developed an intrusive fear of contamination from rat germs, accompanied by compulsive hand washing, after discovering that her husband had engaged in an extramarital affair. Her behaviors were exacerbated during her pregnancy and she "would not allow her husband or daughter to touch her" (p. 362). She was intensively preoccupied with these behaviors and thereby was able to significantly reduce the accessibility of stress-related thoughts. Her behaviors also increased her control over the stressors by transferring all the household duties to her husband. In addition, her ritualistic body cleaning and compulsive need to wash her hands, enabled her to avoid physical contact with her husband and "his" daughter, supposedly for fear of rat-germ contamination.

The effect of availability is associated with the fact that as a child she saw a rat in her family's garage while she was being sexually abused by her brother. Years later, when she found out about her husband's extramarital relationships, she recalled the earlier traumatic experience and the adverse memories associated with it. By intensively preoccupying herself with rat-related thoughts, which may have in fact symbolized disgust felt toward her husband, she blocked the accessibility of stress-related thoughts.

Thus, similar to the psychoanalytic mechanism of displacement illustrated in Freud's (1909/1964) case of little Hans, instead of focusing on the husband's stress-provoking behavior, the woman chose to alienate herself from the painful situation by directing her feelings of disgust toward the available representative of her earlier sexual mistreatment (i.e., the rat).

Bernice's Case Study of Dissociative Fugue (Masserman, 1946): Bernice, a 42-year-old woman, developed dissociative fugue, following several years of severe depression during an unhappy marriage. Bernice was raised in a hostile and abusive family. She was deeply attached to her older sister, who died when Bernice was 17, leaving her depressed for more than a year. Afterward, her parents forced her to study missionary work. At university, she lived with Rose L., an attractive, benevolent, and gifted girl, who introduced her to various friends and encouraged her to develop her neglected talents as a pianist. Bernice became very close to Rose, and this period of happiness was very significant in her life. She fell in love with Rose's fiancé, and became depressed when they finally married and moved away.

After university, Bernice entered into an arrange marriage with a clergyman chosen by her parents. The couple spent six unhappy years in missionary work abroad and then returned with their two children to live in a small town in the United States. During these years, she became increasingly unhappy as her husband busied himself with various church affairs, and felt stifled by the religious prohibitions of the village. Though depressed, Bernice tolerated the situation until the death of her youngest child, whereupon she suddenly disappeared from home without an explanation or a trace. Eventually, she was located in the college town of her youth, over 1,000 miles away.

Bernice forgot her previous identity, and started calling herself Rose, the name of her old university friend. Under her new identity, she started playing and teaching piano and even became the assistant director of a music conservatory. She chose friends who did not question her about her past, and successfully established a new social identity. Bernice continued in this fugue state for 4 years, successfully maintaining her new identity, until a friend who knew both her and the true Rose identified her. Masserman (1946) noted that the patient sincerely and rigorously denied her true identity and failed to recognize her husband and family.

As illustrated above, the patient was under such unbearable levels of stress that she literally ran away from her previous life by leaving home and changing her identity. Her fugue state provided her with an excellent repressive tool that helped her to block the accessibility of stress-related thoughts. In addition, compared with the dull and constricting environment of the small village she had lived in, the college town, which held many happy memories, provided her with the opportunity to fulfill previously abandoned dreams and aspirations. Repression was also facilitated by her rapid success as a pianist and the building of a new social network.

Gupta and Kumar's (2005) Case of Dissociative Identity Disorder: This case concerns a 14-year-old girl who developed this disorder following strained relationships among family members that caused parental separation and the departure of her elder sister, to whom she was strongly attached. The patient's behavior and symptoms were reinforced by the special attention and care she received from her mother. In an attempt to prevent any worsening of the disorder, her mother readily fulfilled her special requests for specific foods and various privileges. The patient gradually improved after meeting with her sister, and was able to fully recover following short-term behavior therapy, in which her mother was instructed to cut down on any special privileges.

As will be elaborated on later, psychoanalytic researchers attribute this disorder to physical and/or sexual abuse in childhood (e.g., see Vissia et al., 2016). However, DID can also develop in the absence of childhood trauma, as in the last case and in other examples (Nakic & Thomas, 2012). Accordingly, it seems that similar to other bizarre behaviors, the underlying cause of DID is a current source of stress rather than a historical one. Childhood trauma may aggravate the individual's current stress and or contribute to the development of this disorder through availability, as will be elaborated on in the "Discussion" section of Part II.

Dissociation is a normal distractive mechanism that enables the child "to avoid the pain of psychological surrender" (McElroy, 1992, p. 839). As noted by Young (1987), "the dissociation into personalities is thought to begin in childhood as a defensive operation, protecting the patient from the intolerable experiences associated with the early abuse" (p. 249). Although this coping response usually remains within the boundaries of normal behavior, in certain extreme cases, children may develop DID. This is illustrated in a case study reported by Spitzer, Skodol, Gibbon, & Williams (1983). The patient's father had placed her in an orphanage at the age of 9, where she suffered severe mistreatment by the staff members. Complaints to her father did not help, and often made the situation worse. In an attempt to cope with this situation, the girl developed an imaginary friend whom she named "Ellen." Unlike her dominant personality ("Sue-Sue"), which was very timid and took her punishment stoically, Ellen was able to resist her abusers. "Ellen frequently yelled at and hit back at her tormentors when they tried to touch her" (Spitzer et al., 1983, p. 39). The girl ceased to practice this behavior after her father remarried and she left the orphanage.

Helen's Case of Anorexia Nervosa: Money, Davies, and Tchanturia (2011) reported the case of 19-year-old, Helen, who suffered from anorexia nervosa. Helen experienced a difficult childhood, during which she witnessed her father abuse her mother. Her parents separated when she was young. Her mother's second partner was also violent, and they separated shortly after Helen was first admitted to an inpatient unit for adolescents with anorexia.

Helen was a successful athlete and began competitive gymnastics at the age of seven. She trained four to five times a week and described this as a way of avoiding her problems at home, behavior which is *described by PBT as normal repression* (see Rofé, 2000, pp. 105–106). At the age of 14, Helen suffered an injury that prevented her from participating in any sport activities for 6 weeks. During this time, she began to lose a significant amount of weight, and eventually developed anorexia. From that point onward, she spent the majority of her time in inpatient wards. The authors note

> until this point, athletics had been Helen's means of escape from home life and the difficult feelings this created, alongside giving her a sense of being in control of an aspect of her life. Exercise had become a way of managing her feelings of anxiety. Without it, Helen needed an alternative way to gain a sense of control in a chronic home life. This became the function of her [anorexia] (p. 115; for additional case of anorexia see Karbasi, 2010).

Money et al. note that in addition to distraction, the patient "perceived the AN [anorexia] as a means of gaining attention from her mum and protecting her from further violence ... AN became a means to manage difficult feelings and ensured that she was looked after. It enabled her to move away from the caring role she felt toward her mother. She craved stability, warmth, and guidance from her mum and found this was more present when she became unwell" (p. 115).

Thus, Helen was subjected to difficult life conditions during her childhood, where she used her athletic training to block the accessibility of stress-related thoughts (i.e., normal repression; see Rofés' review, 2008). When she lost this coping mechanism, as a result of her injury, she experienced intensification in her stress levels, leading to her adoption of anorexia nervosa. This pathological coping mechanism enabled her to both repress stress-related thoughts and to shape her stressful environment to serve her psychological needs.

Spirit Possession: Spirit possession, which can develop following stressful life-events, is a disorder in which patients believe spirits take control their body (see Adityanjee, Raju and Khandelwal, 1989; Ravenscroft, 1965; Seltzer, 1983). Patients utilize their available cultural experiences of spirit possession to develop bizarre behaviors that meet their repressive and controllability demands. Adityanjee, Raju and Khandelwal (1989), in discussing the frequency of this psychiatric syndrome in India, described this mode of coping as follow:

> the possessing spirit through the patient makes various demands on the surroundings, usually on close relatives who humbly comply with them. This sometimes ends a single episode of possession, although the accompanying reinforcement ensures a recurrence in the event of a stressful situation. In these cases, the symptoms of spirit possessions ... help in the release of strangulated effects. Such behavior focuses the attention of the family on the individual, valuable time is gained, and the resulting structural realignment of forces within the family often improves the precipitating condition. (p. 1609, see also Akhtar, 1988; Claus, 1979; Grisaru & Witztum, 1995; Mischel & Mischel, 1958)

The significant relationship between spirit possession and stress has been reported by a number of researchers (e.g., Hecker, Bamewitz, Stenmark, & Iversen, 2016; Ranganathan, 2013; Sar, Alioglu, & Akyuz, 2014). One example which demonstrates this effect is the case of a 40-year-old mother of four children. She managed to live reasonably well for several years after losing her husband to a sudden illness, until she faced a crisis in her business (Wijesinghe, Dissanayake, & Mendis, 1976). Subsequently, she was possessed by the spirit of her late husband.

> During the trance state, the spirit called out to friends and relatives, imploring them to help the subject in her distress.

> There was a good response to this appeal and her relatives rallied around her, relieving her of many of her financial burdens. This led to a gradual decrease in the frequency of attacks. (p. 137)

This social susceptibility and the relatively high availability of these symptoms may account for why these bizarre behaviors are relatively more common than other neurotic disorders in less-developed countries. Ravenscroft (1965) notes, in describing the Haitian Vodun possession, that although peasants do not necessarily perform ritual acts daily, their perception of the world is dominated by a constant recognition of supernatural forces at work. From a very early age the individual is exposed to parents and relatives who are intensely occupied with gods and their worship. "In his presence they perform the prescribed rituals and experience possession over and over again … a knowledge of Vodun belief is developed through conversations, observation, and participation …" (pp. 163–164). Consequently, since these experiences are prevalent in non-western countries, people are more likely to develop spirit possession, as opposed to other neurotic disorders, when a need for a pathological coping mechanisms arises.

In conclusion, each of the above cases of neurotic disorders are a clear depiction of bizarre behaviors, which fulfill PBT's diagnostic criteria of madness. Hence, in all cases, the symptoms intensively preoccupied the patient's attention and severely disrupted his or her daily functioning (criterion 1). There were radical changes in each patient's behavior in the absence of factors exclusively linked with the disorder (criterion 2). The patient was unaware of the underlying cause of his or her behavioral change (criterion 3). The symptoms were very rare, below 3% (criterion 4). Additionally, all these behaviors are stigmatized by social agencies or medical health centers as bizarre or as a reflection of mental illness. Additionally, in all cases, the symptom served the patient's need for repression and the choice of the specific symptom was determined by the individual's need of controllability, availability of suitable experiences and cost benefit analysis.

Unacceptable Impulses

Neurotic symptoms are not only employed to force a desired change in the environment, but also to control highly stressful inner feelings that result from unacceptable aggressive or sexual impulses. While ordinary stressful life-events may result in depression and/or anxiety, in some cases, as suggested by frustration-aggression theory (e.g., Berkowitz, 1988, 1989; Dill & Anderson, 1995; Gustafson, 1989), they may also cause strong feelings of hostility toward others. Consequently, the individual may experience an unbearable fear of losing control, as well as feelings of guilt. These experiences are particularly likely when the individual has both a rigid value system and poor self-restraint against aggression. In such cases, individuals are likely to adopt bizarre behaviors, which have the unique ability to restrain unacceptable impulses, and thus reduce feelings of guilt and the fear of losing control. In some cases the unacceptable impulse is so strong that individuals are unable to restrain its manifestation. These individuals employ bizarre behaviors that provide justification for the implementation of the unacceptable impulses. These pathological coping mechanisms are described below.

Restraining the Impulse via OCD

An example of an unacceptable impulse is a strong, conflicting, love–hate feelings toward a close relative. One type of mad behavior that is usually associated with such unacceptable impulses is OCD (e.g., Hollander, 1999a, 1999b; Horowitz, 2004; Miller, 1983; Stein & Hollander, 1993; Stein, Hollander, DeCaria, & Trungold, 1991; Whiteside & Abramowitz, 2005). OCD can reduce the likelihood of uncontrolled, impulsive behavior by offering one of two coping mechanisms, which psychoanalysis terms "reaction formation" and "isolation" (see Fenichel, 1946; Freud, 1936; Freud, 1905, 1926). PBT incorporates both of these concepts, but contrary to psychoanalysis, they are conceptualized as rational deliberate reactions.

Karen — An Example of Reaction Formation: In reaction formation, illustrated in a case study by Neale and his colleague (1982), the individual reduces the fear of losing control by obsessive thoughts and compulsive acts of love that counteract the unacceptable impulses. The patient, Karen, was a 30 year-old married mother of four children who was subjected to two sources of stress: a chronically unhappy marriage and disciplinary issues managing her children. Her husband became incapacitated due to a serious heart condition, leaving Karen to take full responsibility for the household chores and family errands. "Her days were spent getting the children dressed, fed, and transported to school; cleaning; washing; shopping; and fetching potato chips, dips, and beer whenever Tony [her husband] needed a snack" (p. 2). Karen detested her children due to their difficult disciplinary problems, which she had to cope with alone, and particularly because they constituted an obstacle in fulfilling her desire to leave the marriage. Karen became increasingly depressed by her life situation.

Karen began to experience intrusive, repetitive thoughts related to her children's safety. Often she imagined that a serious accident had occurred, and was unable to keep these thoughts out of her mind. Her daily activities became seriously disrupted by an extensive series of counting rituals. For example, Karen came to believe that if she purchased the first product on the shelf, something horrible would occur to her oldest child. If she selected the second item, a disaster would come to her second child, and so on for all four children. Additionally, the patient attributed significant meaning to the children's ages. Her compulsive rituals were generalized to several other activities, such as the pattern in which she smoked cigarettes and drank coffee (e.g., if she smoked one cigarette she continued to have at least another four in a row, believing that one of her children would be harmed if she did not do).

It seems that these counting rituals enabled her to *repress stressful thoughts* relating to her marital life. Most importantly, she intuitively chose this behavior primarily because *it reduced her fear of losing control over unacceptable feelings of hostility* toward her children. As noted by Neale et al. (1982), "instead of injuring the children, she spent a good deal of time every day performing irrational responses aimed at protecting them" (p. 12). Furthermore, although Karen's bizarre rituals did not physically distance her from the original stressors (i.e., husband and children), they were time consuming enough to provide temporary relief. As noted by Neale et al. (1982), the symptoms ensured that she would be away from her home for extended periods of time. If she went to her neighbor's house for coffee, it would be at least 2 hours before she could consume enough cups and smoke enough cigarettes to satisfy the rituals. Grocery shopping, which she did by herself, was also turned into a long, complicated process (p. 13).

Another factor that affected her specific choice of symptoms was the *availability* of rituals in her "premorbid" state. "Her family was deeply religious, and she was raised to be a devout Roman Catholic … The formal rituals of the church played an important role in her life" (p. 3). The high prevalence of OCD among religious subjects (e.g., Abramowitz, Deacon, Woods, & Tolin, 2004), and the excessive religious themes in their obsessive thoughts and compulsive rituals (e.g., Greenberg & Witztum, 1994; Raphael, Rani, Bale, & Drummond, 1996; Rasmussen & Eisen, 1992; Steketee, Quay, & White, 1991), can be viewed as a deliberate exaggeration of the available behavioral repertoire for pathological coping purposes.

This case also meets PBT's criteria of madness (1) the OCD symptoms heavily occupied her attention and severely disrupted her daily functioning; (2) their onset was spontaneous, in the absence of an event that could account for the severe behavioral change; (3) although the patient rationalized her behavior as protective measures for her children, she was clearly unaware of the underlying causes of her symptoms; (4) her symptoms are rare (the total prevalence of OCD in the general population is less than 2%); (5) the mental health system would have classified her OCD's symptoms as bizarre (e.g., see Erdelyi, 1985; Shevrin &Dickman, 1980). Additionally, the onset of the patient's symptoms was preceded by stress and she suffered from an intense level of depression.

McAndrew's Case (1989) — An Example of Isolation: Isolation is another coping mechanism that has the same aim as reaction formation: combating the fear of losing control. However, in isolation this goal is obtained by extremely obsessive, hostile thoughts, which appear senseless, and not to mention, contrary to PBT's basic assumption that madness serves the individual's best interest. The use of the coping mechanism of isolation is illustrated in the case study of a 26-year-old woman who, like Karen, was unhappy in her marriage and resented her children. Her husband was "very strict, aggressive … insensitive to her needs … [and] physically abused her" (p. 317), and her difficult children frustrated her as she lacked adequate disciplinary skills to parent them. The patient had reached a state of helplessness, feeling "stuck in a bad marriage" (p. 314). Consequently, she not only experienced severe depression, but intense anger directed at her husband and children, accompanied by feelings of guilt and a fear of losing control. Bizarre aggressive cognitions that lacked the appropriate affect of anger heavily occupied her attention. "I'm having terrible thoughts about stabbing my children. (crying). That's terrible — isn't it? I've been having thoughts of hurting others too … I love my kids. How could I have these horrible thoughts of hurting them?" (McAndrew, 1989, pp. 312, 316).

Lewis (1981) notes that Freud was puzzled by the fact that while obsessive patients perceive their forbidden thoughts as "crazy," they remain powerless to stop them from penetrating into the conscious mind. As noted by Lewis (1981)

> In any rational system, knowing that ideas are crazy should be adequate to demolish them, but in the obsessional neurosis the patient's intellect is powerless to do more than observe his 'craziness.' (p. 101)

However, while psychoanalysis considers obsessive neurosis irrational, PBT views it as a rational coping mechanism. Patients deliberately produce obsessive thoughts that are devoid of anger, termed by Freud "isolation," thereby they become unaware of their own hate-laden cognitions. As described below, this coping mechanism increases patients' control over their unacceptable impulses for the following reasons (1) given the artificial production of the obsessions and the lack of a suitable emotional base (e.g., anger), these cognitions are less likely to motivate impulsive behavior than the original emotionally charged thoughts; (2) obsessive thoughts intensify patients' self-awareness that they may cause harm to others. Consequently, patients take appropriate preventative measures to reduce the likelihood of inflicting harm, such as removing potentially harmful objects; (3) they may share their anxiety-provoking thoughts with close family members so that they may supervise their behavior; (4) obsessive thoughts reduce guilt, because, unlike the emotionally charged impulse which motivated the adoption of this coping mechanism, these thoughts are experienced as foreign to the self. This feeling of extraneousness stems from the absence of corresponding emotions and the patient's unawareness of his or her conscious involvement in producing the obsessive thoughts.

In reference to the above case study, the high distractive value of the obsessive symptoms, which enabled the above patient to repress her original aggression toward her children, was reflected by her inability "to force them out of her head" (p. 312). The patient noted that when she tried to suppress these cognitions "the thoughts get worse and I get a headache or my heart starts pounding" (p. 312). The patient reinforced these distractive measures even more by adopting compulsive-behaviors as well. "I have to keep busy all the time … check things … clean my house very often. I'm meticulous and very slow doing things" (p. 316).

With regard to controllability, the obsessive thoughts of stabbing her children heightened the patient's awareness to their potentially dangerous nature. As a result, she took appropriate preventative precautions, thereby reducing the danger of losing control. As noted by the patient

> I can't look at violence on TV because I feel I could do something … I have to check things and make sure I know everything is all right. I make sure the guns are locked up many times during the day. (pp. 314–316)

The obsessive thoughts motivated her to express concern and love toward her children, further minimizing the possibility of dangerous impulsive behavior. The patient's symptoms were also aimed at increasing the supervision of others. For example, she stated, "I had my sister and my mother stay with me so I wouldn't do anything … I must call or be around other people. Someone would intervene if I was about to hurt my kids" (pp. 313–316).

The absurdity of these thoughts, and the sense that they were alien to the self, enabled the patient to attribute them to sources beyond her control, thereby alleviating her feelings of guilt ("someone like the devil must be making me have these thoughts," p. 313). Moreover, although the focus on the obsessive thoughts unusually increases patients' level of anxiety, this emotional discomfort is readily reduced by distractive/neutralizing activities, such as ritualized internal dialogue, reading and forming a counter image, which patients perform soon afterward (see Freeston et al., 1997; Rachman, 1976; Salkovskis & Westbrook, 1989). Thus, although obsessive thoughts are emotionally and cognitively disruptive, the overall experience is not as highly disruptive as the original state before adopting the symptoms. In fact, without the pathological coping mechanism, the anxiety and depression would be so intense as to be beyond the patient's tolerance level.

The principle of availability also affects the choice of OCD's isolation. As noted by Rachman and De Silva (1978) unacceptable obsessive thoughts are not unique to neurotic patients but characterize a large majority of normal people. However, while normal people disregard the sporadic unacceptable thoughts, which are spontaneously triggered by their impulses (see Rachman, 1976, p. 438), patients who have a need to repress and control their anxiety-provoking impulses, concentrate on these thoughts, and exaggerate them to an absurd degree. Although this may be the most common form by which isolation is adopted, clinical evidence indicates that patients may create obsessive thoughts on the basis of other personal experiences, such as films (e.g., lurid death scenes; see case 1 Salkovskis & Westbrook, 1989) and reading materials (e.g., see case study by Bevan, 1960). Almost simultaneously with the adoption of this coping mechanism, patients become unaware of their self-involvement in the deliberate exaggeration/production and maintenance of these thoughts due to sophisticated self-deceptive processes (see "Part II").

Other Forms of Impulse-Restraint

OCD is not the only coping measure that patients employ to cope with unacceptable impulses. For example, Abse (1959, p. 282) described a case of conversion disorder concerning a man who became a paraplegic after his wife left him for another man. The patient had a strong urge to pursue his wife and kill both her and her lover, but his symptoms prevented him from carrying it out. In a similar case study (Carson et al., 1988, p. 203), a female subject, who physically attacked her father using her right arm, developed a marked tremor and partial paralysis in that arm and hand. Carson et al. (1988) suggested that the paralysis represented a symbolic punishment of the "guilty party," while preventing reoccurrence of the aggressive behavior. Subjects may also turn to unusual phobias to cope with unacceptable impulses. For example, a 24-year-old male patient, who experienced anxiety-provoking homosexual fantasies while having sexual relations with women, developed a morbid fear of syphilis, inhibiting him from having any sexual relations (Coleman, 1984).

Implementation of Unacceptable Impulses

Sometimes subjects are unable to sufficiently restrain their unacceptable impulses. In such cases, they may develop DID, a rational coping mechanism, which absolves them of their responsibility and guilt. Spanos, Weekes, and Bertrand (1985) explain, in their socio-cognitive model of DID, that this disorder "provides a viable and face-saving account for personal failings and problems" (p. 364; see also Spanos, 1996; Spanos, Weekes, Menary, & Bertrand, 1986). For example, Spitzer et al. (1983) described the case of a 37-year-old married woman suffering from DID. Approximately one afternoon per week, she would shift into another personality named Ellen, meet a stranger at the bar in a neighboring town, and spend the afternoon with him in a motel. Typically, she would disparage his performance afterward and would always refuse to meet him again. Occasionally she would even fantasize about killing the man after sexual intercourse. These thoughts made her feel uneasy, prompting a shift back to her dominant personality, who would then hurry home to cook dinner. The patient felt guilty and was angry at "Ellen" — who on several occasions manifested herself at home and told her husband about her affairs. While psychoanalytic advocates would attribute this seemingly uncontrolled sexual behavior to the unconscious, according to PBT the woman deliberately adopted the alternative personality to enable her to act upon her impulses while transferring the responsibility for her actions to forces beyond her control. In agreement with the socio-cognitive model, DID may also be used as a vehicle to execute violent acts, including burglary, murder, or rape (e.g., see Moskowitz, 2004a, 2004b; Perr, 1991; Steinberg, Garver, Moeller, Raese, & Orsulak, 1993), while attributing their causes to sources beyond the individual's conscious control.

There are also individuals who act on their unacceptable impulses but then use bizarre ritual behaviors to reduce the guilt over the anxiety provoking behavior. Sherman (1938, pp. 226–227) described a 14-year-old boy who washed his hands frequently during the day and often stayed in the bathtub for two or three hours. On a number of occasions, he dabbed iodine on his hands and face, telling his parents that he had scratched himself and wanted to prevent infection. The boy refused to play ordinary games with other children because he did not want to soil his hands. During therapy, it was discovered that the boy experienced excessive guilt over masturbation, which according to Sherman was the consequence of a rigid, unforgiving upbringing (e.g., his parents told him that masturbation could result in a terrible disease). The boy described the masturbation behavior as a "dirty habit," which may account for his choice of excessive cleaning as a measure of coping with feelings of guilt and anxiety.

The carrying out of anxiety-provoking impulses may also manifest in psychotic disorders, such as filicidal mothers who claimed they heard voices telling them to kill their children (Valença, Mendlowicz, Nascimento, & Nardi, 2011). The explanations these mothers gave for their actions clearly show that their criminal acts were goal-directed behaviors that improved their quality of life. One mother said, "my husband dropped me out and left me on my own to look after the children … I thought I would not be able to bring up the three children without a father" (Valenca et al., 2011, p. 552). The second mother confessed, "I don't know what happened … I just did it … it occurred to me that the suffering of bringing up a child with difficulty had just begun … I thought that I would not have money enough to pay for schooling and that at school they would mistreat my child … I thought that they would abuse him because he was dark skinned" (p. 552). While the mothers did hear voices telling them to kill their children, one needs to consider findings demonstrating that visual (e.g., Mintz & Alpert, 1972) and auditory (e.g., Hoffman & Hampson, 2012; Jones, 2010; Lavigne & Woodward, 2018) hallucinations may be the consequences of vivid imaginations and self-talk.

Principle of Availability in Bizarre Behaviors

As was shown, the choice of a specific mad behavior is affected by the individuals' unique experiences that can meet their coping needs in a manner analogous to a consumer's decision to purchase a particular product. Additional evidence supporting this claim is reviewed below.

Medical Conditions

Clinical evidence suggests that subjects may utilize their current or past injuries or illnesses to cultivate a neurotic disorder that meets their pathological coping needs. For example, a high prevalence of some initial organic illness or physical injury has been reported among patients who subsequently developed conversion disorder (e.g., Carden & Schramel, 1966; Jones, 1980; Merskey & Buhrich, 1975; Miller & Forbes, 1990; Spierings, Poels, Sijben, Gabreels, & Renier, 1990; Volkmar, Poll, & Lewis, 1984; Whitlock, 1967). Volkmar et al. (1984) have found that children with conversion symptoms had a significantly higher prevalence of hospitalization than a control group in the year prior to their psychiatric evaluations. Conversion symptoms are "commonly placed in some organ that was the site of previous injury or disability" (White & Watt, 1981, p. 216; see also Mucha & Reinhardt, 1970; Weinstein, Eck, & Lyerly, 1969). For instance, Ironside and Batchelor (1945) reported that a significant number of military aircrew members, who developed ocular hysteria, had a prior history of eye trouble. Similarly, Brady and Lind's (1961) patient developed hysterical blindness rather than other conversion symptoms, because, while in the army, he developed an eye infection that resulted in partial loss of vision in one eye. Likewise, as noted by Merskey and Buhrich (1975) "patients who have epileptic fits may learn the pattern of their attacks and, when it is convenient to solve a conflict with this technique, they may use their knowledge of organic fits in order to develop hysterical ones" (p. 65). Accordingly, Blanchard and Hersen (1976) described a case study of a 22-year-old, female patient who had a history of grand mal seizures for seven or eight years. Later, shortly after her marriage, when she was subjected to frustrating life-events, she developed hysterical seizures.

Utilization of physical symptoms as a coping mechanism is also observed in other neurotic disorders, such as hypochondriasis (e.g., Noyes et al., 2004). As noted by Salkovskis and Warwick (1986), "it is significant that past experience of true organic disease in self or a family member has been identified as a predisposing factor for hypochondriasis" (p. 597; see also case study by Davison & Neale, 1986, pp. 148–150). Availability may also account for the significant relationships between panic disorder and pulmonary diseases (e.g., Brenes, 2003; Mikkelsen, Middelboe, Pisinger, & Stage, 2004; Nascimento et al., 2002; Roy-Byrne, Craske, & Stein, 2006; Shavitt, Gentil, & Mandetta, 1992; Valença et al., 2006). Respiratory diseases (e.g., asthma) are more prevalent among panic/agoraphobic disorders patients (Shavitt et al., 1992; Yellowlees & Kalucy, 1990), and they often precede the onset of these disorders (e.g., Verburg, Griez, Meijer, & Pols, 1995; Zandbergen et al., 1991). Overall, this evidence suggests that patients with respiratory disease are more likely to develop panic disorder, when this is suitable for their coping demands, since they are familiar with the symptoms that characterize this disorder.

Behavioral Repertoire

Patients may intensify their available behavioral repertoire to pathological levels for coping purposes. Accordingly, it seems likely that increased dieting practices in recent years have motivated people to transform this socially accepted behavior into eating disorders. For example, Polivy and Herman (1987) attributed the dramatic increase of this disorder (see also Lucas, Beard, O'Fallon, & Kurland, 1991; Mitchell & Eckert, 1987) to "the intensified quest for a slim physique and to the dieting that such a quest seems to require" (pp. 636–637). Patton (1992) reported that dieters who developed depressive symptoms were more likely to progress to a state of disordered eating. In a study of 61 school-girls approaching the peak age incidence for anorexia nervosa, dieting was associated with an 8-fold risk increase of later eating disorders (see also Hill, 1993).

Kaffman and Sadeh's (1989) study of anorexia nervosa in the Israeli kibbutz movement demonstrated such a phenomenon. They related the 800% increase of the disorder within the kibbutz, over a period of 25 years, to the growing emphasis placed on the kibbutz women's external appearances. The authors noted, "a change in the norms regarding the importance of feminine sliminess and beauty … Today, in nearly every kibbutz the cosmetician, the hairdresser, the beautician, as well as the dietitian play an important part in the life of the woman" (pp. 34–35). Similarly, the higher prevalence of eating disorders among women has been explained by the fact that women are more preoccupied with weight and dieting than men (e.g., Stice, 1994). Studies also suggest that due to the higher value placed on their appearance, homosexual males and males whose occupation requires strict weight control and a thin appearance (e.g., dancers, actors, models, and athletes) are more likely to develop eating disorders than other males (e.g., Carlat, Camargo, & Herzog, 1997; Stice, 1994).

The escalation of a normal behavioral repertoire to pathological levels occurs in OCD as well. For example, the high rate of compulsive cleaning among women can be attributed to the fact that "in our culture most women are responsible for running the household (i.e., cleaning)" (Emmelkamp, 1982, p. 167). Similarly, the high prevalence of OCD among religious subjects (e.g., Abramowitz et al., 2004), and the excessive religious themes in their obsessive thoughts and compulsive rituals (e.g., Greenberg & Witztum, 1994;

Raphael, Rani, Bale, & Drummond, 1996; Rasmussen & Eisen, 1992; Steketee et al., 1991), can be viewed as a deliberate exaggeration of the available behavioral repertoire for purposes of pathological coping. For example, the high proportion of washing symptoms reported among Hindus suffering from OCD, may be the result of their religion's emphasis on purity and cleanliness (Khanna & Channabasavanna, 1988).

Similarly, Hoffnung, Aizenberg, Hermesh et al. (1989) reported that in a study of 50 obsessive-compulsive patients, "a substantial portion of the patients who were presented with OC [obsessive compulsive] symptoms in the religious realm were from the ultra-orthodox ('Haredi') community of Israel" (p. 141). As noted by Hoffnung et al. these symptoms were "predominantly distortions and exaggerations of religious rituals" (p. 141). One of the patients, a 35 year-old married woman, suffered from obsessive observance of religious laws. She was born into a modern-orthodox Jewish family, but over the years she became increasingly meticulous in her religious observance, and then she married an ultra-orthodox man. Her religious background indicates that she must have had a strong religious behavioral repertoire, which was later inflated to a bizarre level for the purpose of a coping strategy. One example of bizarre behavior was her observance of Jewish dietary laws. The severity of her symptoms extremely limited her effectiveness in the kitchen. "Eventually, she attempted to function in her kitchen with her eyes closed so as not to become involved in these questions [of dietary laws] and even injured herself on one occasion after having walked into a wall" (p. 142).

Individuals' behavioral repertoires affect the development of agoraphobia and panic disorder as well. Studies show that among the general population, many people experience one or more panic-like attacks that do not meet the criteria for panic disorder (Brown & Deagle, 1992; Telch, Brouillard, Telch, Agras, & Taylor, 1989; Whittal & Goetsch, 1995). Although the emotional and behavioral characteristics of these cases (e.g., dizziness, palpitations, shaking, and sweating) are similar to those of panic patients, they are of a lesser magnitude. While PBT agrees that these individuals are at a higher risk for developing panic disorder (see Whittal & Goetsch, 1995), it points that this heightened risk is not the result of uncontrolled mechanisms, such as conditioning, maladaptive cognitive interpretation or physiological mechanisms. Rather it stems from the individual's decision to inflate his or her behavioral repertoire of intense arousal to a bizarre level, as in agoraphobia and panic disorders.

Once a pathological coping strategy is adopted it becomes part of the patient's behavioral repertoire, even if the response is later abandoned. Patients are likely to reinitiate this available behavioral repertoire when re-confronted with an unbearable level of stress, thus accounting for relapses of pathological episodes. As reported by Folks, Ford and Regan (1984) "a sizable percentage of patients diagnosed as having conversion disorders have had a prior conversion symptom and/or have concurrent somatization disorder" (p. 294). The authors described the case of a woman suffering from hysterical paralysis who had the same symptoms three years prior. The family members observed a definite pattern of somatizing when the patient was under any acute stress or was feeling neglected by her husband. Similarly, Wolpe (1982, pp. 286–287) reported a case of an agoraphobic woman whose symptoms ceased when she moved to another city to live with her boyfriend and resurfaced when she was reunited with her husband. Likewise, Marks (1987b) described a case study of an agoraphobic woman who "kept up her [therapeutic] progress for 4 years… but then she had some family difficulties, which depressed her, and quickly relapsed" (p. 1163). Thus, relapse in PBT has a different meaning than in the traditional mechanistic theories. While in traditional theories relapse is involuntary and beyond the individual's conscious control, in PBT it is the result of the individual's conscious decision.

Family

Modeling after family members is an important factor in the availability of neurotic symptoms. Effects of modeling do not have to be displayed immediately following the observation of the deviant behavior. Rather, a child may latently learn a behavior (e.g., Campanella & Rovee-Collier, 2005) and utilize it later, when the need for a pathological coping mechanism arises. This is consistent with findings that show 70% of conversion disorder patients had parents who suffered from illnesses in the same organs that were affected by their hysterical symptoms (Mucha & Reinhardt, 1970; see also Koon, 1983; Siegel & Barthel, 1986; Volkmar et al., 1984). In this sense, the increased prevalence of hysteria among relatives of subjects with hysteric disorder (Inouye, 1972) demonstrates the important role of "imitation and learning in the production of the syndrome" (Volkmar et al., 1984, p. 429). This is also reflected in Siegel and Barthel's (1986) study on conversion symptoms among children. They reported that in all of their cases "either the patient, a friend, or a relative who held some emotional significance for the patient had displayed similar physical complaints in the past" (p. 203).

Modeling plays an important role in the adoption of other disorders as well. For example, Pike and Rodin's (1991) study indicates that mothers whose daughters exhibited eating disorders displayed similar behavioral patterns. Similarly, Dell and Eisenhower (1990) reported that 73% of patients with DID had at least one parent who suffered from a diagnosable dissociative disorder, and 36% of the patients' mothers suffered from DID. Likewise, 17%–19% of parents of OCD patients suffer from the same disorder (see Piacentini & Graae, 1997). Although these findings are often attributed to genetic factors, they can equally be accounted for by the principle of availability.

Individuals may be predisposed to choose certain neurotic disorders by observing their familial environments, even if family members themselves do not display the disorder. For example, families of eating disorder patients were more likely to be excessively preoccupied with food and dieting than the general population (e.g., Kaffman & Sadeh, 1989; Stice, 1994). As indicated by Kaffman and Sadeh (1989), "excessive preoccupation with food and diet — whether for reasons of health or esthetics — was noted among 73% of the mothers of the anorexics" (p. 40). Stice (1994) stated that, "families of eating-disordered youth are thought to be hyperconscious of weight and appearance, and thus perpetuate these socio-cultural pressures" (p. 645). The author reviewed evidence showing that in a significant number of cases the onset of eating disorders was associated with pressure from the family to lose weight.

Likewise, OCD may be partly the consequence of the individual's family's overemphasis on cleanliness and orderliness. As indicated by Hoover and Insel (1984), many obsessive-compulsive patients were raised in families characterized by

> super cleanliness, over meticulousness and the likes .... Grandparents, aunts and uncles, as well as parents, had habits, attitudes and standards of cleanliness and performance which went beyond the ordinary, and they suffered considerable anxiety if these could not be fulfilled. (p. 209)

Hence, just as with dieting and eating disorders, subjects with these acquired obsessive-compulsive traits (Emmelkamp, 1982, p. 187; Pollak, 1979) may inflate these personality characteristics to a bizarre level (i.e., obsessive-compulsive disorder) when in need of a pathological coping method. This theoretical position is consistent with Rachman and Hodgson (1980) who, emphasizing the importance of learning processes in the acquisition of obsessive-compulsive traits, noted that, "these dispositions provide fertile soil for the growth of obsessions and compulsions" (p. 46).

Similarly, an overly fearful parent may encourage the development of an overly fearful personality in their offspring (Gerlsma,

Emmelkamp, & Arrindell, 1990; Tearnan, Telch, & Keefe, 1984), which may later be exaggerated to agoraphobia or panic disorders when suitable to the current stressful demands.

Mutual learning experiences may also be the cause, at least partially, for similarity in neurotic disorders among twins who have been raised together. As noted by Carey and Gottesman (1981), "given the theoretical role of modeling in the genesis of fears … higher concordant rate in MZ [monozygotic] twins may be caused by a greater opportunity to imitate each other or to model the fears of a shared friend" (p. 131). Evidence supporting this claim was reported by Marks, Crowe, Drewe, Young, and Dewhurst (1969) in a case study of identical twins, both of whom suffered from obsessive-compulsive disorder. Both brothers developed a compulsive ritual of avoiding dogs, involving many aspects of their lives. At the age of 10, they agreed that butter and milk were dirty and "if contaminated [the co-twin] would scrupulously wash and make the patient do the same before he would accept him" (p. 993). As stated by Marks et al., "the similarity of *content* of the disorder in both twins is probably the result of mutual social interactions between them" (p. 913). Rachman and Hodgson (1980) commented in reference to this case that, "the importance of environmental transmission from the co-twin to the patient is beyond dispute" (p. 40).

Thus, it seems likely that when these individuals are confronted with intolerable levels of stress, they may copy or exaggerate familial behaviors (i.e., dieting or cleaning) to a neurotic level. Accordingly, given that John Nash did not have a family history of schizophrenia, it seems probable that the paranoid disorder of Nash's son was the result of modeling rather than genetic predisposition. As noted by Nash with regard to his son's psychiatric disorder, "of course, I've been a bad example" (Nasar, 1998, p. 382).

Peer Group

Peers displaying neurotic behaviors may also serve as models for imitation when their symptoms meet the individual's coping needs.

For example, in their investigation of contagious hysteria among West Bengali women, Nandi, Banerjee, Bera, Nandi, and Nandi (1985) reported that a husband's violence toward his wife usually precipitated her episodes of hysterical seizures. As soon as the victim fell into a fit, other women suffering from similar stressors began to have hysterical seizures as well (for additional examples, see Stevens, 1969, pp. 34–35; Ullmann & Krasner, 1975, pp. 253–254). Similarly, various studies indicate that the effect of peers on the selection of symptoms, expressed through modeling or suggestion, may play a significant role in the development of eating disorders (see reviews by Polivy & Herman, 2002; Stice, 1994). Accordingly, Striegel-Moore, Silberstein, and Rodin (1986) pointed out that "a college woman who purges almost always knows another female student who purges, whereas a woman, who does not purge, rarely knows someone who does" (p. 256).

Media

In the last few decades, there has been a dramatic increase in the prevalence of eating disorders in western society (e.g., Hoek, 1993; Hoek & Van Hoeken, 2003; Lucas et al., 1991; Pope, Hudson, & Yurgelun-Todd, 1984; Shisslak, Crago, Neal, & Swain, 1987; Striegel-Moore et al., 1986; Willi, Giacometti, & Limacher, 1990). Moreover, while these disorders were once rare among the lower classes (e.g., Bruch, 1973, p. 13; Garfinkel & Kaplan, 1986, pp. 270–271; Nagel & Jones, 1992) and in non-western countries (e.g., Hoek et al., 2005; Keel & Klump, 2003), they have now spread to equally affect all ranks of western society (see Culberg & Engström-Lindberg, 1988; Mitchell & Eckert, 1987; Pope, Champoux, & Hudson, 1987; Whitaker et al., 1989) and increasingly in non-western societies as well (e.g., Miller, 2006; Pate, Pumariega, Hester, & Garner, 1992).

One of the central reasons for the increasing risk of developing eating disorders is the influence of mass media, which has increased the awareness of these disorders (e.g., Calogero,

Davis, & Thompson, 2004; Lucas et al., 1991; Murray, Touyz, & Beumont, 1990; Polivy & Herman, 2002; Spettigue & Henderson, 2004; Striegel-Moore et al., 1986). As a result, individuals tend to choose these behaviors when they are suitable for their coping needs. As noted by Striegel-Moore et al. (1986):

> The bestseller *Beverly Hills Diet Book* … advocated a form of bulimia in which binges are 'compensated' for by eating massive quantities of raw fruit to induce diarrhea … In addition to the mass media making available what one might call manuals for 'how to develop an eating disorder,' females more directly teach each other how to diet and how to binge, purge, and starve. (p. 256)

Accordingly, Murray et al. (1990) found that mass media was the major source of knowledge about anorexia and bulimia nervosa. Similarly, upon examining the underlying causes of sex differences in eating disorders. For forty-nine percent of their subjects "some type of media (television and/or printed media) was their only source of information" (p. 89). Andersen and DiDomenico (1992) reported that women's magazines contained 10.5 more articles and advertisements regarding weight loss and anorexia nervosa than men's magazines. The effect of mass media has also been observed in non-western countries, where westernization has increased the prevalence of eating disorders (e.g., see Elal, 2003; Miller, 2006).

Largely as a result of mass communication, the risk for such disorders, which was once reported as being a disorder of the upper social classes (e.g., Bruch, 1973, p. 13; Garfinkel & Kaplan, 1986, pp. 270–271; Nagel & Jones, 1992a), has spread to all ranks of society. Not only has dieting become an integral part of the individual's behavioral repertoire, but there has also been an increase in the awareness of eating disorder symptoms and their potential coping value. Therefore, it is not surprising that a shift towards an equal distribution or higher prevalence of these disorders among lower socio-economical classes has occurred (see Culberg & Engström-Lindberg, 1988; Mitchell & Eckert, 1987; Pope, Hudson, & Yurgelun-Todd, 1987; Whitaker, Davies, Shaffer et al., 1989).

Some investigators downplay the effect of mass media on the development of eating disorders, claiming that only a small minority of those who are exposed to the media develops these disorders (e.g., see Kaye, Strober, & Klump, 2002; Polivy & Herman, 2002). However, as with advertisements, which only persuade people who need and are willing to pay for the advertised product; only those who have a need for pathological coping mechanisms, and are ready to pay the cost involved, will be affected by the "commercial."

As with eating disorders, a marked increase in the incidence of DID has occurred in recent years (e.g., Lilienfeld et al., 1999; Mai, 1995; Merskey, 1995; North, Ryall, Ricci, & Wetzel, 1993; Uchinuma & Sekine, 2000). Although some researchers deny an actual increase (e.g., see Fahy, 1988; Kihlstrom, 2005; Piper, 1994), there seems to be enough evidence to reject this claim (e.g., Spanos, 1994, 1996; Uchinuma & Sekine, 2000). In accounting for these findings, Spanos et al. (1985) noted that

> popular movies and television shows like 'The Three Faces of Eve' and 'Sybil', and a number of popular biographies like 'Sybil' … provide detailed examples of the symptoms and course of multiple personality. Moreover, these sources usually make the role of multiple personality appear relatively attractive … . (p. 363)

Soon after the publication of The Three Faces of Eve, the authors were "inundated with telephone calls and letters from people who had diagnosed themselves as multiple personalities and who presented themselves in terms of this diagnosis" (Spanos et al., 1985, p. 364). Similarly, evidence reviewed by Spanos (1996) reveals that 53% of DID patients read books or articles, attended lectures, or watched movies about this disorder. "In short, the notion of DID and the symptoms associated with this disorder are well known in our culture" (Spanos, 1996, p. 242). Mai (1995) also reported that a substantial majority of members of the Canadian Psychiatrists Association agreed that publicity has affected the prevalence of DID. These findings can account for the rarity of DID in non-western societies (e.g., Adityanjee et al., 1989, Varma, Bouri, & Wig, 1981) and for its growing prevalence in these countries (e.g., see Uchinuma & Sekine, 2000).

Vocation and Education

Other sources of availability are vocational and educational experiences. According to Ziegler, Imboden, and Meyer (1960), the ability to simulate conversion symptoms is positively correlated with the patient's level of medical sophistication. Patients associated with the medical field, such as physicians, nurses, and neurologists' secretaries, developed symptoms simulating "complicated disease entities" (p. 903). Levy and Jankovic (1983) reported the case of a woman in her mid-20s, with training in both paramedical care and psychology, who developed a unique form of conversion symptoms (e.g., aphasia, pseudo-seizures and profound unresponsiveness). The patient utilized her educational and vocational background to develop a disorder that required advanced knowledge of both medicine and psychology. As a result, her symptoms were so rare, requiring such sophisticated knowledge in medicine, that the doctors had to develop special methods to diagnose the patient's bizarre behavior as a conversion disorder.

Knowledge in medicine may stimulate the selection of other types of behavioral disorders as well. For example, evidence reviewed by Spanos (1996, p. 242) shows some DID patients were exposed to information about this disorder in professional settings. Thus, 17% of patients had training in the mental health field, 17% more aspired to become mental health professionals, and 28% had extensive psychiatric or medical knowledge. Similarly, patients with functional cardiac disorder (a subtype of panic disorder, Buller, Mair, & Benkert, 1987), displayed more dramatic symptoms than the group that had actually experienced myocardial infarction. According to Margraf and Ehlers (1991), "one explanation for this finding could be that functional patients were 'better informed' than patients with myocardial infarction, and therefore knew where the pain had to be" (p. 312). Thus, their vast knowledge regarding myocardial infarctions rendered the symptoms available to them. Additional data that demonstrates the effect of vocation on the choice of a specific mad behavior are the case studies of Charles Cullen, Mordechai Vanunu and Andre Lubitz, discussed above.

Suggestions

Individuals suffering from intolerable levels of stress may be tempted to choose a particular neurotic disorder as a coping mechanism, such as DID, through suggestions given by a therapist (e.g., Ganaway, 1995; Jaroff, 1993; Read & Lindsay; 1994; Spanos, 1996; Spanos & Burgess, 1994). Accordingly, Spanos et al. (1985) reviewed clinical data indicating that, "therapists sometimes encourage patients to adopt the multiple personality role, provide them with information about how to enact that role convincingly, and, perhaps most important, provide 'official' validation for the different identities that their patients enact" (p. 363). Spanos (1996) reviewed experimental evidence which demonstrates "that the interviewing procedures used routinely to diagnose MPD convey all of the information required to allow even psychiatrically unsophisticated subjects to enact the cardinal symptoms of multiplicity" (p. 240). Similarly, Jaroff (1993) reported that, "in many cases the therapists conclude, and eventually convince the patients through suggestion, that the repressed memories of childhood abuse have caused them to 'dissociate'. As a result, they appear to develop multiple personality disorder" (p. 50). Likewise, Read and Lindsay (1994) referred to evidence indicating that "on average patients eventually diagnosed as having DID receive

6 to 7 years of mental healthcare before that diagnosis is made" (p. 420). One very extreme example where the therapist in fact manufactured the diagnosis of MPD is the case of Sybil (Rieber, 1999). In reanalyzing the case, Rieber concluded that, "in the final analysis Sybil is a phony multiple personality case at best" (p. 10).

The suggestions of other authoritative individuals may have similar effects. Fenichel (1934, pp. 160–163) described a 17-year-old man, who developed an unusual avoidance phobia, based on preaching he heard in church. His pastor delivered a sermon, in which he advised young men to avoid contact with those who masturbate. Soon afterward, he began avoiding boys whom he knew masturbated, particularly a certain boy, whom he knew did so often. The patient developed a phobia toward meeting the boy and named him "The Avoided," using this nickname in order to avoid using the boy's real name. The phobia later spread and gradually came to necessitate avoidance of the boy's family and friends. An additional example of suggestion, reported by Dollard and Miller (1950), concerns a woman with marital problems, who developed compulsive counting of heartbeats and breaths shortly after a conversation with her aunt, who told her about her own fear of heart trouble.

Unique Personal Experiences

Patients tend to adopt symptoms with which they are familiar through various channels of information (e.g., media and family). In some cases, however, people utilize their personal experiences to create idiosyncratic symptoms. For example, Emmelkamp (1982, p. 161) describes a 22-year-old woman who suffered from obsessive thoughts of choking. When the subject was 11 years old, she nearly choked to death on a piece of candy. Five years later, she developed a compulsive ritual of checking objects that she might swallow. Emmelkamp, who rejects the conditioning theory of OCD, attributes the patient's behavior to "some serious difficulties in her work" (p. 161) at the onset stage, as there was no other observable event that could plausibly account for the sudden behavioral change. In some cases, patients may use their unique experiences to create psychological disorders that symbolically represent their stressors, as demonstrated by the previously reviewed case by Brandt and Mackenzie (1987). As a child the patient saw a rat in her family's garage while being sexually abused by her brother. Years later, when she discovered her husband's extramarital relationships she developed phobia of contamination from rat germs, which symbolically represented her disgust toward her husband.

Another example of the utilization of an emotionally loaded stimulus for symptom production is found in the autobiographical account of Leonard (1927). The triggering stimulus was a train that acquired its emotional significance when, at age two, Leonard was terrified by a "thundering locomotive." As was noted earlier, it is very unlikely that Leonard repressed this event in the psychoanalytic sense. In fact, Leonard rehearsed rather than repressed the event. This emotionally loaded experience remained latent in his memory for many years, without causing him emotional or behavioral disturbances, until the age of 36, when he was confronted with a severe form of stress. The stress stemmed from his wife's suicide and being ostracized by his community, which blamed him for her death. Coincidentally, while in a state of extreme depression and anxiety, Leonard saw a moving freight train that, due to his desperate search for a coping strategy, reminded him of the traumatic childhood episode. Leonard utilized the coincidental encounter with the train while being in extreme emotional distress to develop panic attack. Apparently, this decision was largely affected by his strong belief in psychoanalysis, with which he was highly familiar. The moving train and the retrieval of the "repressed" episode — where he was almost run down — allowed Leonard to imagine the same state in a much more extreme way (see Leonard, 1927, p. 304). This facilitated the intentional production of the panic attack and, more importantly, enabled Leonard to more easily create a state of unawareness regarding his active involvement in producing the panic attack, by deceiving himself to believe that his behavior was controlled by his unconscious, as will be specified later.

A further example refers to a woman who developed an extreme chocolate phobia which expanded to any object or place associated with chocolate (Rachman & Seligman, 1976). The onset coincided with the death of her mother, upon whom she was extremely dependent. Her behavior could not be accounted for by any environmental event. Intensive behavior therapy did not help to extinguish her phobia. The patient noted that a bar of chocolate was present in the room that had contained her mother's dark colored coffin, and this "may have contributed to the association which she had between death and chocolate" (p. 336). While the color of the chocolate may have been a factor in the development of the phobia, it is likely that chocolate was also selected because of its symbolic meaning. Prior to her mother's death, the patient enjoyed eating chocolate and derived pleasure from it. It may well be that the "loss" of chocolate, which she associated with her mother's coffin, symbolically represented the loss of the beloved mother.

Principle of Availability in Non-Bizarre Behaviors

In addition to bizarre behaviors, stress and depression may lead to other forms of behavioral deviations, such as *suicide* (Bonner & Rich., 1990; Chiu, 1989; Clum, Luscomb, & Patsiokas, 1991; Conrad, 1992; Landau & Rahav, 1989; Pfeffer, 1988; Rich, Warstadt, Nemiroff, Fowler, & Young, 1991; Rudd, 1990) or *substance abuse* (Brown, 1987; Forney, Forney, Sheets, Sitorius et al., 1990; Gorman, 1988; Kumpfer & DeMarsh, 1985; Margolis, 1992; McKirnan & Peterson, 1988; Merikangas & Gelernter, 1990; Quick, Horn, & Quick, 1986;

Schinke, Moncher, Palleja, Zayas, & Schilling, 1988). Here too, availability plays a major role in determining the type of deviant behavior selected.

For example, personal contact with suicidal individuals (see Conrad, 1992; Pfeffer, 1988) or indirect exposure to events of suicide (e.g., mass media or literature; see Goldney, 1989; Ishii, 1991; Lester, 1983a; 126–127; Pfeffer, 1988; Stack, 1988, 1993) may provide a suicidal model and, thus, increase the probability of this behavioral option. In light of this, the high incidence of suicide among individuals from families with a history of suicide may be primarily due to availability rather than by the suggested genetic model (e.g., Mann, 1987; Mitterauer, 1990; Roy, Segal, Centerwall, & Robinette, 1991). Moreover, availability influences not only the decision to commit suicide, but it can determine the means of suicide as well. This is consistent with Lester's (1988a, 1988b) observations that the choice of a particular method of suicide is affected by the availability of that method. For example, in Thailand, where many citizens work in agriculture, ingesting pesticides and fertilizers are commonly used as methods of suicide; in Hong Kong, jumping from a building is more likely. Likewise, it has been shown that strict gun-control laws and lower firearm availability are associated with a lower rate of suicide by firearms (Leenaars & Lester, 1996; Lester, 1993, 1996).

The principle of availability may also account for the adoption of alcohol or drug abuse as a coping response. Research indicates that association with other substance abusers, such as peers (e.g., Hawkins, Lishner, Catalano, & Howard, 1985; Menon, Barrett, & Simpson, 1990; Ong, 1989) and family members (Hawkins et al., 1985; Kosten, Rounsaville, Kosten, & Merikangas, 1991; Kumpfer & DeMarsh, 1985; Mathew, Wilson, Blazer, & George, 1993) or accessibility to the substance itself (Jones-Webb et al., 1997; Tarter & Edwards, 1987), increases the likelihood for the selection of this type of behavior.

An additional factor is the behavioral repertoire of normal drinking which may be intensified to a pathological level in times of stress. Behavioral repertoire may partially account for the higher prevalence of alcoholism among men (see Robbins, 1989), in light of the fact that normal drinking behavior is more common among men than women (e.g., Berkowitz & Perkins, 1987; Engs & Hanson, 1990; Robbins, 1989).

Conclusions

Three major conclusions can be derived from the case studies of neuroses and evidence reviewed above. First, neuroses are fully consistent with PBT's theoretical position: they fulfil PBT's criteria of madness, develop in response to stress, the major function of these behaviors are repression and the choice of a specific symptoms is determined by controllability demands, availability and cost-benefit analysis. Second, there are no significant differences between neurosis, criminal insanity and schizophrenia in terms of diagnosis, etiology and the manner by which they develop. Third, this data constitutes strong blow to the traditional conception of schizophrenia as a brain disease, which later was expanded also to neurosis.

Gender Differences

Neuroses

Neurotic disorders, such as conversion disorder, agoraphobia, panic disorder, eating disorders, and DID, are far more prevalent among women than among men. **OCD** is the only neurosis in which the occurrence is identical between genders or perhaps even higher among men (American Psychiatric Association, 2000). While these differences may be partially accounted for by the principle of availability, a major factor is the lower social tolerance for weakness in men. Men are expected to be "independent, masterful, assertive, and instrumentally competent" (Eagly & Wood, 1991, p. 309). They also tend to "repress emotions that might be associated with vulnerability" (Good, Sherrod & Dillon, 2000, p. 64). Socialization processes encourage men "not to be sissies" (Sanborn, 1990, p. 151) and not "to express their desires for emotional support during stressful situations, because it would be perceived as an inappropriate feminine coping strategy" (Eisler & Blalock, 1991, p. 50; see also Brody & Hall, 1993; Fischer, 1993).

Such disorders may also damage the patient's ability to work. Men tend to avoid neurotic disorders, such as agoraphobia and conversion disorder, mainly because these behaviors increase the risk of unemployment, a prospect which is seen as far more threatening to men than women (e.g., Artazcoz, Benach, Borrell, & Cortes, 2004; Broman, Hamilton, Hoffman, & Mavaddat, 1995; Hammarstrom & Janlert, 2002; Levenstein, Smith, & Kaplan, 2001; Loganathan & Murthy, 2011). As noted by Sanborn (1990), men "overvalue their business powers to the exception of everything else, and this puts them at risk if their business falls apart" (p. 152).

OCD is equally "attractive" for the two sexes (*DSM-IV*-TR, American Psychiatric Association, 2000), because it is not subject to the cost involved in unemployment and social disapproval. Unlike other neuroses (e.g., conversion disorder and agoraphobia), which provide patients with less flexibility in concealing their symptoms when the manifestation is inconvenient for them, OCD patients can restrict their rituals to certain times or places without being perceived as malingering. As noted by Rachman and Hodgson (1980), "a compulsive cleaner or checker can abbreviate, extend, curtail or postpone a compulsive act" (p. 15). These authors described several case studies demonstrating how OCD poses a minimal threat of unemployment for working individuals. One example is the case of a compulsive handwashing woman who succeeded, through careful planning and considerable effort, to disguise her problem at work: she continued to work successfully and without any apparent problems for a number of years, restricting her cleaning rituals to the evenings, in the privacy of her own home.

OCD minimizes social embarrassment, as patients usually display their symptoms in solitude, mostly at home, or inhibit them in the presence of others (e.g., Clarizio, 1991; Newth & Rachman, 2001; Rachman & Hodgson, 1980). Even when patients feel the need to display their symptoms in public, they can reduce their personal embarrassment by providing a socially accepted rationale for their deviant behaviors. For example, Rachman and Hodgson (1980) described a compulsive hand washer who rationalized her behavior by saying that it helped her to prevent illness. When pressed about the exaggerated nature of her actions, she "customarily added that it was 'better to be safe than sorry', and always insisted that her behavior was rational" (p. 19, see also case study by Rofé, 2010).

Schizophrenia

While earlier studies reported that the incidence of ***schizophrenia*** is the same for men and women, some recent studies show that the rate tends to be higher in men (American Psychiatric Association, 2000; Ochoa, Usall, Cobo, Labad, & Kulkarni, 2012). Because schizophrenics usually have few social ties, it seems unlikely that the cost of social embarrassment could account for gender differences. Although other explanations have been suggested (e.g., Blanz, Schmidt, Detzner, & Lay, 1994; Donoghue et al., 2014; Patton, Riecher-Rössler, & Häfner, 1994), the gender differences might partly be due to the poor performance often observed in the premorbid and high-risk populations in the workforce (Cohen, 1993; Terzian, Andreoli, de Oliveria, de Jesus, & McGrath, 2007). Consequently, since social pressure to work is greater for men than for women (e.g., Shankar, Kamath, & Joseph, 1995; Terzian et al., 2007; Thara & Joseph, 1995), and high-risk individuals have poor working skills (e.g., Salokangas & Stengård, 1990; Thara & Rajkumar, 1992), these men either might not find suitable jobs or fail to keep them if they do (see the aforementioned case of Jennifer). Accordingly, while in neuroses the cost of being unable to work often prevents men from adopting these behaviors, with schizophrenia the stress resulting from their inability to work precipitates the onset of this disorder among high-risk men. This may be advantageous for men as they can attribute their professional failure to their illness. This may explain the earlier onset of schizophrenia in men, occurring between the ages 18–25 (Ochoa et al., 2012) when individuals normally go to work or strengthen their vocational skills for better jobs in the future (e.g., Zimmer-Gembeck & Mortimer, 2006). The late onset of schizophrenia in women, at 25–35 (Ochoa et al., 2012), may be because women at these ages realizing that their prospects for marriage are low or because these "women face a lot of problems especially in relation to marriage, pregnancy childbirth, and menopause" (Thara & Kamath, 2015, p. S249).

Drug Therapy: Fixing or Damaging the Brain

PBT's new understanding of psychological disorders has important implication for therapy, as it enables the integration of all therapeutic methods pertaining to mad behaviors into one theoretical framework. Since this issue requires extensive discussion, it will be addressed in a separate section in Part III. However, considering the fact that the scientific reputation of the disease conception of schizophrenia is also based on the conviction that antipsychotics restore brain functioning, research and clinical data which negate this belief are reviewed in the context of Part I. Two case studies are presented in this section in order to demonstrate the harmful consequences of antipsychotics, in contrast to the successful results of psychological interventions.

Antipsychotics

Antipsychotics have been widely recognized as the primary treatment for schizophrenia and they are recommended by the American Psychiatry Association (Lehman et al., 2004), the Schizophrenia Patient Outcomes Research Team (PORT; Lehman et al., 2003), and the National Institute for Clinical Excellence (2002). This recommendation should be reevaluated when examining both their efficacy and their harmful effects.

Efficacy: Research indicates that antipsychotics primarily reduce schizophrenics' positive symptoms (i.e., delusions and hallucinations), and have little or no effect on the negative symptoms, which as stated before, constitute the source of patients' stresses (e.g., Artaloytia, Arango, Lahti, Sanz et al., 2006; Green, 2016; Haddad & Correll, 2018; Miyamoto, Miyake, Jarskog et al., 2012). Although some researchers reported that antipsychotics also affect negative symptoms, such as avolition–apathy and alogia (Subotnik et al., 2014), these outcomes do not include social and cognitive deficits, which are the core problems of schizophrenia. Antipsychotics alone or adjunctive antidepressants have no effect on problem solving, social competence, or social cognition (e.g., Bellack, Schooler, Marder, Kane et al., 2004; Green, 2016; Kucharska-Pietura & Mortimer, 2013; Sergi, Green, Widmark, Reist et al., 2007; Vernon, Grudnikoff, Seidman et al., 2014; Usall, López-Carrilero, Iniesta et al., 2014. Accordingly, researchers have concluded that "the results do no engender optimism for the possibility that antipsychotic drugs can specifically facilitate social recovery" (Kucharska-Pietura & Mortimer, 2013, p. 335).

In the same way, psychiatrists tend to be pessimistic about the prospect of recovery in schizophrenia (Ng, Pearson, & Chen, 2008). Research examining the efficacy of antipsychotics after 3 years of treatment, found that 33% of patients achieved long-lasting symptom remission, 13% had long-lasting functional remission (a positive effect on occupational/vocational functioning, independent living, and active social interaction), 27% experienced long-lasting adequate quality of life, and only 4% achieved complete recovery, defined as simultaneously achieving long-lasting symptomatic functional remission and an adequate quality of life (Novick, Haro, Suarez, Vieta, & Naber, 2009). When patients were treated with antipsychotics in conjunction with psychosocial interventions, 36% maintained full symptom remission for 6 months, while the rate of recovery was 10%. However, after a period of 1 year, symptom remission was reduced to 22% and only 1% met the criteria of recovery (Ventura et al., 2011). Antipsychotics had little impact on the schizophrenics' overall satisfaction of life (Fervaha, Agid, Takeuchi, Foussias, & Remington, 2014), and in some cases, prolonged drug therapy aggravated the individual's psychological state. A 20-year longitudinal study shows that patients who did not take antipsychotics for prolonged periods, were less psychotic and experienced more periods of recovery than those who were on medications continuously (Harrow, Jobe, & Faull, 2012; see also Harrow & Jobe, 2013).

Harmful Effects: Even if antipsychotics had a significant recovery effect, it is doubtful whether this benefit would outweigh the heavy toll they take on patients using these drugs, as they have serious harmful effects on psychophysiological systems. These effects include akathisia, sexual dysfunction (e.g., Kane et al., 2009; Olfson, Uttaro, Carson, & Tafesse, 2005; Peluso, Lewis, Barnes, & Jones, 2013), and increased risk of metabolic syndrome, comprised of obesity, dyslipidemias, glucose intolerance, insulin resistance (or hyperinsulinemia), hypertension, which contributes to cardiovascular disease (e.g., Casey et al., 2004; Mittal et al., 2017; Scigliano & Ronchetti, 2013; Yogaratnam, Biswas, Vadivel, & Jacob, 2013), and sudden cardiac arrest (Ray, Chung, Murray, Hall, & Stein, 2009).

A high percentage of patients (42.2%–57.7%) are treated with multiple medications (Faries, Ascher-Svanum, Zhu, Correll, & Kane, 2005; Suokas, Suvisaari, Haukka, Korhonen, & Tiihonen, 2013), compounding the adverse effects of the drugs. The negative synergistic effects of these drugs can lead to decreased cognitive function (especially with prolonged use; e.g., Elie et al., 2010; Wolf, Leucht, & Pajonk, 2017; Xiang, Weng, Leung, Tang, & Ungvari, 2007), a decline in verbal learning and memory, poor cognitive performance, difficulty in thinking and concentration, and even death (e.g., Fakhoury, Wright, & Wallace, 2001; Husa, Rannikko, Moilanen, Haapea et al., 2014; Tiihonen, Mittendorfer-Rutz, Torniainen et al., 2016; Tiihonen, suokas, suvisaan et al., 2012).

Long-term treatment through antipsychotics has also been correlated with smaller brain tissue volumes and larger cerebrospinal fluid volumes (e.g., Fusar-Poli et al., 2013; Ho, Andreasen, Ziebell, Pierson, & Magnotta, 2011; Torres et al., 2013; Veijola et al., 2014). Adverse alterations of brain structure and decreased cognitive functioning associated with antipsychotics were also observed in animals (Konopaske et al., 2007, 2008; Terry & Mahadik, 2007). Thus, "although antipsychotics relieve psychosis and its attendant suffering, these drugs may not arrest the pathophysiologic processes underlying schizophrenia and may even aggravate progressive brain tissue volume reductions" (Ho et al., 2011, p. 8; see also Moncrieff, 2013). Some researchers have also found that antipsychotics, widely used for patients with severe depression, might be associated with alteration of the cerebrospinal fluids Amyloid-B and total tau, which are thought to be predictive of Alzheimer's disease (Clarke, Hartmann, Jones, Ballard et al., 2011; Gøtzsche, 2014).

It may be worthwhile to note that while some researchers reported that negative effects of antipsychotics are more prominent with first generation antipsychotics (Kiviniemi et al., 2013), others have found that the second generation is associated with a greater frequency of metabolic and cardiovascular disturbances (Peluso et al., 2013; Scigliano & Ronchetti, 2013). Some have found that both types of drugs had a similar effect in increasing various side effects, including the risk of sudden cardiac arrest (Leucht, Cipriani, Spineli, Mavridis et al., 2013; Ray, Chung, Murray, Hall et al., 2009). Whitaker (2010) noted in this respect that the "wonder drug" glow around the second generation psychotropic has long since disappeared. He views the camping for the top-selling atypical antipsychotics as "one of the more embarrassing episodes in psychiatry's history, as one government-funded study after another failed to find that they were any better than the first-generation anti-psychotics" (p. 303).

Clinical Examples

The Unfortunate Fate of John Cronholm Versus The Happy End of Mr. X

In order to demonstrate the anti-humanistic approach of the medical system and the horrible damages that antipsychotics can inflict, two case studies of schizophrenia are reviewed below. The first case illustrates the totalitarian power of the medical system and the disastrous effects of antipsychotics. The second case describes how one patient avoided this unfortunate fate when his hospitalization was discontinued and he was instead referred to psychoanalytic therapy.

The first case, reported by Leon (1990), concerns a 28-year-old schizophrenic, John Cronholm, who was hospitalized several times starting at the age of 19. John attended university and was successful academically during his first semester. He stopped going to class during the second semester, and progressively developed schizophrenic symptoms. After several years of unsuccessful drug treatment, Cronholm's condition deteriorated and the patient refused both medication and continued hospitalization. Nevertheless, he was hospitalized against his will and forced to take medication. As a result, the patient experienced severe side effects from different antipsychotic medications. He developed a variety of dysfunctions in his extrapyramidal motor system, including tremors, motor restlessness and pacing, and muscle spasms of the limbs, which caused his arms and legs to twist to one side. Despite these negative effects and his continued protests, he was forced to continue medications, albeit at a lower dosage to reduce side effects. Although the antipsychotics' harmful effects were reduced, he never recovered from his "illness." In discussing this case, Leon (1990) raised the ethical question of "how far health professionals and other social agents can go in forcing someone to take medications against their will, even if there is clear improvement in their condition with the medication. Do patients have a right to their mental illness?" (p. 333).

A happier ending was seen in the case of Mr. X, discussed previously. This case refers to a 31-year old, married, university lecturer, diagnosed as schizophrenic, whom psychiatrists deemed incurable. As specified earlier, Mr. X's breakdown occurred due to his mother's disappointment in his marriage to a non-Jewish woman. The patient was not eating, not sleeping, and continually hallucinating. ECT was strongly but pessimistically recommended. "He had been held together by the fantasy that if only he were good enough, then his parents would accept him." However, when he realized that his intellectual achievements as a Ph.D. and a lecturer at a prestigious college did not please his parents, "his defenses unraveled" (p. 14). An additional contributing factor was "fear of punishment for his sexuality and intense guilt about masturbating, feeling that "his body and his penis really did not belong to him" (p. 15). The major components of the therapy that enabled Mr. X to recover from his psychological problems were as follows:

1. ***Therapeutic Alliance and Support from His Wife:*** Mr. X's therapist, Karon, was supportive and optimistic, and told the patient

that he could telephone him at any time. In emphasizing the importance of this issue, Karon noted, "the therapist must create a therapeutic alliance by becoming helpful, tolerating incoherence, tolerating not understanding, and being realistically optimistic" (p. 4). Mr. X's wife also contributed to his recovery by supporting and defending him. As noted by the patient "when I needed her, she saved my life. The doctors said, 'Shock him'. My family said, 'Shock him', but she had the courage to defy them and see that I got real treatment" (p. 21).

2. ***Behavior Therapy*:** In order to motivate Mr. X to eat, Karon scheduled a few sessions at an "all-night restaurant." Initially, Mr. X only watched the therapist eat, then in the next session he took some coffee, and finally he ate breakfast. Similarly, to overcome his sexual inhibitions and his complaint of not being able to read, he was asked to buy a copy of Playboy magazine and try to read it. The therapist then talked with him about the normality of sexual curiosity and interest. Within a few sessions, he was able to read, while protesting that it was a terrible "pandering magazine."
3. ***Stress Management and Lifting of Repression*:** Mr. X's therapy focused on increasing his awareness of his current stressors and strengthening his ability to resolve them by rational means. These effects were obtained through the *distortion of his idealization his mother***.** The therapist increased Mr. X's awareness, especially in regards to the harmful effects his mother had on his feelings of inadequacy, guilt, and worthlessness. He was encouraged to adopt an antagonistic attitude toward his mother, and thereby disconnect his self-worth from her expectations. The therapist systematically utilized various memories from Mr. X's childhood to shatter the idealization of his mother. For example, the patient recalled how when he was 5-years-old his mother used to dress him in white clothes, send him out to play, and then punish him for getting dirty. Mr. X believed that his mother's reactions were justified and that it was his fault. The

therapist used this memory to break down his mother's image, explaining that

> of course, any parent knows that if you put a little boy in all white clothes in a hermetically sealed room, he would still manage to get dirty in an hour or less. I pointed out how his mother set him up for this, that any child would get dirty, and that she probably enjoyed punishing him. (p. 16)

Another example concerns the scar on Mr. X's hand which was the result of his mother holding his hand to stove burner to teach him not to steal after he took a toy from a store when he was 5 years old. After a session focused on the irrationality of such a response, Mr. X's hallucination of burning in hell disappeared. The negative portrayal of his mother in this episode and in other memories had curative effects as it undermined Mr. X's idealization of his mother.

Through therapy Mr. X was able to fully recover, and he returned to work at his intellectually demanding job 4 months later. Twenty years later, he sent the therapist a note thanking him for "giving me my life back" (Karon, 2008; see also Silver, 2008).

Not only does this case challenge the validity of medical models, as it is hard to see how they would be able to explain Mr. X's full recovery from a brain disease through therapy alone, but it also emphasizes their faulty therapeutic intervention. Had his wife not intervened while he was in the hospital, Mr. X might have suffered the same unfortunate fate as John Cronholm.

Although the recovery was achieved through psychoanalytic therapy, this case is not brought as support of psychoanalysis. First, as stated, studies refute the existence of Freud's repression, including the idea that the lifting of repression is a necessary condition for a genuine recovery (e.g., see a review by Rofé, 2008). Second, psychoanalysis is unable to explain schizophrenia, both because it attributes its cause to early fixations that produced defects in ego and because of its inability to address the neurological findings that this disorder is seemingly a brain disease (e.g., see Willick, 2002).

Thus, it seems that the therapeutic success of Mr. X was not the result of the psychoanalytic therapeutic method, which supposedly uncovers repressed childhood traumas. Rather, this effect seems to be the result of stress management, where the therapist increased the patient's awareness of his stressor and confronted him with evidence that neutralized the stress. As will be elaborated on later in Part III, PBT uses the term lifting of repression whenever a therapeutic procedure increases the patient's awareness of his or her current stressors, in order to counteract the distractive value of the symptom. While the issue of therapy will be discussed in much more detail in Part III, two additional observations should be made in this context.

1. Studies have shown that psychoanalysis is usually ineffective with schizophrenic patients, and significantly increases the risk of suicide (see review by Mueser & Berenbaum, 1990). In line with these findings, the Schizophrenic PORT has concluded that "there is no evidence in support of the superiority of psychoanalytic therapy to other forms of therapy, and there is a consensus that ... [It] can be harmful to persons with schizophrenia" (Lehman, Steinwachs, & the Survey Co-Investigators, 1998, p. 13). Psychoanalysis may be harmful, especially for patients who suffer from significant cognitive deficits and a severe lack of social skills, which usually results from genetic flaws. Under these conditions, insight-oriented therapy designed to increase patients' awareness of traumas, real, or fictitious, can aggravates their emotional state, as they are inherently unable to cope with the situation.
2. A full recovery has also been achieved through therapeutic methods that enhanced the schizophrenic's ability to cope with his current stressors. As will be described in Part III, Bradshaw

(1998) reported a case study of a 26-year-old single woman, with a similar background to John Cronholm, who fully recovered through cognitive therapy, which addressed the patient's current stressful situation.

In conclusion, medical models use the outcomes of drug therapy as one of the strongest pieces of evidence in their campaign to demonstrate that schizophrenia is a brain disease. Yet, it is difficult to see how the disease model can integrate cases of complete recovery in the absence of drugs. Additionally, not only does the evidence of drug therapy not support such theoretical claims, but the harmful effects of drugs further negate any purported benefits. As noted by Peter Tyrer (2012), the Editor of the British Journal of Psychiatry,

> it is time to reappraise the assumption that antipsychotics must always be the first line of treatment for people with psychoses. This is not a wild cry from the distant outback, but a considered opinion by influential researchers...and the reasons for the change in view are... an increasing body of evidence that [show that] the adverse effects treatment are, to put it simply, not worth the candle (p. 168).

Similarly, Williams (2012), summarizing relevant studies, stated that

> the use of antipsychotics helps reduce the positive symptoms of psychosis and the associated distressing emotions for many people in the short term (during the first six weeks or so). The long-term use of antipsychotics increases the likelihood of the development of a chronic psychotic condition and significantly reduces the likelihood of recovery, as well as carrying the high likelihood of causing other serious physical, cognitive, and emotional impairments ... (p. 58; see also Whitaker, 2015).

Antidepressants

Efficacy: In contrast to antipsychotics, antidepressants have beneficial effects on nearly all neurotic disorders, including **panic disorder, agoraphobia** (e.g., Furukawa, Watanabe, & Churchill, 2006; Mavissakalian & Ryan, 1998; Westenberg, 1996), **OCD** (e.g., Abramovitz, 1997; Cottraux, Bouvard, & Maud, 2005; Dell'Osso, Nestadt, Allen, & Hollander, 2006; Dougherty, Rauch, & Jenike, 2004), **DID** (e.g., Kluft, 1987; Loewenstein, 1991; Putnam & Loewenstein, 1993; Miller, 2000) **eating disorders** (e.g., Bacaltchuk, Hay, & Mari, 2000; Ferguson & Pigott, 2000; Vaswani, Ramesh, Kalra, & Sagar, 2005), and **conversion disorder** (e.g., Cybulska, 1997; Pu, Mohamed, Imam, & El-Roey, 1986; Voon, 2006; Voon & Lang, 2005).

Discontinuation of antidepressants (e.g., Doyle & Pollack, 2004; Mavissakalian & Guo, 2004; Mavissakalian & Perel, 2002; Mavissakalian & Ryan, 1998) or anti-panic medication (see review by Taylor, 2000) increases the risk of relapse among panic and agoraphobic patients. Similar effects were found regarding the discontinuation of drug therapy for OCD patients (e.g., Bystritsky, 2004; Koran, Bullock, Hartston, Elliot, D'Andrea, 2002; Pato, Murphy, & DeVane, 1991; Ravizza et al., 1998; Marks & O'Sullivan, 1988) and bulimic patients (see Kotler & Walsh, 2000). In a similar fashion, continuous use of antidepressant medication for panic disorder (Mavissakalian & Perel, 1999), OCD (e.g., Fineberg, Pampaloni, Pallanti, Ipser, & Stein, 2007; Ravizza et al, 1998), and bulimia nervosa (e.g., Kotler & Walsh, 2000; Peterson & Mitchell, 1999) reduced the risk of relapse.

Many studies show that the same medication may be effective for disorders of different symptomatology. For example, clomipramine, fluoxetine, fluvoxamine, monoamine oxidase inhibitors, and tricyclic antidepressants are effective in the treatment of ***OCDs*** (e.g., Abramovitz, 1997; Demal, Zitterl, Lenz, Zapotoczky, & Zitterl-Eglseer, 1996; Park, Jefferson, & Greist, 1997; Piccinelli, Pini, Bellantuono, & Wilkinson, 1995; Van Balkom et al., 1994),

agoraphobia **and** ***panic disorders*** (e.g., Alexander, 1991; Black, Wesner, Bowers, & Gabel, 1993; Burrows, Judd, & Norman, 1993; Gelder, 1992; Klerman, 1992; Westenberg, 1996). Similar results were reported for ***eating disorders*** *as well* (e.g., Hoffman & Halmi, 1993; Wolfe, 1995).

Harmful Effects: Drug therapy has far fewer harmful effects for neurotic patients than for schizophrenic patients. The main negative effects of antidepressants, which are used as the major medical intervention for such patients, are weight gain and sexual dysfunction (e.g., Bet, Hugtenburg, Penninx, & Hoogendijk, 2013; Bijlsma et al., 2014; Rothschild, 2000). It is possible that the negative effects of these drugs would be significantly worse if administered intensively, as is common in psychiatric hospitals.

Theoretical and Practical Implications

Historically, medical interventions in schizophrenia became universally accepted, despite their disastrous consequences, because of the strong conviction that this disorder is the result of brain disease. The horrible outcomes of lobotomy (e.g., De Mille, 1962; Hakola et al., 1993; Mashour, Walker, & Martuza, 2005) and insulin shock (e.g., Doroshow, 2006) did not damage the scientific statues of medical models, but only motivated advocates to search for seemingly safer medical interventions. Therefore, it is unlikely that presenting evidence of the serious damage caused by antipsychotics to patients' cognitive and physiological systems will have any effect in changing the common belief that schizophrenia is a brain disease. Advocates of this model will continue to search for neurological mechanisms which they believe cause this disorder, overlooking the previously mentioned findings that negate this belief. Moreover, researchers will continue to suggest new medical interventions that supposedly lack harmful effects, without examining first the possible long-term toxic effects of these drugs.

One example is a growing number of researchers who claim, based on correlational studies, that schizophrenia is caused by inflammation, which is part of the body's immune system. This claim is strengthened by studies demonstrating that anti-inflammation drugs are an effective treatment for schizophrenia, especially as adjuvant therapy to antipsychotics (e.g., Cho, Lee, Kwak et al., 2019; Mongan, Ramesar, Föcking et al., 2019). These findings are not different than the conventional correlational studies between schizophrenia and neurological impairments reviewed earlier. Therefore, the same research and clinical data reviewed in the Introduction and Part-I, which refute the conception of schizophrenia as a brain disease, are applicable to these studies as well. Furthermore, it seems unlikely that the fate of these new drugs will be different from that of antipsychotics. However, in the meantime, until research confirm this claim, the drug companies will continue to prosper.

Accordingly, it is PBT's goal to provide a theoretical and scientific platform for a social movement which will lead to the recognition of schizophrenia as a psychological disorder, thereby minimizing the use of drug treatment. Such understanding will then lead to the conclusion that the major therapeutic intervention should be psychological, rather than medical, as will be elaborated on in Part-III. Although antipsychotics and-inflammatory drugs may sometimes be helpful, as they reduce the patient's emotional distress, these medications should be minimalized and only be employed on a short-term basis. Medication should be used as an adjunct therapy to psychological intervention, whose function is to enhance the patient's coping ability.

The term "antipsychotics" may seem misleading not only because of their disastrous long-term consequences with little prospect for recovery, but also because they are employed in the treatment of psychological disorders that do not have psychotic symptoms, such as **panic disorder** (e.g., Wang, Woo, & Bahk, 2014), **OCD** (e.g., Dold, Aigner, Lazenberger, & Kasper, 2013; Masi, Pfanner, & Brovedani, 2013; Matsunaga, Nagata, Hayashida,

Ohya et al., 2009; Zhou, Zhou, Chen et al., 2019), eating disorders (Fernández, & Cano, 2005; Mehler-Wex, Romanos, Kirchheiner, & Schulze, 2008; Pisano, Catone, Pascotto, & Gritti, 2014), and **PTSD** (Han, Pae, Wang at el., 2014).

It seems likely that the short-term effects of antipsychotics in the treatment of schizophrenia occur, because these drugs reduce patients' levels of depression (e.g., DeBattista & Hawkins, 2009; Kasper & Akimova, 2013; Kato & Chang, 2013; Philip, Carpenter, Tyrka, Whiteley, & Price, 2009). Antipsychotics augment the effect of antidepressants in the treatment of major depression (Cha, Luo, Ahmed, Becirovic et al., 2019) even more than lithium (Dold, Bartova, Kautzky et al., 2018) and are effective in the treatment of acute bipolar depression (Bartoli, Dell'Osso, Crocamo et al., 2017). These findings may explain why antipsychotics reduce the risk of suicide (Kaneda, 2007; Keck, Strakowski, & McElroy, 2000; Reutfors, Clapham, Bahmanyar et al., 2016). Similar effects were found with respect to anti-inflammatory drugs (e.g., Allison, Sharma, & Timmons, 2019; Fiedorow, Cyranowski, Liu, & Swartz, 2019). Considering these studies, it may be more accurate to rename these drugs as "augmentative antidepressants", rather than antipsychotics.

Accordingly, it seems that while on these medications both schizophrenics and neurotic patients tend to abandon their pathological behaviors. The drugs alleviate patients' emotional distress, making these behaviors superfluous. Thus, drugs may have an indirect curative effect, either because they relieve patients' level of their depression, thereby allowing them to search for more adaptive solutions to their stressors, or because of positive compensation events that occur while the patient is using the drug. However, relapse is likely regardless of whether patients remain on drugs or discontinue this treatment (e.g., see Emsley, 2018 and studies reviewed by Williams, 2012) as often patients cannot cope with the stress in the long-term without improving their coping abilities (see case study by Bradshaw, 1998 in Part-III). This theoretical position is consistent with Haddad and Correll's (2018) statement, in a review which summarizes key meta-analytic findings regarding antipsychotic efficacy, that "the management of schizophrenia always requires a comprehensive individualized treatment plan that includes appropriate psychological support and interventions, as well as pharmacological treatment" (p. 315). Thus, while drugs may be useful when combined with psychological methods that address patients' stressful conditions, they may lead to disastrous consequences when one follows the medical models' belief that patients suffer from brain disease, and therefore neglects the employment of psychotherapy. As noted by the Unabomber (1995), in his manifesto

> instead of removing the conditions that make people depressed, modern society gives them antidepressant drugs. In effect, antidepressants are a means of modifying an individual's internal state in such a way as to enable him to tolerate social conditions that he would otherwise find intolerable.

Discussion

Diagnostic Advantages

One of the fundamental requirements of a scientific theory is the clear definition of the object of its inquiry. Although Freud made an invaluable contribution to the understanding psychological disorders by making bizarre behaviors the focus of his investigation, his theory did not allow him to provide clear empirical criteria for defending his diagnostic approach, as indicated by evidence reviewed in Part I. Consequently, with the deterioration of the scientific status of psychoanalysis, *DSM-III's* task force decided to remove this diagnostic method, seemingly because of the lack of empirical criteria for his diagnostic concepts (e.g., see Bayer & Spitzer, 1985). Instead, although the task force claimed to be atheoretical, in reality, the committee members, comprising solely of psychiatrists (e.g., see Pilecki et al., 2011), implicitly turned the *DSM* into a medical book (e.g., see Burstow, 2005; Follette & Houts, 1996; Pilecki et al., 2011). As a result, the *DSM* became "an expanding list of disease, from a few dozen disorders in the first edition to well over 200" (Grinker, 2010, p. 169; see also Warelow & Holmes, 2011).

Given the international scientific reputation of the *DSM*, this dramatic shift in the perception of behavioral disorders was not limited to the diagnostic system. It also had far-reaching effects on research and treatment approaches. Through the shift of scientific efforts toward medical models and away from other competing theories, these models succeeded in expanding their scientific reputation and have resulted in a dramatic increase in the consumption of psychiatric drugs.

One of PBT's major theoretical contributions to this field plagued with discords is the empirical definition of madness. Contrary to both *DSM* (American Psychiatric Association, 1976) and medical models (e.g., see Wakefield, 1999), who undermine the possibility of common empirical criteria for neuroses, PBT provides seven (five major and two secondary) diagnostic criteria, which can differentiate between bizarre behavioral disorders and non-bizarre deviant behaviors. These diagnostic criteria have three main advantages over the *DSM's* current diagnostic system. **First**, unlike the *DSM*, which has reached its diagnostic decisions through the consensus of one group of experts who were theoretically biased and possibly even motivated by personal interests (see Pilecki et al., 2011), PBT's diagnostic categories are based on notable clinical and research data. **Second**, the *DSM*, which was originally designed to be a neutral diagnostic system, did not emerge out of a scientific theory that provides insight into the underlying causes of psychological disorders. This is a fundamental deficit since as noted by Wakefield (1999) "the use of theory-neutral criteria goes against a common position in philosophy of science that scientific progress generally goes hand-in-hand with greater theory-ladenness of basic classificatory concepts" (p. 1002). Accordingly, PBT's diagnostic approach is an improvement on the *DSM*, as it has already demonstrated its ability to account for the development and treatment of neurosis and psychosis using one set of theoretical concepts (Rofé, 2000; 2010; Rofé & Rofé, 2013; see also Part III).

Third, following the removal of Freud's cataloging system, the *DSM* created heterogeneous diagnostic categories in which bizarre and non-bizarre deviant behaviors were classified in the same diagnostic category. One example is the *DSM-III's* diagnostic category of *anxiety disorder*. This category classifies OCD, which is composed of bizarre behaviors — such as the compulsive cleaner who washes her hands 200 times per day but leaves her legs and feet unwashed for months (Rachman & Hodgson, 1980, p. 65) — together with PTSD — which is understandable behavior in response to extreme trauma (see Burstow, 2005), only because both display observable anxiety. Another example is the *DSM-5's* new diagnostic category, *Psychological Factors Affecting Other Medical Conditions*. This category contains physical diseases, such as diabetes, cancer, and coronary disease — which are exacerbated by stress — together with the neurosis of conversion disorder (e.g., hysterical blindness, leg paralysis, and psychogenic movements), which lacks any physiological basis (American Psychiatric Association, 2013). In an attempt to rationalize this decision, the *DSM's* authors note that they did not want to define conversion disorder as a psychological disorder because this would reinforce the concept of "mind-body dualism" (309). Thus, although the *DSM-5* acknowledges that conversion disorder is medically inexplicable, this disorder is classified together with physical diseases, which have clear medical cause, to distance the diagnosis from the psychoanalytic conjecture of mind-body dualism (Carella, 1974). This is a clear demonstration of a biased decision made by the *DSM's* authors to avoid supporting the psychoanalytic conception in this matter. While such anti-psychoanalytic conclusions may be a legitimate scientific perspective, this approach can be problematic when it lacks objectivity and is used solely to undermine a competing theory. This claim is especially true it is promoted by a biased scientific body with an interest in promoting the pharmacology industry (see Lacasse, 2014; Pilecki et al., 2011).

Parsimonious Theoretical Approach

The principle of parsimony, also known as Ockham's razor, is a philosophical principle used to assess the scientific value of a given theory (e.g., Baker, 2007; Braithwaite, 2007; Epstein, 1984; Sober, 1981). According to this principle, simplicity should be a major factor in the evaluation of competing theories. When comparing rival theories, the theory with the fewest assumptions must be selected over a more complex theory (e.g., Baker, 2007; Braithwaite, 2007; Epstein, 1984; Sober, 1981). "The essence of this point, in its proper context, is to start from the simplest possible explanation and make it more complex only if, and when absolutely necessary" (Braithwaite, 2007, p. 1). PBT satisfies this requirement by explaining a large variety of behavioral disorders, including schizophrenia, criminal insanity, and neurosis, which exhibit completely different symptoms, using just a few simple concepts. In their critique of psychoanalytic theory, advocates of medical models reject the possibility that an alternative theory could follow Freud's parsimonious approach (e.g., Wakefield, 1999). PBT proves that this skepticism is unfounded. Evidence reviewed in Part I demonstrates that PBT can serve as an overarching umbrella theory, under which data pertaining to the various bizarre behaviors (schizophrenia, criminal insanity, and neuroses) can be integrated. This theoretical achievement has been made possible by (1) maintaining Freud's basic idea concerning bizarre behaviors, while providing empirical diagnostic criteria for this concept; (2) rejecting the axiomatic assumption, common to all traditional theories of psychopathology, that behavioral disorders are determined by irrational factors; 3) viewing bizarre behaviors as coping mechanisms which certain individuals adopt when confronted with intolerable levels of stress, which can be the result of environmental events, unacceptable impulses, a deficit of coping skills, neurological impairments or some combination of these factors.

One additional contributing factor is the new conceptualization of repression. On the one hand, PBT maintains Freud's idea that neurotic patients repress the underlying causes of the dramatic change in their behaviors, expanding this claim to schizophrenia as well. On the other hand, it rejects the psychoanalytic doctrine of repression which views it as an unconscious process (Cramer, 2001; Wilson & Dunn, 2004). Repression is redefined as a conscious, deliberate distraction, as originally suggested by Freud (see Erdelyi, 2006; Erdelyi and Goldberg, 1979). However, PBT's most significant change to psychoanalysis is that repression is seen as the consequence rather than the cause of madness: patients intuitively choose mad behaviors in order to block the accessibility of stress-related thoughts.

Another unique aspect of PBT is the use of economic concepts for explaining the large variability of mad behaviors, originally termed by Freud (1913) "choice of neurosis". Research and clinical data reviewed above indicate that there is little difference between a consumer's decision process when purchasing products and the decision process used to choose a specific behavioral madness. In both cases, this choice is determined by three principles: needs, availability of suitable "merchandise," and cost-benefit analysis. These principles enable PBT to account for:

1. Variability within each disorder: why one patient develops hysterical blindness while another develops hysterical paralysis, or why schizophrenic patients with similar backgrounds develop completely different symptoms?
2. Variability between different types of disorders: why people develop neuroses, criminal insanity, or schizophrenia?
3. Variability in the prevalence of mad behaviors among different social groups: gender, sociocultural, and religiosity differences, and the recent increase in the prevalence of eating disorders and DID.

Methodological Considerations

As stated previously, the main reason for the widespread belief that schizophrenia is a brain disease is the absence of a psychological theory that addresses the significant relationships between schizophrenia and genetic/brain impairments. However, one additional major factor for this misinterpretation of the data is the inappropriate methodology used by medical models. Taking for granted that all schizophrenics have brain disease, medical models focused their research on correlational studies and on examining the brain function of patients with brain impairments. Then, they have generalized their conclusions also to schizophrenics with no evidence of genetic/neurological defects. PBT challenges the validity of this belief not only by providing a new theory that replaces the medical model of the genetic/neurological interpretation, but by changing the method of investigation.

One technical change is to first examine cases with no evidence of genetic/neurological flaws and then generalize conclusions derived from these cases to explain correlational findings. A more radical methodological argument is that medical models have never truly investigated schizophrenia. Given the numerous evidence reviewed in Part I, demonstrating that schizophrenia is a response to stress just as with other types of bizarre behaviors, it becomes obvious that brain research has nothing to do with schizophrenia. These studies have only examined the major underlying cause of stress experienced by one group of schizophrenic patients. In this regard, as with key notions in Freud's theory (e.g., bizarreness, repression and common etiology), PBT follows Freud's opinion that case study should be the major research tool of mad behaviors, including schizophrenia.

Not only Freud, but many other researchers as well view case study as critically important in examining complex issues, particularly in the early phases of the development of a new theory, when key variables and their relationships are being explored (Bowers & Favolden, 1996; Brewin & Andrews, 19; Flyvbjerg, 2006; Gibbert et al., 2008; Zaidah, 2007). It is difficult to see, especially at this stage of investigation, which alternative methods can examine PBT's suggestions concerning the psychological functions of bizarre behaviors and the underlying mechanism for choosing a specific mad behavior, better than case study.

Case studies are certainly better than animal studies used by behaviorists and medical models for the understanding of psychological disorders. Animals are unable to exhibit human-like bizarre behaviors; such behaviors seem to be a unique innovation of the human mind. For example, though harsh environmental conditions (e.g., electric shocks) may induce extreme behavioral dysfunction among animals which mimics human behavior, as shown in a number of studies on "experimental neurosis" (see Mineka & Kihlstrom's review, 1978), and learned helplessness (Seligman, 1974, 1975), these behaviors do not resemble the seemingly nonsensical behaviors seen in psychosis and neurosis. As noted by Mineka and Kihlstrom (1978), given the unusual, stressful conditions to which the animals were subjected during experimental neurosis, it would have been surprising if the animals did not display emotional disturbances. Moreover, there is no evidence that animals, exhibit a variety of deviant behaviors, when exposed to the same stressful situation. While animal deviant behaviors can be experimentally produced in the laboratory, no bizarre behaviors can be artificially produced in human beings Accordingly, it seems that while animals may promote our understanding of the development and treatment of simple phobias and depression, they cannot assist in understanding the development of neurosis and psychosis. This claim is especially applicable to schizophrenia, which animal models have been used to understand the underlying cause of this disorder (e.g., see Faatehi, Basiri, Nezhadi et al., 2019; and a review by Marcotte, Pearson, Srivastava, 2001). As noted by Skrabanek (1984):

> [It is] startling when one reads about attempts to use animal models of schizophrenia. It is an understatement to

> write that 'the fact that schizophrenia is a thought disorder complicates the creation of animal models … ' A paranoid rat? A hallucinating guinea pig? A thought insertion in the ass? (p. 22)

Conclusions

During the 20th century, the explanation and treatment of psychological disorders was dominated by two major theoretical empires, psychoanalysis and medical models. While psychoanalytic theory was limited primarily to neuroses, medical models dominated the explanation of psychotic disorders. With the decline of psychoanalysis, medical models expanded their theoretical scope to include the entire field of behavioral disorders. However, as stated above, they reached this respectable scientific position not by the strength of their data but because no psychological theory could provide more valid explanation for mad behaviors.

Clinical and research data reviewed in Part I demonstrates the superiority of PBT over the medical models in reference to four major topics **(1) Diagnosis of psychological disorders:** PBT's diagnostic criteria showed that neuroses and psychoses share common empirical characteristics, which differentiate them from other deviant behavior; **(2) Variability of symptoms:** unlike medical models, which are unable to explain the variability of symptoms even within the same psychological disorder, PBT's three principles for the choice of symptoms allow us to account for all variances of the symptoms within each disorder, as well as between different disorders; **(3) Integrative abilities:** contrary to medical models, which focus only on a specific disorder and their own data, overlooking the theoretical and empirical data by rival theories, PBT is capable of integrating research and clinical data contributed by all schools of thoughts in this field, which are seemingly incompatible with each other. This includes data regarding the development of these disorders, along with data relating to the phenomenon of unawareness and the treatments of these disorders, as will be demonstrated in the next two parts of this book.

In conclusion, PBT maintains Freud's clinical intuition that a sharp distinction between bizarre and non-bizarre behaviors is necessary for the understanding of human deviant behavior. PBT also adheres to his claim that bizarre behaviors should be explained by one set of theoretical concepts, as they share a similar etiology. However, in contrast to Freud, PBT is able to satisfactorily and empirically explain the causes and mechanisms behind these behaviors. Thus, it seems the victory trumpeted by advocates of medical models that "previous claims to have formulated general theories of the etiology of all mental disorders … have consistently proven unsatisfactory and degenerated into the ideological masked as scientific theories" (Wakefield, 1999, p. 969), has been premature.

Part II

Unawareness

Introduction

According to psychoanalysis, people possess an autonomous unconscious entity, which under certain circumstances may spontaneously induce radical change in their behavior which seriously disrupt their daily functioning (see Bonanno & Keuler, 1998; Gross, 1978). Freud proposed this idea in order to explain neurotic and psychotic patients' unawareness of the underlying causes of the dramatic shift in their behaviors and their inability to resume normal functioning (see review by Rofé, 2008). However, it is difficult to accept this proposal for the explanation of unawareness of mad behaviors for the following reasons:

First, the Freudian unconscious is incompatible with clinical evidence, reviewed in Part I, indicating the coexistence of awareness–unawareness. One example is the case studies of the Unabomber and Charles Cullen, who were unaware of their own underlying motives for murdering innocent people and yet carefully planned the murders and took appropriate precautions to successfully elude arrest for many years. Another example is of patients with conversion disorder, who can regulate the presentation of their symptoms in order to reduce potential harm (e.g., see Leary, 2003; Nicol, 1969), and even stop this behavior when the cost exceeds the benefit (see Blanchard & Hersen, 1976; Goldblatt & Munitz, 1976). Similarly, Mischel and Mischel (1958) noted with regard to spirit possession,

> even in the most extreme examples observed, the individual seemed to retain sufficient consciousness and control to permit him to behave without injury to self or others; that is without stumbling over objects or mishandling implements (p. 253).

Second, according to Freud's theory, the unconscious is an evil cognitive entity that has the potential to inflict serious behavioral disorders that harm the individual's well-being (see Rofé, 2008). This conception is incompatible with PBT's theoretical position, supported by many clinical examples reviewed in Part I, that schizophrenia, criminal insanity and neuroses, are goal-directed behaviors that actually improve the individual's quality of life.

Third, the unconscious is strongly linked with Freud's concept of repression in three respects, which are critical for the understanding of mad behaviors: (1) it preserves the repressed traumatic experiences for an indefinite period of time (Lynn, Knox, Fassler, Lilienfeld et al., 2004; McNally, 2003; Wachtel, 1977); (2) it determines the specific type of bizarre behavior that individuals develop in accordance with the specific repressed traumas (e.g., Fayek, 2005; Fenichel, 1946; Freud, 1915b; Wachtel, 1977); (3) a genuine recovery from mad behaviors necessitates lifting the repression, through which the patient is made aware of the repressed traumatic materials (e.g., see Bergmann, 1992; Blum, 2003; Eagle, 2000; Grünbaum, 2002; Kluft, 1995). However, as explained in Part I, numerous studies refute the soundness of these three basic aspects of repression and the existence of repression in general (see review by Rofé, 2008), findings which indirectly invalidate the Freudian unconscious as far as the development and treatment of madness are concerned.

In order to avoid these problems and yet preserve the main psychological function of the Freudian unconscious (i.e., explaining patients' unawareness of the underlying causes of their mad behaviors), PBT suggests that this effect is the consequence of two types of psychological process. One process results in the individual's unawareness of the stressor, which as stated in Part I is obtained through the repressive value of the symptom. The high distractive value of the symptom blocks the accessibility of stress-related thoughts. The second process, which constitutes the main topic of Part II, concerns the patient's unawareness of the mechanism that makes the decision to adopt a specific mad behavior and is responsible for its actual display. In this regard, PBT claims that this state of unawareness is a joint production of unconscious and conscious processes. The choice of a specific mad behavior is intuitive and is the result of unconscious processes. However, the decision to actually adopt this behavior and thereafter to redisplay or inhibit it is conscious. The consciousness is the only cognitive system which decides to accept or reject suggestions made by the unconscious, as well as to maintain, modify, or stop it. Patients become unaware of their conscious involvement in the display of this behavior through a variety of cognitive processes, to be specified shortly.

This new concept of unawareness has a number of advantages: (1) it is not susceptible to the earlier three problems that challenges the validity of the Freudian unconscious; (2) it helps resolve a number of fundamental theoretical disagreements regarding certain mad behaviors, as will be elaborated on in the discussion section of this part; (3) it enables PBT to understand how the mechanism of therapeutic change occurs and to integrate the various therapeutic interventions pertaining to mad behaviors under one theoretical umbrella, as will be elaborated on in Part III.

Part II starts by explaining the intuitive choice behind mad behavior. Subsequently, it discusses the manner by which patients become unaware of their conscious involvement in the display and maintenance of this behavior.

The Intuitive Choice of Madness

Decision-making processes can be based either on analytic or intuitive thinking. Analytic thinking occurs when an individual consciously examines various options and relevant information before reaching a decision. In contrast, intuitive choices are unconscious or with little conscious effort, automatic, rapid and impulsive (e.g., see Dane, Baer, Pratt, & Oldham, 2011; Evans, 2008; Glöckner & Witteman, 2010; Hogarth, 2010; Kahneman, 2003; Pretz, 2008; Sarmány-Schuller, 2010). An intuitive decision is "often experienced in the form of feelings (not words) … *we know, but we do not know why* [italics added]" (Hogarth, 2001, pp. 9–31). "A defining property of intuitive thoughts is that they come to mind spontaneously, like percepts" (Kahneman, 2003,

p. 699; see also Sinclair, Ashkanasy, & Chattopadhyay, 2010; Sadler-Smith, 2008). Intuitive decisions are often made during stressful situations "when an in-depth analysis is not possible and the decision-maker must move quickly to a plausible solution" (Sayegh, Anthony, & Perrewe, 2004, p. 183; see also Roghanizad & Neufeld, 2015). Such decisions are based on the individual's experiential resources stored in the long-term memory and usually are no less rational than conscious deliberate decisions (e.g., Glöckner & Witteman, 2010; Motl, Krieshok, & Multon, 2018; Sayegh et al., 2004). Sayegh et al. noted, "theories of rationality have come a long way since Descartes proclaiming the superiority of cognitions. We now acknowledge that the human mind and the nature of our existence are defined by more than our ability to reason … [rationality] is partly defined through our ability to experience emotions … especially under crisis conditions …" (p. 196). Similarly, the unconscious processes are no longer perceived as a "dumb entity" as in Freud's theory (Loftus & Klinger, 1992), but rather are "highly intelligent and adaptive" (Bargh & Morsella, 2008, p. 73; see also Bargh, 2014; Gigerenzer, 2007). Although analytical thinking may initially be more precise than intuitive thinking, this advantage disappears with the accumulation of experience (Sahm & von Weizsacker, 2016).

Abnormal reactions to intolerable levels of stress should be reevaluated according to this new outlook on the unconscious processes. When exposed to extreme levels of stress, a specific mad behavior would be intuitively experienced as the most effective method for relieving the individual's emotional tension. The specific reaction selected is unique to each individual and is based on his or her current or past experiences. Gut feelings that a particular behavior can effectively reduce emotional distress may motivate individuals to consciously implement it as a coping mechanism.

This claim is consistent with experimental studies from the field of economics, which indicate that people under stress tend to spontaneously choose a product that provides short-term gratification, despite negative long-terms consequences (Shiv & Fedorikhin, 1999,

2002). It also fits with Nash's response to the question of how he, a mathematician devoted to reason and logical proof, could believe that extraterrestrials were sending him messages. "The ideas I had about supernatural beings came to me the same way that my mathematical ideas did. So I took them seriously" (Nasar, 1998, p. 11). Nash's insinuation that madness may be an intuitive rational decision is also reflected in his autobiography, written after his recovery.

> At the present time, I seem to be thinking rationally again in the style that is characteristic of scientists. However, this is not entirely a matter of joy as if someone returned from physical disability to good physical health. One aspect of this is that rationality of thought imposes a limit on a person's concept of his relation to the cosmos. For example, a non-Zoroastrian could think of Zarathustra as simply a madman who led millions of naive followers to adopt a cult of ritual fire worship. But without his "madness" Zarathustra would necessarily have been only another of the millions or billions of human individuals who have lived and then been forgotten (Nash, 1994).

Nash implies that though his mad behaviors generally would, in terms of classic scientific thinking, be considered irrational or a reflection of illness, in fact they were completely rational and served important psychological goals. His brilliant insight that his mad behaviors were produced by the same mode of thinking with which he invented his game theory, coincides with the assertion of Nash's colleagues that "his approach to the solving of mathematics problems was highly intuitive" (Capps, 2011, p. 158). The unique commonality between these two supposed poles of rationality, namely madness and solving mathematical problems, is that solutions in both are obtained through intuitive thinking, which constitutes the core of the creative process (e.g., see review by Burnett & Francisco, 2013 and Dörfler & Ackermann, 2012).

Three Stages of Unawareness: Creation, Preservation, and Stabilization

As stated earlier, while the choice of a specific mad behavior is an intuitive/unconscious process, the decision to actually adopt this behavior and to redisplay, inhibit, or stop it altogether, is a conscious process. From this perspective, unawareness observed among these individuals is the consequence of two major psychological processes: (1) cognitive processes that cause forgetting of the knowledge of self-involvement (KSI) or their true reason (TR) for acting bizarrely; (2) self-deceptive processes that enable patients, following the forgetting of KSI/TR, to develop a self-deceptive belief that rationalizes the radical change in the individual's behavior.

The new concept of unawareness discussed in the following comprises three stages. The first stage — creation of unawareness — involves a state in which patients forget the KSI/TR. The second stage — preservation of unawareness — concerns a state in which patients develop self-deceptive beliefs that rationalize the presentation of these behaviors. The third stage — stabilization of unawareness — describes a deceptive cycle wherein the consciousness repeatedly displays the mad behavior and yet remains unaware of doing so.

I. *Creation of Unawareness: The Forgetting of KSI/TR*

This section describes the psychological processes by which patients become unaware of their KSI or their TR for acting bizarrely, immediately after the adoption of this behavior. This effect is achieved through a variety of cognitive processes that disrupt the encoding of KSI/TR in the long-term memory, along with a number of memory-inhibiting mechanisms that cause this information to be forgotten.

Encoding-Disrupting Factors

1. ***Brief exposure to KSI/TR*:** A critical variable that determines the likelihood of a patient forgetting their KSI/TR immediately after adopting the mad behavior is the duration of their exposure to this information. Evidence indicates that the duration of exposure to a stimulus is critical in determining the strength of the memory formed and the likelihood of subsequently forgetting this information (e.g., see DiNardo & Rainey, 1991; Memon, Hope, & Bull, 2003; Mensink & Raaijmakers, 1988). In individuals who adopt bizarre behaviors, their exposure to the KSI/TR is necessarily brief, as the decision to do so is made spontaneously with little conscious consideration.

One example of this process can be seen in the case of an unhappily married man whose wife became pregnant despite their agreement not to have children (Malamud, 1944). On the way to the hospital to visit his wife and the newly born child, the man was slightly injured in a car accident and spontaneously developed hysterical blindness. The man did not have an opportunity to contemplate his KSI/TR, as he spontaneously decided to develop the symptom.

A second example is the case previously mentioned by Brady and Lind (1961) of a 40-year-old man who suddenly developed hysterical blindness, in an attempt to cope with the unbearable demands of his wife and mother-in-law. Similarly, Masserman (1946) describes a 40-year-old woman who suffered through several years of severe depression during an unhappy marriage. The woman remained tolerant of her situation until the death of her favorite child, after which she suddenly developed a dissociative fugue. In another case (Abse, 1959), a man spontaneously developed total paralysis of his legs after his wife left him for another man. The husband had a strong impulse to pursue and kill his wife's lover, but the sudden paralysis prevented him from carrying out this impulse. In all of the earlier cases, patients' conscious exposure to the KSI/TR was inevitably brief as the decision to act bizarrely was spontaneous.

Another example is Leonard (1927), who experienced a sudden panic attack when he saw a freight train from afar and imagined the train was going to run him over. The reason this behavioral option was intuitively chosen were specified in Part I. What is relevant in this context is the fact that the unconscious choice and its implementation were spontaneous and without prior contemplation. Thus, as in the earlier examples, the encoding of the KSI/TR would have been weak as a result of the brief exposure to this information.

2. *Impaired cognitive functioning*: Many studies indicate that the adverse emotional states of anxiety and depression cause cognitive impairments, especially attention deficits (e.g., Erickson et al., 2005; Kemp et al., 2010; Mialet, Pope, & Yurgelun-Todd, 1996; Rief & Hermanutz, 1996). The cognitive system is thrown into a state of disarray, resulting in a decreased efficacy of information processing. Subjects' emotional distress interferes with memory encoding processes, resulting in poor learning and memory (e.g., Christopher & MacDonald, 2005; Krames & MacDonald, 1985; Mialet et al., 1996; O'Brien, Sahakian, & Checkley, 1993; Roberson-Nay et al., 2006; Rose & Ebmeier, 2006). The ruminating thoughts of depressed patients act as distracters, interfering with the performance of cognitive tasks by using up available short-term memory space and reducing cognitive efficiency (e.g., Abas, Sahakian, & Levy, 1990; Breslow, Kocsis, & Belkin, 1980; Krames & MacDonald, 1985; Mialet et al., 1996; O'Brien, Sahakian, & Checkley, 1993). Accordingly, given PBT's assumption that madness is adopted when individuals are faced with an intolerable level of stress, the encoding of KSI/TR is likely to be disrupted at the point when they consciously decide to implement the intuitively chosen symptom. The distraction is likely to be high, especially at the decision-making stage of symptom adoption, because a marked emotional arousal is experienced when an important decision has to be made (e.g., Baradell & Klein, 1993; Janis & Mann, 1977; Rau, 1996; Schaeffer, 1989).

3. *Symptom distractibility*: Research shows that memory encoding can also be disrupted by distractive factors that are irrelevant to the memory task (e.g., Tremblay, Nicholls, Parmentier, & Jones, 2005; Wolach & Pratt, 2001). In this regard, the behavioral change when adopting madness is so dramatic and unusual that it is likely to consume the patient's full attention. The individual's attention becomes so intensely focused on these extremely powerful and distractive stimuli that the encoding of rival stimuli, such as KSI/TR, is seriously disrupted. This suggestion is consistent with the theoretical position of Van Pelt (1975) who noted that neurotic symptoms cause "*super concentration of the mind*, [inducing] a state of what may be called *accidental hypnosis* … A patient suffering from psychoneurosis behaves in every way as though under the influence of a post-hypnotic suggestion …" (Van Pelt, 1975, pp. 28–29; see also Bliss, 1980, 1983, 1984; Frankel, 1974).

Furthermore, according to social cognitive theories of hypnosis, individuals become unaware of their intentional display of the hypnotic state by becoming fully absorbed in their goal-directed fantasies (see review by Lynn, Kirsch, & Hallquist, 2008). Therefore, considering PBT's claim that both neurotic and psychotic patients consciously implement their intuitive choice as a coping mechanism, it can be argued that as in hypnosis, mad patients become unaware of their KSI/TR by intentionally focusing on the actual display of the symptom. A clinical example demonstrating the overwhelming effect that symptoms may have on the individual's attention can be seen when DID patients alter their personalities. As noted by Bliss (1980), a dissociative identity disorder (DID) patient "creates personalities by blocking everything from her head, mentally relaxes, concentrates very hard …

clears her mind, blocks everything out and then wishes for the person, but she isn't aware of what she's doing" (p. 1392).

An additional example demonstrating the powerful distractive effect of neurotic symptoms can be seen in Leonard's (1927) autobiographical account of his initial panic attack. The encoding of KSI/TR was seriously disrupted, since as shown in the following, Leonard's attention was dominated by his panic-related symptoms, such as extreme catastrophic thoughts, loud shouting, and exaggerated motor behaviors.

> Then on the tracks from behind … comes a freight-train, blowing its whistle. Instantaneously diffused premonitions become acute panic. The cabin of that locomotive feels right over my head, as if about to engulf me … The train feels as if it were about to rush over me … I race back and forth on the embankment. I say to myself (and aloud): "it is half a mile across the lake — it can't touch you, it can't; it can't run you down … I rush back and forth on the bluffs: My God, won't that train go, my God, won't that train go away!" I smash a wooden box to pieces, board by board, against my knee to occupy myself against panic … (pp. 304–307)

It seems obvious that such extreme preoccupation with symptom-related thoughts, especially when accompanied by intensive activities, such as running back and forth, shouting aloud, and smashing wood, which demand a vast amount of attention, will disrupt the encoding of the KSI/TR from the short-term memory to the long-term memory.

4. *Directed forgetting*: Studies in which subjects are instructed to forget given information, demonstrate that people have the ability to forget information by deliberately disrupting its encoding process (e.g., Anderson, 2005; Golding, 2005; Gottlob, Golding, & Hauselt,

2006; Hourihan & Taylor, 2006). Thus, given patients' interest in being unaware of their conscious self-involvement, they can hinder the encoding of their KSI/TR by intentionally directing their attention away from this information.

Retrieved-Inhibiting Mechanisms

The encoding-disruptive factors significantly weaken the transformation of the KSI/TR into long-term memory, but may not be sufficient to cause the forgetting of this knowledge completely. A complete failure to recall this information becomes possible due to a number of mechanisms that inhibit its retrieval.

1. *State-dependent memory*: One of the major factors causing everyday forgetfulness has been termed in psychological literature as "state-dependent memory." Studies that have examined this issue report that any change between the original learned conditions and a memory test may hinder the ability to recall the information (e.g., Blaney, 1986; Emmerson, 1986; Houston, 1991, pp. 309–311; Jafari-Sabet & Jannat-Dastjerdi, 2009). For example, retrieval becomes difficult when the individual's cognitive or emotional condition is different from what it was when the information was acquired (e.g., Bower, 1981; Clark, Milberg, & Ross, 1983; Eich, 1995; Eich, Macaulay, & Ryan, 1994; Kunzendorf & Wigner, 1985; Pearce et al., 1990). This effect is also applicable to the change in patients' psychological state following the adoption of the mad behavior.

The distraction and controllability value of the chosen symptom should cause a radical reduction in the individual's emotional distress immediately after its initial display. This extreme emotional change facilitates the forgetting of the KSI/TR. As noted by Leonard, "upon the sudden relief … perhaps a hundred feet away, I forgot — and forgot for fourteen years — all the factors that were associated with the Locomotive" (p. 309; see also case studies no. 2 and 3 of amnesia following attacks of spirit possession, Grisaru & Witztum, 1995 and Ravenscroft, 1965, p. 172). An additional precipitating forgetfulness factor is the radical change in the patient's cognitive state: the individual becomes preoccupied with different thoughts and behaviors than he or she was prior the adoption of the bizarre behavior. In some cases, there may also be environmental changes, as is typical with dissociative fugue, in which patients abandon their previous identity (e.g., see case study by Masserman, 1946).

Thus, based on the aforementioned studies, the abrupt changes in the patients' emotional, cognitive, and environmental states should inhibit the retrieval of the anxiety provoking KSI/TR.

2. *Suppression*: Experimental studies show that people can intentionally inhibit retrieval of unwanted memories by reducing allocation of processing resources to this information (e.g., Anderson & Green, 2001; Anderson et al., 2004; Shane & Peterson, 2004). These findings are consistent with the psychoanalytic concept of suppression, defined as the conscious effort to forget undesirable material (e.g., A. Freud, 1936). Accordingly, it seems likely that patients can intentionally suppress the retrieval of KSI/TR by directing their attention away.

3. *Distraction*: Distraction affects the individual's cognitive processes, not only during the encoding stage, but also when retrieving the encoded information. This claim is demonstrated in studies that have examined the existence of repression in a laboratory setting. Initially, the bulk of research seemingly supported Freudian repression, as subjects forgot anxiety-provoking materials more than they forgot neutral stimuli. However, more controlled studies later revealed that contrary to Freud's theory, this difference was due to distraction rather than repression (e.g., see Holmes, 1974). Thus, since the awareness of KSI/TR would endanger the maintenance of the patients' pathological coping mechanism, it seems plausible that the patient will focus intensely on their dramatic change in behavior to block accessibility of this anxiety-provoking information.

4. *Hypnotic amnesia*: Research pertaining to hypnotic amnesia shows that this phenomenon is the consequence of active distractive maneuvers through which the subject deliberately ignores relevant target cues and attends exclusively to other matters (e.g., Bowers & Woody, 1996; Spanos, 1996; Spanos, Weekes, Menary, & Bertrand, 1986; Wagstaff & Frost, 1996). Hence, given the powerful distractive effects of mad behaviors, patients can induce an amnesic hypnotic-like state by actively focusing on their deviant behaviors, thereby blocking the retrieval of KSI/TR.

II. *The Preservation of Unawareness: The Self-Deception Belief*

The memory-inhibiting factors are effective only for the first episode of the mad behavior or as long as the mad symptoms are active. However, they are insufficient for maintaining the patient's state of unawareness immediately afterward. Once patients become aware of the radical change in their behavior, they may become preoccupied with questions posed by themselves or by others regarding the causes of their unusual behavioral change. This is consistent with Nisbett and Wilson's (1977) suggestion that people search for explanations when they are unaware of the etiology of their behavior (e.g., see case studies by Kraines, 1948, p. 183; Leonard, 1927, p. 308).

Self-probing is less likely among typical schizophrenic patients, who as elaborated on in Part I suffer from severe attention and cognitive deficits. These patients use a simple type of coping mechanism that disrupts their information processing system. Patients may talk to themselves and/or produce nonsensical verbalizations, thereby disrupting any rational thought processes, as demonstrated in the aforementioned case study of Jennifer Plowman (see Schwartz, 2000, pp. 370–411), during an intake interview.

> Men need sex. I have sex 10,000 times. That window is in the room because you want patients to know the color of the world. I know the president… I don't know why I am here. I'm fine (Schwartz, 2000, p. 373).

Self-probing is evident in more sophisticated patients whose information processing systems remain intact. These patients develop self-deceptive belief that can rationalize the radical behavioral change, and thus prevent any self-probing that would threaten the maintenance of their pathological coping mechanism. As described in the following, the self-deceptive belief is not arbitrary, rather, this belief is a plausible explanation, which is based on evidence patients observe during or immediately after their first episode of mad behavior. As specified in the following, this theoretical position can explain why some patients develop a self-deceptive belief that they suffer from illness, such as bulimic patients, while others with similar deviant behaviors, such as anorexics, develop a self-deceptive belief in accordance with which they deny that their behavior is abnormal.

Self-Deceptive Belief of Illness

After the creation of unawareness, most neurotic patients are faced with two types of evidence. One type is ***an extrospective observation*** of a deviant behavior (e.g., panic attacks), and the second is ***an introspective experience*** of loss of control (e.g., the inability to move a limb). As a result, patients ***diagnose*** themselves as physically or mentally ill, thus attributing the deviant behavior to forces beyond their control. This is consistent with evidence that lack of control is one of the strongest experiences felt amongst neurotic patients, such as those who choose to develop panic disorders (e.g. McNally et al., 1995). Assigning their problems to outside forces provides considerable emotional relief, an additional factor motivating patients to ascribe their symptoms to illness.

One example of this psychological process is illustrated in Leonard's (1927) autobiographical account soon after the experience of his panic attack. Initially, after observing a dramatic change in his behavior (extrospective evidence) and experiencing a loss of control (introspective evidence), he thought that he had been stricken with sunstroke (p. 308). However, he soon dismissed this idea. "I know from the symptoms it cannot be sunstroke. But I do know I am in a critical condition" (p. 308). At a later stage, he stated "I knew I was a 'case.' I knew my terrors were phobic" (p. 323). Although Leonard intuitively chose this diagnosis due to its distraction and controllability values, he paid lip service as part of his self-deceptive process by saying "I refused by iron thinking to consider the diagnosis of insanity" (p. 323). Moreover, when he was taken to his parent's home soon after the initial incident, he lay on the davenport, shaken with terror and said in a low voice, "father and mother, this looks like the end. I guess I am dying" (Leonard, 1927, p. 308). Apparently, he successfully tricked himself into this belief by focusing intensely on his extremely negative physiological sensations that often result from a high level of stress and by interpreting them in a catastrophic way, as suggested by the cognitive theory of panic disorder (e.g., see Barlow, 2004; Bouton et al., 2001; Clark, 1986).

Hence, after the creation of unawareness as a result of the aforementioned psychological processes, Leonard observed two types of evidence: a dramatic negative change in his behavior, which he intentionally intensified, and lack of control. These observations enabled Leonard to preserve his state of unawareness by deceiving himself that he was ill, without deciding whether he suffered from a mental or physical illness.

In another example, Kraines (1948) described the case a woman who was obsessed with thoughts of death of her boyfriend and immediate family. The patient was experiencing cognitive confusion because she could not specify the cause of her symptom. She stated, "these thoughts make me hysterical. I love them; why should I wish such terrible things to happen? It drives me wild, *makes me feel like I'm crazy* …" (p.183; see also Carson, Butcher, & Coleman, 1988, p. 192; italics added).

The deceptive self-diagnosis of illness is sufficient to preserve unawareness of self-involvement, enabling the symptoms to fulfill their repression and controllability functions. Nevertheless, most patients build an additional barrier to preserve the state of unawareness by producing **a self-deceptive *explanation concerning the etiology of their "illness."*** Subjects formulate a plausible and socially acceptable explanation for their symptoms, to the extent that their cultural background or experiences enable them to do so. This is consistent with Nisbett and Wilson's (1977) theoretical position that when people are unaware of the underlying causes of their behavior, they employ implicit cultural theories to account for their responses. For example, Leonard utilized his broad knowledge of psychoanalysis to develop a self-deceptive explanation regarding the nature of his illness:

> I was my own physician … I knew I was a "case." I knew my terrors were phobic … I even knew they were somehow infantile in ultimate causes. A matter of infantile regression. The source of that conviction is psychologically noteworthy … I was … already familiar with abnormal psychology-even as I have since read, first and last … the chief men in the field, their books and technical journals in half a dozen languages … even to eight German volumes of Freud (pp. 323–324).

Leonard developed a ***self-deceptive explanation*** that his panic attack was "a matter of infantile regression." In fact, Leonard was no different than patients in less-developed countries, who employ concepts from their culture, such as spiritual possession, to deceive themselves into preserving a state of unawareness when adopting bizarre behavioral deviations (e.g., see Csordas, 1987; Grisaru & Witztum, 1995; Kua, Sim, & Chee, 1986; Ravenscroft, 1965; Seltzer, 1983; Varma, Bouri, & Wig, 1981; Wijesinghe, Dissanayake, & Mendis, 1976).

Due to the increasing popularity of medical models (e.g., Reich, 1982; Telch, 1988), patients from Western cultures may frequently attribute their symptoms to medical causes. For example, in a case study of obsessive neurosis reported by McAndrew (1989), a woman experiencing aggressive thoughts toward her children, acknowledged her behavior as bizarre (i.e., self-deceptive belief of illness), by noting that she had "terrible thoughts," being unable "to force them out of her head," "and feelings that she was "going crazy" (p. 312). Although the patient managed to preserve her state of unawareness by her self-diagnosis of illness, she built an additional barrier of a self-deceptive explanation by suggesting that her symptoms might have been "premenstrual syndrome" (p. 316). She arrived at this conclusion after seeing a television program about a woman with premenstrual syndrome who had stabbed her children. In another case, O'Kearney (1993) described a 24-year-old woman, in her final year of medical school, who suffered from obsessive ruminations of extreme aggression. The patient reported that she had suffered intrusive thoughts at a younger age as well, and linked the latest onset of ruminations to minor illnesses such as "a short duration gastric upset" (p. 358).

Patients may also selectively focus on suitable information to strengthen their self-deceptive explanation. As noted by Peterson and Djikic (2003), "we are always pursuing the limited goals we construe as valuable, from our particular idiosyncratic perspectives. We pay attention to, and remember, those events we construe as relevant, with regards to those goals. We do not and cannot strive for comprehensive, 'objective' coverage" (p. 88). Accordingly, "the hysteric misinterprets evidence and selectively attends to only a certain part of the overall evidence" (Bass, 2001, p. 139). For example, conversion disorder patients utilize the presence of organic illnesses and physical injuries prior to their disorder (e.g., Blanchard & Hersen, 1976; Jones, 1980; Merskey & Buhrich, 1975) to strengthen the belief that their symptoms are caused by biological factors (see also Stone & Sharpe, 2006). As noted by Weinstein, Eck, and Lyerly (1969), these patients "stressed their injuries in the belief that they were etiologically significant" (p. 337; see also case studies by Brown, Poliakoff, & Kirkman, 2007; de Vignemont, 2009).

Likewise, panic patients are likely to utilize adverse physiological sensations resulting from their stressful situations (e.g., see Barlow, 2004; Bouton et al., 2001; Clark, 1986; Klein, 1993) and their available physiological deficits (e.g., respiratory deficits; see the principle of availability in Part I) in deceiving themselves that they suffer from heart disease, and thus to account for their seemingly uncontrollable panic attacks (e.g., Clark, 1986, 1988; Eifert, 1992; Ley, 1989; Margraf & Ehlers, 1991; McNally, Hornig, & Donnell, 1995; Pauli, Marquardt, Hartl, Nutzinger, & Strian, 1991). Similarly, given that hyperventilation symptoms are voluntary (Ley, 1989), subjects can deliberately intensify their adverse physiological sensations experienced as a result of stress (Wolpe & Rowan, 1988) in order to facilitate both the display of panic and the development of the self-deceptive explanation of organic etiology (e.g., see a case study by Spitzer, Skodol, Gibbon, & Williams, 1983, pp. 7–10). Panic patients may even be more knowledgeable about the symptoms related to myocardial infarction than those who actually suffer from the disease (Margraf & Ehlers, 1991). This allows them to mimic the disease, develop a suitable self-deceptive explanation for it, and validate it by concentrating on and reinforcing adverse physiological sensations.

An additional source of information that strengthens patient's self-deceptive explanation is **therapy**. Patients' participation in therapy and the selection of a specific intervention may be partly motivated by the need to develop a convincing self-deceptive explanation (e.g., see Csordas, 1987). Pattison and Wintrob (1981) noted in reference to spiritual possession, that the "concordance of belief systems of subject and healer concerning the causes and appropriate treatment of illness is usually the primary determinant of choice of healer" (p. 17). To these ends, a therapist may endorse the patient's deceptive self-diagnosis of illness, and provide a wealth of "scientific" information that can facilitate the development of a self-deceptive explanation.

Furthermore, as noted by Marmor (1962), patients have a general readiness to accept the therapist's suggestions as a "scientific" explanation of their symptoms. Patients treated by analysts of all these schools may not only respond favorably, but also believe strongly in the insights they have been given. Admittedly, even "inexact" interpretations have been noted to be of therapeutic value! Moreover, depending upon the point of view of the analyst, the patients of each school seem to bring up precisely the kind of phenomenological data that confirm the theories and interpretations of their analysts (p. 289; see also Heine, 1953). As noted by Fisher and Greenberg (1977), empirical evidence consistently shows that

> A patient's belief interpretations and his consequent anxiety reduction do not depend on the accuracy of the interpretations. Investigators have found that individuals will enthusiastically accept bogus interpretations as accurate descriptions of their own personalities (p. 364; see also Grünbaum, 1984, p. 135, 211, 265; Marmor, 1962, p. 289).

In this context, it is worth mentioning clinical data indicating that DID may be produced in the therapist's office, where therapists "implicitly encourage" (Spanos, Weekes, & Bertrand, 1985, p. 364) patients to develop this disorder (see also Jaroff, 1993; Read & Lindsay, 1994; Rieber, 1999). In such cases, patients also internalize the psychoanalytic beliefs that their symptoms are the result of repressed childhood abuse, and may even confabulate abusive memories (e.g., Acocella, 1999; Giesbrecht, Lynn, Lilienfeld, & Merckelbach,

2008, 2010; Lilienfeld et al., 1999; Merckelbach, Horselenberg, & Schmidt, 2002; Read & Lindsay, 1994; Spanos, 1994, 1996). Consequently, when DID patients decide to adopt the therapists' suggestion as a coping mechanism, they are likely to focus on the implicit belief that the other personality is the result of a "repressed" childhood trauma, thereby hindering further self-probing regarding the true causes of their symptoms.

Patients' tendency to adopt their therapist's belief system has been attributed to the analysts' ability to "induce, alter, and control their client's self-insights" (Bandura, 1969, p. 94). As Gross (1978) has indicated, even when the therapist's suggestions seem to the patient to be unsound and without merit, "the analyst keeps coming back with so much triangulation of the idea that the patient finally accepts the interpretation, even if it is potentially false. It is a form of brainwashing" (p. 208).

This is consistent with a growing number of studies indicating that false memories can be implanted in the individual's cognitive system through the therapist's suggestive effort, to the extent that patients may come to believe the authenticity of these "memories" (e.g., Ceci & Loftus, 1994; Gutheil, 1993; Lindsay & Read, 1994; Loftus, 1993; Loftus & Hoffman, 1989; Mantell, 1988; Zaragoza & Lane, 1994). *However, while therapists may play a vital role in motivating patients to confirm their theoretical views, it seems that their persuasive capabilities have been overemphasized, failing to take into account patients' interest and readiness to be deceived.*

Given PBT's assumption that self-deceptive belief satisfies an important psychological need, one would expect patients to refuse to change or abandon a therapy that strengths their beliefs, even if they realize that the intervention has been ineffective. Indeed, hypochondriacs are reluctant to accept referrals to psychiatric services and continue to request to be treated by physicians, even after medical intervention proves ineffective for their problems (see Salkovskis & Warwick, 1986; Warwick & Salkovskis, 1990;

see also case study by Davison & Neale, 1986, pp. 148–150). Similarly, patients may spend years in psychoanalytic therapy, despite the lack of therapeutic success (see Erwin, 1980; Gross, 1978) mainly because it enables them to deceive themselves that they have no control on their "illness". As noted by Leonard (1927), who spent several years in psychoanalytic therapy without satisfactory results, despite "a thousand circumstances that would have robbed many men of faith … I have even now not lost all faith in the method, nor all faith that it may yet work out in this case. But the *fact* is that it has not" (p. 414; italics added).

Self-Deceptive Belief of Denial

The fact that some patients deny their behavior is deviant is seemingly incompatible with PBT's claim that self-deceptive belief is a logical inference derived from external observation and subjective experience with which patients are confronted immediately after the creation of unawareness. It is also unclear why this seemingly illogical belief is characteristic of certain types of psychological disorders, such as **anorexics** (e.g., see Melamed, Mester, Margolin, & Kalian, 2003; Vandereycken, 2006a, 2006b), **some OCD patients** (e.g., compulsive cleaners, see Foa, 1979; Kozak & Foa, 1994; Rachman & Hodgson, 1980), **criminal insanity** (e.g., the Unabomber and Charles Cullen) and **schizophrenia** (e.g., Cella, Dymond, Cooper, & Turnbull, 2012; Gerretsen et al., 2013; Langdon & Ward, 2009; Lysaker, Buck, Salvatore et al., 2009; Voss et al., 2010).

Traditional theories of psychopathology regard the "deniers" as suffering from greater severity of illness than the "admitters" (e.g., Amador & Paul-Odouard, 2000; Kozak & Foa, 1994; Melamed et al., 2003; Vandereycken, 2006a, 2006b). Medical models also claim that denial damages the prospect of recovery by hindering the adherence to medications or psychotherapy (e.g., Lien, Chang, Kao et al., 2018; Siebert, 2000).

However, as was elaborated on in Part I, in schizophrenia denial is a rational coping mechanism that enhances patients' self-esteem, and reduces their intolerable level of stress. This may explain the fact that nullifying denial among schizophrenic patients leads to poorer well-being, depression, low self-esteem, hopelessness, and suicidal behavior (e.g., Acosta, et al., 2013; Balhara & Verma, 2012; Crumlish et al., 2005; Ekinci, et al., 2012; Lysaker et al., 2007; Melle & Barrett, 2012; Murri et al., 2016; Kao & Liu, 2011). Furthermore, as noted by Pryor, Johnson, Wiedrman, and Boswell (1995) with respect to anorexia nervosa, "denial does not appear to be a reliable sign of poor prognosis, nor do deniers differ systematically from admitters with regard to the onset or general presentation of their illness" (p. 301). Kozak and Foa (1994) arrive at a similar conclusion with respect to OCD. This evidence challenges the validity of traditional explanations of denial.

Moreover, as specified below, the self-deceptive belief of denial is not less rational than the self-deceptive belief of illness. Both types of beliefs are logical inferences that are based on evidence to which patients are exposed immediately after the creation of unawareness. They develop different beliefs because they are confronted with different piece of extrospective and introspective evidence. This theoretical position is demonstrated with regard to anorexia nervosa, OCD, criminal insanity and schizophrenia.

1. ***Anorexia nervosa*:** Unlike the illness group, anorexic patients **observe *a socially acceptable behavioral change*** of dieting immediately after creation of unawareness. Often, the symptom is an integral part of the individual's behavioral repertoire for which he or she was praised before its exaggeration to bizarre levels. **Social reinforcements** that are normally given for these behaviors are likely at least during the initial stage of this disorder. For example, Branch and Eurman (1980) found that in the beginning family and friends admire those who suffer from anorexia for their appearance and self-control (see also

Porzelius, Berel, & Howard, 1999). Since patients are unaware of the underlying causes of their behavioral change, they are likely to interpret this ***extrospective evidence*** in positive terms. Such an interpretation is especially likely because patients simultaneously experience ***introspective evidence of emotional relief*** resulting from the repression and controllability effects of the symptom. As noted by one anorexic patient "I enjoy having this disease and I want it" (Bruch, 1978, p. 2).

Similarly, a father of an anorexic patient noted, "when she is not eating and her weight is falling, she appears in good spirits" (Bruch, 1973, p. 90). This denial is also strengthened by the ***internal experience of a sense of control***. Having control over their weight and body size provides anorexics with a considerable sense of achievement and gives them a life goal, which replaces their emptiness and helplessness (Bruch, 1978). *Weight loss constitutes a source of self-worth and helps combat feelings of inadequacy* (Garner, Vitousek, & Pike, 1997; Vitousek & Hollon, 1990). Edelstein (1989) similarly noted that anorexia satisfies patients' compulsive need to master their vital drive of hunger (see also Huebner, 1993).

Since denial of illness is a rational conclusion that fits the extrospective and introspective evidence to which anorexic patients are subjected, they must invent self-deceptive explanations to justify their abrupt behavioral change. Accordingly, as noted by Garner (1986), "the apparently bizarre eating patterns and the resolute refusal of adequate nourishment become plausible given the anorexic patient's conviction that thinness is essential for her happiness or well-being" (p. 302). Anorexics must also overestimate their body size or fatness (Benninghoven, Raykowski, Solzbacher, Kunzendorf, & Jantschek, 2007; Skrzypek, Wehmeier, & Remschmidt, 2001; Waldman, Loomes, Mountford, & Tchanturia, 2013) to preserve "a non-pathological image of their body by negating their severe underweight" (Benninghoven et al., 2007, p. 56).

However, anorexics abandon the denial strategy in favor of a self-deceptive belief of illness when their bodily conditions seriously deteriorate. Indeed, as reported by Greenfeld, Anyan, Hobart, Quinlan, and Plantes (1991), the tendency to adopt a belief of illness is greater among patients with the greatest weight loss, and longest in-patient stays. Moreover, when anorexic behavior is accompanied by bulimic symptoms, patients are more likely to choose the strategy of illness, rather than denial (see Pryor et al., 1995), possibly because binge eating is socially unacceptable and is associated with the sense of loss of control (*DSM-IV-TR*, American Psychiatric Association, 2000). This theoretical perspective, which views anorexics' denial of illness as a rational behavior with intact cognitive functioning, is consistent with research showing that these patients display no impairments when perceiving other women's bodies (Benninghoven et al., 2007). As noted by Skrzypek et al. (2001) in a review article on anorexics' body image, "the findings suggest that body image disturbance is not due to any perceptual deficit, but is based on cognitive-evaluative dissatisfaction" (p. 215; see also Waldman et al., 2013).

2. ***OCD***: OCD patients, like those suffering from anorexia, are often faced with **extrospective** (e.g., excessive cleaning or praying) and **introspective evidence** (emotional relief resulting from both the socially accepted behaviors and the repression and controllability effects of the symptom) that enable a rational individual to deny that he or she suffers from illness. Sherman (1938) described a 14-year-old boy who developed compulsive washing, using the coping mechanism of undoing to counteract the guilt he felt for masturbation. He washed his hands several times a day and frequently stayed 2 or 3 hours in the bathtub. On a number of occasions, he dabbed iodine on his hands and face, telling his parents that he had scratched himself and wanted to prevent infection. The patient also used a boric acid solution to wash his eyes every evening. When asked to

explain his excessive cleanness "he stated that he realized that he washed more than other boys, but that in his case there were real reasons." *Thus, the patient observed the socially accepted behavior of washing, as well as the reduction of guilt feelings, which the act of cleaning symbolically brought about.* Consequently, since the patient was unaware of the underlying cause of his behavior, he must have denied that he suffered from illness. Moreover, as a rational person, in an attempt to explain the radical change in his behavior, the patient "believed that his skin was of such a texture that it retained dirt and germs, and he therefore was forced to wash and scrub himself" (p. 226. See also a case study by Rachman & Hodgson, 1980, p. 19).

Like with obsessive cleaning, those who exhibit excessive prayer rationalize their bizarre behavior as a preemptive measure against potential danger (e.g., accidents or terror activities; see, Rofé, 2010) or view it as part of a religious ceremony (Rachman & Hodgson, 1980, p.19). **An additional introspective experience** that leads OCD patients to develop a self-deceptive belief is controllability, as the denial strategy reduces their fear of losing control over their unacceptable impulses (e.g., Denys, De Geus, Van Megen, & Westenberg, 2004; Horowitz, 2004, pp. 169–186; McAndrew, 1989). For example, in the previously mentioned case study by Neale, Oltmanns, and Davison (1982), Karen chose her OCD symptoms mainly because she feared she would lose control over her unacceptable, aggressive impulses toward her children. "Instead of injuring the children, she spent a good deal of time every day performing irrational responses aimed at protecting them" (p. 12). Similar to the earlier cases, Karen used self-deceptive explanation to rationalize her seemingly senseless compulsive counting rituals. "She agreed that her rituals did not afford them direct protection but felt that the rituals were helpful in the same way prayers are. She concluded that her rituals were irrational only to the extent that prayers are irrational" (Rachman & Hodgson, 1980, p. 19).

3. ***Insane criminal behaviors***: Similar to anorexic and OCD patients, criminally insane individuals base their denial of illness on two pieces of evidence: ***Extrospective observation*** of their radical behavioral change which they subjectively interpret as socially acceptable, and ***introspective experience*** of emotional relief resulting from the repression and controllability values of the behavioral change. For example, as elaborated on in Part I, the ***Unabomber*** (Graysmith, 1996) perceived his criminal acts as a social mission (extrospective observation), due to the delusional belief he employed to rationalize his antisocial behavior. He also derived significant emotional relief from his criminal acts (introspective observation) which, as discussed in Part I, resulted from the repressive functions of his criminal behavior and the enhancement of his self-esteem. Furthermore, like anorexics and compulsive cleaners who are initially rewarded for their deviant behaviors, the Unabomber enjoyed his celebrity status and thrived on the attention he received in the media, which is typical amongst serial killers (Haggerty, 2009). Thus, the Unabomber was aware that he consciously committed the murders, but was unaware of his underlying motives due to the aforementioned factors, that according to PBT, are involved in the creation of unawareness of the KSI/TR. These include the encoding-disruptive factors and the retrieval-inhibiting mechanisms, specified earlier.

   Similarly, when ***Charles Cullen*** (Graeber, 2013) committed his first murder, he focused on the belief that he was helping people by ending their suffering. It is also likely that the initial patients he killed were terminally ill, leading him to extrospectively ***observe*** his actions as benevolent and compassionate. This evidence, together with his ***introspective observation*** of emotional relief resulted by the repressive and controllability values of his criminal act, caused him to deny that his actions were iniquitous. However, like anorexics who transform their self-denial into a self-deceptive belief of illness when faced with incompatible evidence, Cullen abandoned the denial strategy when confronted, in the "60 Minutes" interview, with the fact that he had killed patients who were not terminally ill. He noted that he felt overwhelmed at the time and said "it felt like I needed to do something and I did. And that's not an answer to anything." In other words, he used a self-deceptive belief of illness, namely that his murders were out of his control, thus maintaining his unawareness of the underlying cause of his behavior.

The same analysis can be applied to account for the aforementioned case of ***Mordechai Vanunu***, the Israeli nuclear spy (Toscano, 1990). Vanunu is an interesting case because his self-deceptive belief of denial was based not only on his own extrospective and introspective observations but also on the misleading positive feedback he derived from the sympathy of notable people, including Nobel Laureates and the American astronomer, Carl Sagan (Toscano, 1990, p. 291). To some extent, the support Vanunu received from these notable people is similar to the therapist's affirmation of patients' self-deceptive belief of illness discussed previously. In both cases, the deceptive information by respected agents is used to strengthen the individual's self-deceptive explanation of his or her deviant-bizarre behavior.

4. ***Schizophrenia***: Most schizophrenics base their denial of illness on **two introspective observations**. The first is the delusional or imaginary visions or voices (i.e., hallucinations), which are perceived as a real phenomenon following the creation of unawareness. The second experience is the significant emotional relief attained by the repression and controllability effects of these bizarre behaviors. As a result of these experiences, patients rationally develop a self-deceptive belief of denial. For example, Percy King, who suffered from paranoid schizophrenia, believed pursuers with some "astounding, unheard of, utterly unbelievable occult powers" controlled him (White, 1964). As discussed earlier, King's delusions and hallucinations can be seen as a rational coping mechanism which dominated his attention through intuitive processes in response to guilty feelings over

his sexual impulses and his deep sense of incompetence. While he initially may have been momentarily aware that these experiences were illusory, they were perceived as real phenomena immediately after the creation of unawareness of KSI/TR. Once King became unaware of the KSI/TR, he utilized his experiences, such as sexual sensations and hospitalizations, as "proof" to further validate his self-deceptive belief of denial. Freeman, Garety, Kuipers, Fowler, and Bebbingtom (2002) noted with regard to schizophrenia that the confirmatory evidence of beliefs can be obtained in a number of ways

> individuals will look for evidence consistent with their belief …; attentional biases will come on-line, as is found in emotional disorders: threat will be preferentially processed …; threatening interpretations of ambiguous events will be made; and such biases are likely to be enhanced by a self-focused cognitive style … Memory biases, which may be associated with emotional disorders (e.g. intrusive trauma memories), will lead to frequent presentations in mind of the individual of the evidence for delusion (p. 338).

III. *Stabilization of Unawareness*

The creation of unawareness — namely forgetting the KSI/TR — and the preservation of this cognitive state, obtained through self-deceptive belief, relate only to the initial presentation of symptoms. However, this behavior is often manifested not just once but many times, such as with the serial killings of the Unabomber and Cullen or with the recurrence of panic attack in panic disorder patients (see Seligman, 1988). Since the consciousness is the sole cognitive system responsible for the reactivation of the bizarre behaviors, as assumed by PBT, it is necessary to clarify **(a)** which situations cause patients to consciously reactivate their symptoms?

and **(b)** how patients succeed in remaining unaware of KSI/TR, despite repeated displays of this behavior.

Symptom Reactivation Situations

Stress

One situation that causes patients to reactivate their symptom is exposure to stress. This reaction enhances their ability to repress stress-related thoughts and allows them to exercise control over the stressor. For example, Blanchard and Hersen (1976) described a case of a 14-year-old girl who developed aphonic hysteria following a quarrel with her mother from which she spontaneously recovered in several weeks. However, any subsequent arguments with one of her sisters or severe scolding by her mother reduced her voice to a whisper. A full relapse occurred when the mother sharply questioned the patient about her sexual relationships with her cousin. In another case, the reactivation of the subject's conversion symptom coincided with a variety of environmental stressors. "Among these were his role as 'housewife,' difficulties with his 18-year-old son, being discharged from the National Guard after 20 years of service, and his strong opposition to his youngest daughter's marital plans" (Blanchard & Hersen, 1976, p. 124). Similarly, Benzick (2001) mentions a case of a 17-year-old female who suffered from pseudo-seizures, and whose symptom worsened in the presence of the stressor (her father). In another case study of hysterical seizures, the patient displayed her symptom usually when being beaten by her husband (Nandi, Banerjee, Bera, Nandi, & Nandi, 1985).

Wijesinghe et al. (1976) described a 35-year-old woman who developed spiritual possession, which meets PBT's criteria of bizarre behavior. The first episode occurred at the age of 23, when her husband's drinking became a serious problem. The symptom was displayed when the drunken husband assaulted the patient and her children.

> These attacks recurred during the next 10 years — first being precipitated by quarrels with the husband, and later also by culture-bound stimuli. The husband's drinking has become less of a problem to the family in the past 3 years as he has had to reside at the worksite and can only visit the family during weekends. Apparently in consequence of this, her attacks have become less frequent and in the past two years she has had none — although she believes she is still susceptible to possession (p. 137) .

Mathews, Gelder, and Johnston (1981) noted, with respect to agoraphobia, that, "it has often been suggested that both onset and fluctuations are related to changes in interpersonal relationships or to environmental stress" (p. 39). Similarly, as claimed by Marks (1987a)

> agoraphobia that has been stable for some time can be exacerbated suddenly by as many factors as those which might have precipitated the original episode. Remission, too, may coincide with similar sudden life events ... Any stressful situation might intensify agoraphobia. Depression often aggravates agoraphobia to the point of major disability; after the depression clears the handicap reverts to its previous lower level (p. 338).

In the same manner, clinical data suggests that the intensity of obsessive rumination tends to fluctuate in accordance with the patient's level of depression (e.g., see case study by Rachman & Hodgson, 1980, p. 257).

Another example concerns DID. As noted by Bliss (1984), "the 'spontaneous' transformation of the alert patient into another personality usually occurs when the patient encounters a stress with which he or she cannot cope" (p. 137; see case study by Spitzer et al., 1983, pp. 37–41). Similarly, La Via and Brewerton (1996), noted, "switching often occurs in response to environmental stress and/or internal psychological triggers, usually evoking traumatic memories" (p. 232).

No evidence is available with regard to psychotic disorders but it seems likely that the same rules also apply to these cases. Thus, Percy King, who suffered from delusional disorder and associated his unacceptable impulses with an invisible group of pursuers, probably reactivated his delusions whenever he experienced feelings of guilt due to homosexual fantasies or masturbation. Other stimuli that could have motivated these behaviors were stress-related thoughts, especially those that intensified his low self-esteem. Similarly, it seems probable that the repeated criminal acts of the Unabomber and other serial killers, such as Cullen, coincided with stress-related thoughts that intensified their level of depression.

Likewise, as specified in Part I, Nash's schizophrenic symptoms were largely associated with his constant attempts to block the accessibility of stress-related thoughts. Additionally, the fact that the removal of stress or increasing patients' coping skills resulted in complete recovery (e.g., Bradshaw, 1998; Karon, 2008), indicates that the maintenance of schizophrenic symptoms is due to the patient's intolerable level of emotional distress.

Belief-Challenging Conditions

The second situation that causes the reactivation of symptoms is formation of belief-challenging conditions. Given PBT's assumption that the self-deceptive belief is necessary for preserving unawareness of KSI/TR, it is expected that challenging this belief will cause reactivation of the symptom. Failure to do so may invalidate the belief, and therefore threaten the patient's ability to maintain the symptom. In an experimental study by Levy and Jankovic (1983), a hysterical patient displayed a variety of dramatic pseudo-neurological symptoms when given a placebo she believed was the substance that intensified her symptoms. The patient was obliged to consciously display her symptom because failing to do so would sabotage her self-deceptive belief and, consequently, the maintenance of her pathological coping mechanism.

In another experimental study (Grosz & Zimmerman, 1965; Zimmerman & Grosz, 1966), a patient suffering from hysterical blindness scored below the chance level, when asked to indicate the presence or absence of visual stimuli. The experimenter manipulated the patient's behavior through a collaborator by telling him that the doctor thought he could see and that a truly blind person would identify a higher number of correct responses. As one would expect, in the subsequent visual test, the subject's correct responses increased to chance level. Here too, when thc self-deceptive belief was threatened, the patient adjusted his symptomatic behavior accordingly.

This theoretical position can be applied to specific bizarre phobias, as well as to panic disorder and agoraphobia. Thus, when individuals with bizarre phobia are confronted with their object of fear, such as chocolate (Rachman & Seligman, 1976) and trains (Leonard, 1927) or when a compulsive hand washer touches a contaminated object, such as dirt (Rachman & Hodgson, 1980, p. 173), they must display fear, or invent a self-deceptive excuse for not doing so. Failing to do so will invalidate the belief and necessitate the abandonment of the symptom. This is illustrated by Leonard who, in order to visit his fiancé, had to board a train, to which he previously reacted with panic. "She wants me... 'I must think of her'... I walked to the station — precisely as one walks to the electric chair ... The slogan that sang in my ears was only: 'You are going to your death'..." (Leonard, 1927, p. 347).

Patients may intentionally expose themselves to situations that challenge their belief in order to obtain "proofs" for strengthening their self-deceptive belief. For example, the morning following his initial panic attack, when he came to the deceptive diagnosis that he was in critical condition and about to die, Leonard noted that:

> In the morning, though feeling strangely weak in body, I start out on a little walk down the street. Within a hundred

> feet of the house I am compelled to rush back, in horror of being so far away... a hundred feet away... from home and security. I have never walked or ridden, alone or with others, as a normal man since that day (p. 308).

Likwise, patients may make a seemingly genuine attempt to face their fear and then use to use the "failures" to revalidate their beliefs. In one such example, a patient noted that:

> Times more than I can recall I have gone into restaurants or dining rooms, ordered a meal and left it untouched, impelled by my desire to escape the crowd ... (or) have bought tickets to theaters, concerts, fairs or what not, merely to give them away when the critical moment arrived… (Marks, 1987a, p. 326).

Similarly, since panic disorder patients deceive themselves into believing they suffer from heart or pulmonary disease (Clark, 1986; Margraf & Ehlers, 1991; McNally et al., 1995), they must display panic attack when they experience increased bodily sensations through a variety of chemical substances (e.g., adrenaline, sodium lactate, and caffeine) or by employment of procedures that affect respiration (e.g., strenuous exercise, experimental hyperventilation, and CO_2 inhalation; see Abrams, Schruers, Cosci, & Sawtell, 2008; Barlow, 2004; Nutt & Lawson, 1992; Rapee, 1995). Failure to display panic may sabotage their deceptive belief of physical illness. A threat to the deceptive belief, and thus the igniting of panic attacks, can also occur with decrease in heart or respiratory rate, due to relaxation procedures (e.g., Barlow, 1988, pp. 148–151).

The idea that the provocation of panic attacks in panic disorder and agoraphobia, or the recrudescence of compulsive rituals in OCD, may be due to belief-challenging conditions is incompatible with the traditional explanation, which attributes these effects to conditioning or irrational thinking (e.g., Bouton et al., 2001; Clark, 1986; Emmelkamp, 1982, 1987). However, as will be specified in the discussion of this part of the book (see also a review by Rofé & Rofé, 2015), these theories suffer from serious problems that challenge their validity. Moreover, as will be demonstrated later, PBT is the only theory which can resolve these difficulties and integrate the relevant data pertaining to these disorders into its theoretical framework.

Demand Characteristics

The third condition that may cause patients to redisplay their symptoms is that of demand characteristics, which refer to expectations of how a patient with a specific disorder is expected to behave. Accordingly, patients suffering from psychogenic movement must routinely display their symptom at a certain frequency and activate it soon after waking from sleep. Failure to do so would challenge their self-deceptive belief of illness, and may result in others either thinking they are faking their symptoms or that their "illness" is not serious. The same claim is true for individuals displaying hysterical paralysis or blindness. They must consistently behave like people suffering from true paralysis or blindness.

Demand characteristics may also explain experimental studies on impression-management among schizophrenic patients. Findings show that schizophrenic patients can effectively present themselves as "sick" or "healthy" to suit their needs. For example, when patients' open ward status was questioned, they convincingly presented themselves in an interview as "healthy" and eligible for open ward living. When their residency status was questioned, they convincingly presented themselves as "sick" and ineligible for discharge (Braginsky & Braginsky, 1967, 1971; Braginsky, Braginsky, & Ring, 1969; Braginsky, Grosse, & Ring, 1966).

The Need for Self-Deceptive Proofs

The fourth condition that may precipitate the display of bizarre behavior is the need for self-deceptive proofs. In this regard, a sharp distinction must be made between schizophrenics with disorganized speech and delusional patients. Those with disorganized speech renounce their rationality, which has little importance for their existence by deliberately disrupting their thinking processes, thus preventing the self-production of threatening thoughts and blocking the accessibility of such stimuli. In contrast, the delusional patients who are unwilling to pay this heavy cost of renouncing rationality, as they are endowed with better cognitive abilities, choose to cope with their problems by developing seemingly senseless beliefs that serve their needs of repression and controllability. The cognitive dissonance that this choice produces motivates patients to reactivate their "senseless" beliefs (i.e., delusions) whenever they are confronted with a situation that can provide "proof" consistent with their belief, and thus resolve their cognitive dissonance.

This theoretical position can shed light on bulk of studies termed in the literature as "jumping to conclusions" (JTC; see Dudley, Taylor, Wickham, & Hutton, 2016; Falcone et al., 2015). This phenomenon refers to situations where delusional schizophrenics hastily arrive at false conclusions on the basis of little evidence. For example, when Nash suspected that Cohen, a PhD student, was rifling through his trash, he jumped to the conclusion that Cohen was trying to steal his mathematical ideas (Nasar, 1998, p. 243).

The conventional explanation of JTC is that this phenomenon is the consequence of impaired functioning of the cognitive system, such as dysfunctional informational processing, typically referred as "cognitive biases" (e.g., see review by Gaweda, Staszkiewich, & Balzan, 2017). However, researchers who have examined JTC, have arrived at the conclusion that delusional people have a bias toward gathering data rather than a difficulty in reasoning (e.g., Dudley et al., 1997; Dudley & Over, 2003). Accordingly, JTC can be viewed as a rational cognitive strategy where patients take advantage of situations in which the display of their delusions can provide "proof" that can strengthen and revalidate "senseless" beliefs, and their unawareness of KSI/TR. This explanation is consistent with Dudley and Over's (2003) statement that "the belief that there is some great conspiracy against oneself, and interpreting much of what happens to oneself in terms of this belief, can be as consistent and coherent as any other view of the world that people have" (p. 269). Thus, if someone is laughing, patients can jump to the conclusion that he is part of the plot against them. In this regard, Dudley and Over noted that

> people with delusions who asserted this condition would have little interest in finding some falsifying instances of it, i.e., cases of someone laughing at a joke or for some other innocent reason. They would be convinced that there was a plot against them and be out to find cases where someone was laughing at them because of the plot, thereby confirming the conditional and the existence of the plot itself (p. 271).

Moreover, since schizophrenics' delusions affect their social interactions, they are likely to elicit hostility toward or break contact with others, thus confirming their self-deceptive beliefs (Freeman et al., 2002, p. 338). By providing the opportunity for validation of their self-deceptive belief, such situations trigger the re-manifestation of the paranoids' delusions. Personal weaknesses and imagined threats may serve the same aims (Dudley & Over, 2003). This can be seen, for example, in the case study of Percy King, discussed in Part I. The patient's weaknesses, including his long hospitalization, masturbation, and homosexual desires, triggered the display of persecutory beliefs as they provided him with self-deceptive proofs that he was a victim of invisible pursuers.

In some cases, patients may redisplay their symptoms in imaginary situations that can provide self-deceptive proofs and thus revalidate their delusions. For example, on one occasion, when walking in an unfamiliar part of New York City, King heard someone exclaiming twice: "shoot him!" Thinking that gangsters had mistaken him for someone else, he rushed from the spot, trying to disappear into the crowd. But the gangsters pursued him: "I knew they were pursuing me because I still heard their voices as close as ever, no matter how fast I walked" (White, 1964, p. 79). Thus, King utilized this imaginary event as "proof" that his delusion was real.

Accordingly, because these cognitive manipulations are aimed at validating the patient's delusional beliefs, it is not surprising that the reduction of delusions causes the reduction of JTC (Dudley et al., 2013; Woodward, Munz, LeClerc, & Lecomte, 2009).

Semi-Automatic Self-Deception Processes

Evidence of Conscious Involvement

PBT's assumption that the conscious is the only cognitive system that controls the individual's voluntary behaviors indicates that this system continues to be involved also after the creation and preservation of unawareness. Clinical examples supporting the coexistence of awareness-unawareness were reviewed in the introduction to Part II. These include the Unabomber and Charles Cullen, who despite being unaware of the underlying motives for their criminal behaviors, carefully planned their murders and took appropriate precautions to avoid their arrest. This phenomenon has also been demonstrated in patients with conversion disorder (e.g., Leary, 2003; Nicol, 1969) and spirit possession (e.g., Mischel & Mischel, 1958), who can regulate their behavior in a manner to avoid potential harm to themselves or others. Similarly, subjects with hysterical paralysis fail to display the symptoms when their attention is diverted (e.g., Cassady et al., 2005; Kihlstrom, 1994, p. 382; Merskey, 1995; Spence, 1999) or when awakened during sleep (e.g., Laurema, 1993).

Consciousness involvement is evident in other types of bizarre behaviors as well. For example, when the university authorities threatened to fire Leonard (1927) if he did not resume his teaching duties (p. 328), he adjusted his symptoms to the demands of reality by moving to an apartment nearer to the university. Likewise, although his agoraphobic symptoms did not allow him to travel far from the university, he did break this rule when it was essential for his adjustment needs (pp. 343, 347). Generally, agoraphobic patients develop self-deceptive excuses that allow them to occasionally inhibit their symptom, and thereby alleviate their suffering, without being accused of a discrepancy that would threaten their coping mechanism. For example, they can allow themselves to be away from their homes if given an avenue for quick return, if escorted by their spouse or if sitting near the door at a restaurant (Thorpe & Burns, 1983, pp. 23–24).

Another example suggesting conscious control is the previously reviewed evidence that obsessive-compulsive patients inhibit their symptoms in situations where their exhibition may be socially embarrassing or threatening to their work. Similarly, Varma et al. (1981) reported a case study of a multiple personality patient who could control the switch to her other personality, as it "occurred at her home only, and never during even prolonged visits with relatives" (pp. 114–115). In the same manner, although kleptomaniacs are unable to resist their bizarre impulse to steal, they will generally avoid stealing when immediate arrest is probable (DSM-IV, American Psychiatric Association, 1994).

The Deceptive Cycle

Figure 1 describes the self-deceptive cycle in which patients consciously reactivate their symptoms in response to the aforementioned four situations and repeatedly cause themselves to remain unaware of KSI/TR. Essentially, the same psychological processes involved in the creation and preservation of unawareness at the initial adoption of the symptom, are repeated in each new exhibition of this behavior. At this stage, however, unawareness of KSI/TR occurs at a much faster rate due to two factors, which are absent in the initial adoption of this behavior. One is the automatization of the display which is the consequence of both practice (i.e., repeated display of

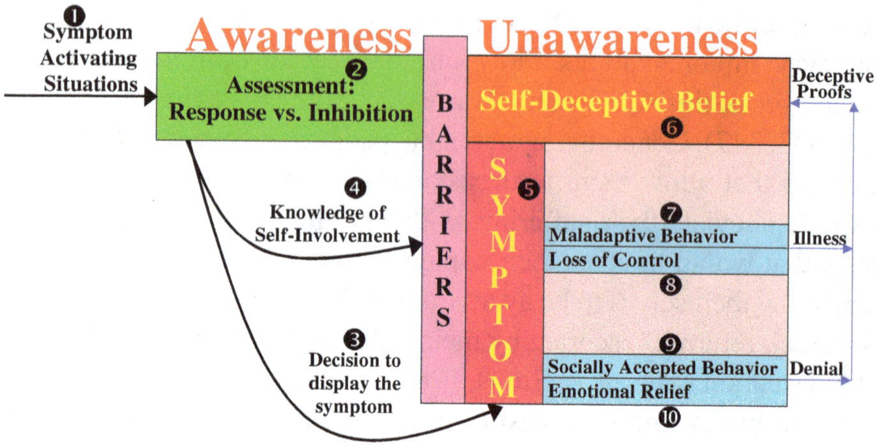

Figure 1. The Deceptive Cycle.

the symptom) and emotional relief (i.e., reinforcement) caused by the distraction and controllability effects of this behavior. Automatization indicates that less attention is allocated to both the decision to reactivate this behavior as well as to its actual performance, and consequently the awareness of KSI/TR. As noted by Lynn et al. (2008) with regard to hypnosis

> once an intention to respond a suggestion is formed, it no longer requires much conscious control. Instead, the response is triggered as an automatic or quasi-automatic operation that intervenes in initiating, correcting, interrupting, inserting, continuing and terminating action (p. 126).

This effect is also demonstrated in the automatic performance of motor skills, which is attributed to the reduced amount of attention allocated to the execution of these behaviors due to practice (e.g., Kihlstrom, 1987; Lewin, 1982; Moore & Stevenson, 1991; Morris, 1981).

The second factor that disrupts the encoding of KSI/TR is the establishment of the self-deceptive belief. Once formed, the belief becomes a powerful distractive tool that hinders the encoding of KSI/TR in manner similar to the display of the symptom.

In Figure 1, No. 1 refers to four situations that stimulate the conscious reactivation of the symptoms: stress, belief-challenging conditions, demand characteristics and the need for self-deceptive proofs. No. 2 relates to the automatic reactivation of the symptoms. Although minimal attention is allocated to the decision to redisplay the symptom, the patient may modify or inhibit the display if rapid assessment indicates potential damage. Nos. 3 and 4 represent the automatic release of the symptom and the patient's minimal awareness of KSI/TR, respectively. Nos. 5 and 6 represent thc self-deceptive belief and the symptom, which constitute the two barriers that block the accessibility of KSI/TR through their powerful, distractive effects. Hence, like hypnosis where the individual becomes unaware of the intentional production of their hypnotic state by focusing on the hypnotic suggestion and their behavioral change (e.g., see Lynn et al., 2008), the intense preoccupation with the symptom and self-deceptive belief enables patients to direct their attention away from KSI/TR.

Two additional memory-inhibiting factors are intentional forgetting and state-dependent memory caused by substantial emotional and cognitive changes. Once unawareness is created following the aforementioned factors, patients are faced with the same psychological state to which they were exposed immediately after the initial display of the symptom. Those with self-deceptive belief of illness are faced with the extrospective observation of maladaptive behavior and introspective experience of loss of control (Nos. 7 and 8, respectively). As a result, they will have additional *deceptive proofs* to revalidate their misleading self-diagnosis and explanation at each new presentation of the symptom. A similar process is performed by patients in the denial group based on their observations of socially encouraged behavior, which in psychoses results from misinterpretation of reality, and the evidence of emotional relief (Nos. 9 and 10). Thus, while one would expect that repeated presentation of the symptom would increase awareness of KSI/TR, in fact given the aforementioned self-deceptive processes, each new presentation of these behaviors reinforces the patient's unawareness of this information.

This deceptive cycle, where the conscious begins with awareness and ends with unawareness, may account for Seligman's (1988) dilemma regarding the resistance to extinction of panic disorder. The author noted that

> A person who has had panic disorder for a decade may have had about 1,000 panic attacks. In each one, on the cognitive account, he misinterpreted his racing heart as meaning that he was about to have a heart attack, and this was disconfirmed. Under the laws of disconfirmation that I know, he received ample evidence that his belief was false, and he should have given it up... But neither theory explains why the beliefs did not extinguish in the face of disconfirmation long ago. (p. 326; see also Eifert, 1992)

Discussion

PBT's concept of unawareness has four major theoretical advantages that distinguish it from rival models, particularly the Freudian unconscious. This is the only model that (1) explains evidence indicating the coexistence of awareness–unawareness among both neuroses, criminal insanity, and schizophrenia; (2) explains why some patients believe that they are ill, while others deny that their behavior is deviant; (3) resolves a number of central theoretical controversies, as will be described in the following; (4) enables, along with other PBT's concepts, to integrate therapeutic interventions pertaining to these disorders, into one theoretical framework, as will be specified in Part III.

Resolving Major Theoretical Disputes

PBT's model of unawareness may help us resolve three theoretical disputes, relating to (1) conversion disorder; (2) DID; and (3) panic disorder and agoraphobia. The first dispute concerns the question of whether conversion disorder is a psychological disorder, as traditionally claimed by psychological theories, or a neurological one, as is argued by neurologists following some studies which seemingly indicate abnormal cerebral function in conversion disorder patients. The second dispute concerns the trauma model of DID, which views this disorder as a coping mechanism for people who were subjected to childhood trauma, as opposed to the socio-cognitive explanation which claims that it is a role enactment. The third issue involves the disagreements regarding the underlying causes of panic disorder and agoraphobia between behavioral, cognitive, and medical theories.

Conversion Disorder

During the last century, it was widely accepted that conversion disorder is a psychological disorder. The main dispute was between psychoanalysis, which attributed it to childhood trauma or unacceptable impulses (Breuer & Freud, 1895; Fenichel, 1946), and behaviorism, which viewed the disorder as a learned behavior or coping mechanism intentionally adopted in response to environmental stressors (e.g., see Blanchard & Hersen, 1976; Rimm & Somervill, 1977; Ullmann & Krasner, 1975). However, in recent years, neurologists have claimed that conversion disorder is a neurological disorder, as patients display abnormal cerebral function (e.g., Fink, Halligan, & Marshall, 2006; Rotge et al., 2009; Van Beilen, Vogt, & Leenders, 2010; see also Reynolds, 2018; Richardson, Isbister, & Nicholson, 2018). For example, patients of hysterical paralysis display an increased activity in the anterior cingulate cortex and associated regions when they attempt to move their affected limb (e.g., de Lange, Roelofs, & Toni, 2007; Marshall, Halligan, Fink, Wade, & Frackowiak, 1997). Similar patterns of neurological changes have been observed among people who were induced into displaying conversion symptoms via hypnotic suggestions (e.g., Deeley et al., 2013; Halligan & Oakley, 2013). These findings have led researchers to claim that conversion disorder should be renamed as *"Functional Neurological Disorder"* (e.g., Stone et al., 2011; see also *DSM-5*, American Psychiatric Association, 2013).

However, neurologists' theoretical position should be rejected for the following reasons: (1) given the weaknesses of psychological theories, advocates of the neurological explanation make the same mistaken assumption, as was made with schizophrenia: correlational findings were interpreted as causality, without indicating, at least on a theoretical level, how these supposed cerebral abnormalities can cause a specific conversion symptom; (2) neurologists focus solely on their own findings, neglecting data which are unexplainable by neurological concepts, such as the large variability of conversion symptoms and the mechanisms by which psychological interventions exert their positive therapeutic effects, as will be demonstrated in Part III. How could these therapies neutralize patients' cerebral deficit? (3) It is difficult to see how neurologists can account for the fact that this disorder is far more prevalent among females and in non-Western countries (see Rofé & Rofé, 2013).

As discussed in Part I, although Freud's concept of repression does not allow us to preserve the name *conversion*, primarily in light of studies which refute the existence of repression (see review by Rofé, 2008), PBT's new concept of repression enables us to maintain this name. Similarly, PBT's concept of controllability preserves behaviorism's suggestion that conversion symptoms are coping mechanisms, which individuals deliberately adopt when subjected to intolerable level of stress. This effect was demonstrated earlier in discussing the case study by Brady and Lind (1961; for additional examples, see Rofé & Rofé, 2013). As was discussed in Part I, PBT's principles of cost-benefited analysis and availability can explain the high prevalence of this disorder and others among women and non-Western countries. PBT's ability to integrate all relevant therapy of conversion disorder in its theoretical system is discussed in Part III.

Regarding aforementioned neurological findings of increase activity in the cingulate cortex of hysterically paralyzed patients, when attempting to move their affected limbs, it seems that this effect occurs because the patient is subjected to two contradictory conscious messages. The first message is the conscious decision to move the affected limb when instructed to do so (Nos. 3 and 4 in Figure 1), which stimulates the brain area responsible for movement. The second message is the simultaneous employment of the self-deceptive belief or hypnotic suggestions to inform the brain of an inability to move the limb. This explanation may account for Van Beilen et al.'s (2010) statement: "I want to move my arm, but I cannot" (p. 156).

PBT's model of unawareness can also resolve the difficulty in distinguishing between conversion disorder, malingering, and fictitious disorder. *DSM-IV-TR's* proposal for solving this problem is its requirement for the diagnosis of the conversion disorder that the "symptom is not intentionally produced or feigned" (American Psychiatric Association, 2000, p. 492). However, this suggestion has been sharply criticized by many researchers (e.g., Kanaan et al., 2010; Krahn, Bostwick, & Stonnington, 2008; Miller, 1999; Stone, LaFrance, Levenson, & Sharpe, 2010). For example, Delis and Wetter (2007) noted that "many clinicians are reluctant to use diagnoses such as Malingering, Factitious, and Conversion Disorder at least in part because of difficulty in objectively assessing the presence or absence of intentionality in the generation of the excessive symptoms" (p. 593). Indeed, the *DSM-5* abandoned the aforementioned requirement, as it now states, "the diagnosis of conversion disorder does not require the judgment that the symptoms are not intentionally produced (i.e., not feigned …"; American Psychiatric Association, 2013, p. 320). However, this resolution provides no diagnostic criteria for distinguishing between conversion disorders and malingering or factitious disorders.

Instead, PBT suggests that conversion disorder be defined as a behavior meeting all five diagnostic criteria of madness, which includes unawareness of the underlying causes for the dramatic change in behavior. Malingering or fictitious disorders are behaviors that do not fulfill these criteria, especially the criterion of unawareness.

Dissociative Identity Disorder

The underlying mechanism of DID is still an open question. In this regard, there is a profound disagreement between the ***trauma model*** (see Bremner, 2008; Dalenberg et al., 2012; Gleaves, 1996; Vissia et al., 2016) and **the *socio-cognitive explanation*** (see reviews by Boysen & VanBergen, 2014; Giesbrecht et al., 2008, 2010; Lilienfeld et al., 1999). The trauma model views DID as a defense mechanism developed in response to sexual or physical abuse. In contrast, the socio-cognitive model claims that DID is a role enactment that is created, legitimized, and maintained by social reinforcements. "Patients with DID synthesize these role enactments by drawing on a wide variety of sources of information, including the print and broadcast media, cues provided by therapists, personal experiences, and observations of individuals who have enacted multiple identities" (Lilienfeld et al., 1999, pp. 507–508).

One factor relevant to this dispute concerns the mechanism involved in producing and manipulating altered personalities. It is unlikely that these behaviors are controlled by a biological mechanism, particularly in light of the fact that patients can manifest their personalities at any time upon request (e.g., Allen & Movius, 2000; Hopper et al., 2002; Savoy, Frederick, Keuroghlian, & Wolk, 2012). The socio-cognitive model provides no explanation regarding the mechanism that controls DID. Advocates only reject the possibility that these behaviors are mediated by the conscious, without providing alternative explanations. For example, Lilienfeld et al. (1999) noted

> The metaphor or concept of role does not imply that role-related behaviors are the product of conscious deception. Instead, role enactments tend to flow spontaneously and are carried out with little or no conscious awareness and with a high degree of 'organismic involvement' (p. 508).

On the opposite side of the barricade, while in the past psychoanalysts have used the concepts of repression and the unconscious to explain this disorder (e.g., see Kluft, 1995; Waiess, 2006), in recent years, proponents avoid these terms apparently because of the increasing number of studies questioning the validity of these concepts. Instead, the trauma model claims that the dissociative individual attempts "to avoid recall of trauma by conscious and unconscious disavowal of the importance, implications, and/or accuracy or reality of the memory" (Dalenberg et al., 2012, p. 553). Thus, both models make no clear statement with regard to the mechanism that controls and manipulates DID.

PBT resolves this controversy by synthesizing ideas from both theories into one framework. On the one hand, it accepts the socio-cognitive claim that DID is a form of role enactment. Moreover, PBT's idea that the choice of a specific mad behavior is made intuitively with little or no conscious effort and is then spontaneously implemented by the conscious, is consistent with the socio-cognitive statement that DID flows spontaneously "with little or no conscious awareness" (Lilienfeld et al., 1999, p. 508). On the other hand, it acknowledges the impressive research and clinical evidence reviewed by the trauma model that stress precedes the onset of DID, and that this disorder, like other types of madness, is a pathological coping mechanism which individuals employ when confronted with an intolerable level of emotional distress.

However, while the integration of these two seemingly incompatible theoretical approaches is undoubtedly important, PBT's major contribution concerns the mechanism that activates this behavior and the manner by which patients become unaware of the underlying causes of their behavior. In this regard, the socio-cognitive experimental studies that demonstrate that DID can be intentionally faked by professional actors (see Boysen & VanBergen, 2014; Giesbrecht et al., 2008) is consistent with PBT's fundamental claim that mad behaviors are controlled by the consciousness. However, these studies do not challenge the validity of the trauma model of DID mainly because subjects were not confronted with an intolerable level of stress, which according to PBT is necessary for activating the psychological processes that create the unawareness of KSI.

PBT also resolves the two opposing approaches concerning childhood abuse. On the one hand, there seems to be little doubt that childhood abuse is prevalent among DID patients (see review by Boysen & VanBergen, 2014; Dalenberg et al., 2012; Gleaves, 1996). These patients also show neurological changes that have been observed in animals who were exposed to stress during their early development (e.g., Hopper et al., 2002; Reinders et al., 2006; Sar, Unal, & Ozturk, 2007; Tsai, Condie, Wu, & Chang, 1999; Vermetten, Schmahl, Lindner, Loewenstein, & Bremner, 2006). In reference to these findings, Hopper et al. (2002) noted that early trauma cause "maturational lag" which in turn may lead to a predisposition to dissociation" (p. 86).

On the other hand, it is difficult to accept the trauma model's claim that child abuse is causally linked to DID. **Firstly**, childhood sexual abuse does not necessarily cause pathogenic effects (e.g., Kendall-Tackett, Williams, & Finkelhor, 1993; Rind, Tromovitch, & Bauserman, 1998). For example, meta-analyses of 59 studies revealed that victims of childhood sexual abuse were on average only slightly less well adjusted than controls (Rind et al., 1998). **Secondly**, as was noted earlier childhood abuse is associated not only with DID, but is also related to a variety of deviant behaviors, such as anxiety and depression (e.g., Bushnell, Wells, & Oakley-Browne, 1992; Yama, Tovey, & Fogas, 1993), panic disorder (e.g., Friedman et al., 2002), conversion disorder (e.g., Kuloglu, Atmaca, Tezcan, Gecici, & Bulut, 2003; Roelofs, Keijsers, Hoogduin, Näring, & Moene, 2002), **OCD** (e.g., Lochner, du Toit, Zungu-Dirwayi et al., 2002) anorexia nervosa (e.g., Oliosi, Dalle, & Grave, 2003; Wentz, Gillberg, Gillberg, & Rástam, 2005), injurious behavior (e.g., Favaro & Santonastaso, 2000), and suicide (e.g., Meadows & Kaslow, 2002; Read, Agar, Barker-Collo, Davies, & Moskowitz, 2001). **Thirdly**, DID may develop in the absence of childhood abuse (e.g., Gupta & Kumar, 2005; Nakic & Thomas, 2012; Spanos, 1994). As noted by Spanos (1994), "most people who suffer even severe child abuse do not exhibit [DID], and many people who have not been abused can easily and quickly be induced to display multiplicity" (p. 158).

Thus, it seems that people who were subjected to childhood abuse are more likely to develop DID, when this is suitable for their coping needs, both because their childhood trauma increases their vulnerability to stress (e.g., see a review by Dalenberg et al., 2012) and because of the availability of their dissociative tendencies crystallized as neurological changes. This, however, does not invalidate the socio-cognitive claim that DID may develop in the absence of childhood abuse. People may adopt this disorder and fabricate childhood experiences, as claimed by the socio-cognitive model (e.g., Acocella, 1999; Giesbrecht et al., 2008; Read & Lindsay, 1994; Spanos, 1994, 1996). While therapists may play a vital role in motivating patients to fabricate childhood trauma (e.g., Loftus, 1993), it seems likely that patients want to be deceived and therefore are inclined to cooperate with therapists' persuasive efforts in order to validate their self-deceptive belief.

It is important to note, when evaluating PBT's explanation of DID, that the validity of a given theory cannot be determined by focusing on a single variable, such as the debate between the trauma model and socio-cognitive explanation, or the biopsychosocial paradigm which emphasizes the neurological features of this disorder (e.g., Chalavi et al., 2015; Şar, Dorahy, & Krüger, 2017). One must simultaneously address other problems as well, such as the increased prevalence of this disorder in recent years, gender differences, its absence in less developed countries, the effect of the media on its prevalence, and the variability of the symptoms (e.g., the fact that DID may manifest with and without criminal acts). PBT is the only theory that can integrate all the relevant data in its theoretical framework.

Panic Disorder and Agoraphobia

Theoretical Dispute: As specified below, the two dominant theories of panic disorder and agoraphobia, which have supposedly received empirical validation, are conditioning theory (e.g., Barlow, 2004; Bouton et al., 2001; Carter & Barlow, 1995) and cognitive theory (e.g., Clark, 1986, 1988). Although other theories have been suggested, such as Klein's (1993) Suffocation False Alarm Theory, they have received little empirical support (see review by Rofé & Rofé, 2015). PBT challenges the validity of both leading theories, arguing that these disorders are just additional examples of bizarre behaviors. Moreover, as is demonstrated below, their findings, as well as additional relevant data that remain unexplained by these theories, can be better integrated within PBT's theoretical framework. Before reviewing PBT, it is essential to first present the hypotheses and main drawbacks of these theories, which are reviewed in more detail elsewhere (see review by Rofé & Rofé, 2015).

Conditioning Theory: Originally, behaviorists applied the Pavlovian paradigm to explain panic disorder and agoraphobia (Wolpe, 1981). Since then, behaviorists have suggested a revised version of this theory, termed interoceptive conditioning (e.g., Barlow, 2004; Bouton et al., 2001; Mineka & Oehlberg, 2008), in light of the fact that these disorders develop in the absence of stimuli which naturally cause fear, termed by this theory "unconditioned stimulus"

(UCS) (e.g., see Jacobs & Nadel, 1985). According to the neo-conditioning theory, the first panic attack, which individuals experience as a result of stress, constitutes the USC. Bodily sensations aroused during this episode constitute the conditioned stimulus (CS). Hene, just like dog phobia, in which the dog (CS) becomes conditioned to bite (UCS), bodily sensations (CS) become conditioned to the first panic attack (UCS). Consequently, patients will automatically experience panic whenever they experience even a weak level of bodily sensations, such as when exercising, drinking coffee or when exposed to CO_2-enriched air. Some of these patients develop agoraphobia rather than panic disorder soon after the experience of the first panic attack, in order to avoid the social embarrassment caused by lose of self-control. As noted by Mineka and Oehlberg (2008) "a substantial subset of people who develop panic disorder go on to develop some degree of agoraphobic avoidance of situations in which they perceive a panic attack might occur and from which escape would be difficult or embarrassing" (p. 569).

Cognitive Theory: This theory accepts the idea that bodily sensations are the key to understanding panic disorder and agoraphobia. However, these disorders are attributed to the catastrophic misinterpretation of bodily sensations which the individual experience following the first panic attack. For example, Clark (1986, 1988) claimed that heart palpitations or dizziness could be misinterpreted by panic patients as evidence of an impending heart attack. These sensations may be triggered by external anxiety-provoking cues, such as a specific location for an agoraphobic who previously had an attack in a similar setting, or internal stimuli (i.e., threatening thoughts). They can also be brought on by intense emotional stimulation, such as excitement or anger, or by innocuous events that result in physiological arousal, such as suddenly standing up from a sitting position (dizziness), strenuous exercise (breathlessness) and coffee consumption (palpitations). Both panic attacks and agoraphobia are attributed to the same psychophysiological process, i.e., misinterpretation of bodily sensations.

Critique: In an attempt to validate the interoceptive conditioning theory, researchers have successfully produced conditioning effects in which the UCS was bodily sensations that were produced by prolonged exposure to CO_2-enriched air, while the CS was a brief exposure to CO_2-enriched air (e.g., Acheson, Forsyth, Prenoveau, & Bouton, 2007). Panic disorder patients, who are supposedly more vulnerable to conditioning due to genetic, temperamental, or experiential vulnerability (e.g., Bouton et al., 2001), demonstrated greater resistance to extinction in comparison with a nonclinical sample (Michael, Blechert, Vriends, Margraf, & Wilhelm, 2007). However, these studies cannot validate the conditioning theory, as there is an enormous gap between panic disorder in everyday life and panic-like effects in the laboratory. For example, unlike laboratory studies, in which the conditioned response is easily extinguished and has no psychological effect on the individual's adjustment (e.g., Harrington, Schmidt, & Telch, 1996; Perna, Cocchi, Politi, & Bellodi, 1997; Prenoveau, Forsyth, Kelly, & Barrios, 2006), true panic disorders severely disrupts the individual's daily functioning and are highly resistant to extinction (see Eifert, 1992; Jacobs & Nadel, 1985; Seligman, 1988). As stated by Jacobs and Nadel (1985), "those afflicted with such problems often fail to show extinction after many years of exposure to the feared stimuli, even in the absence of any aversive consequences" (p. 514). Accordingly, Eysenck (1976) arrived at the conclusion that

> unless this fact can be explained in a satisfactory manner, the theory becomes untenable. Indeed, as the essence of the "neurotic paradox" is precisely the failure of extinction to occur (anxiety fails to extinguish although no reinforcement is offered: behavior which is punished continues to occur), we may say that the Watson theory fails to come to grips

> with the problem which it was designed to solve (p. 254; see also Seligman, 1988, p. 326).

This lack of extinction is typical of other forms of bizarre fears as well (e.g., chocolate phobia; Rachman & Seligman, 1976). The resistance to extinction of panic disorders constitutes a problem for cognitive theory as well.

Cognitive theory is also problematic because panic attacks occur in the absence of catastrophic thoughts. For example, panic attacks are experienced during non-dreaming stages of sleep, when catastrophic thoughts are absent (e.g., Craskc & Barlow, 1989; Craske & Rowe, 1997; Hauri, Friedman, & Ravaris, 1989; Lesser, Poland, Holcant, & Rose, 1985; Ley, 1988; Mellman & Uhde, 1989a, 1989b). Although Schredl, Kronenberg, Nonnell and Heuser (2001) reported that nocturnal panic attacks are closely related to dreams and nightmares, they also found that a subgroup of patients in their study experienced panic attacks in the absence of dreams. Subjects may also display diurnal panic attacks which are not preceded by catastrophic cognitions (e.g., Kenardy, Fried, Kraemer, & Taylor, 1992; Kenardy & Taylor, 1999; Rachman, Lopata, & Levitt, 1988; Zucker, Taylor, Brouillard, Ehlers et al., 1989). Additionally, studies have found cases of "non-fearful panic disorder" or "non-cognitive panic", which occur in the absence of fear or catastrophic cognitions (e.g., Barlow, Brown, & Craske, 1994; Beitman, Lamberti, Mukerji, DeRosear et al., 1987; Beitman, Mukerji, Russell, & Grafing, 1993; Bringager, Gauer, Arnesen, Friis et al., 2008; Fleet, Martel, Lavoie et al., 2000; Kushner & Beitman, 1990; Rachman, Levitt & Lopatka, 1987; Rachman, Lopatka & Levitt, 1988).

In an attempt to defend their theory, cognitivists have argued that fearful thoughts are sometimes "missing" because the catastrophic misinterpretation of bodily sensations takes place so quickly that panic patients may not be aware of their existence (e.g., see Clark, 1988; Rachman et al., 1987). McNally (1990) noted, however, that patients would remember thoughts of having a heart attacks, even if they were momentary. Furthermore, this claim renders Clark's theory untestable. As noted by McNally (1990), if patients could become unaware of such self-producing catastrophic thoughts, "then what would constitute evidence against the hypothesis that catastrophic misinterpretation necessarily precedes panic attacks?" (p. 407; see also McNally, 1999, p. 8).

An additional problem is why certain stressful situations, such as when a person learns that he possesses a deadly health problem (e.g., AIDS, a massive coronary thrombosis), do not increase the rate of panic disorder (Perdices, Dunbar, Grunseit, Hall, & Cooper, 1992; Wolpe & Rowan, 1988). Sanderson and Beck (1989) stated, in response to this criticism, that in the case of AIDS, "death is not imminent. Misattribution theory predicts that panic will occur only when the individual believes that death is imminent (i.e., patients believe that they are dying right now)" (p. 582). Nevertheless, it is hard to accept that a prognosis of prolonged physical, painful deterioration resulting in death is insufficiently frightening to cause catastrophic thoughts, and hence panic. Moreover, if Sanderson and Beck's argument is valid, then one would expect that cardiac patients with advanced heart disease would display a high rate of panic disorder. However, contrary to this expectation, studies indicate that patients with false heart attacks ("cardiac neurosis") or atypical angina display a greater frequency of panic disorder and other related symptoms (e.g., heart palpitations, fear of dying, and trembling) than patients with myocardial infraction (Beitman, Mukerji, Russell, Grafing, 1993; Margraf & Ehlers, 1991).

It is also difficult to see how cognitive theory can be applied to agoraphobia in light of data indicating that agoraphobic patients rarely report catastrophic thoughts during confrontation with their phobic stimuli, despite experiencing intense anxiety (Williams, Chambless, & Ahrens, 1997).

Furthermore, cognitive theory provides no explanation of the mechanisms which make patients think irrationally or non-adaptively. While psychoanalysis attributes this effect to the unconscious (e.g., De Poderoso, Julian, & Linezky, 2005; Shilkret, 2002), conditioning theories to learning experiences (e.g., Bouton et al., 2001; Davey, 1989a), and biological models to adverse neurochemical factors (e.g., Barlow, 2004), cognitivists provide no explanation for why a minority of people suddenly begin to think irrationally.

Neither conditioning nor cognitive theories are able to explain why in many cases patients develop agoraphobia in the absence of a panic attack (Fava, Rafanelli, Tossani et al., 2005; Hayward & Wilson, 2007). As claimed by Wittchen, Nocon, Beesdo, Pine et al. (2008) in a substantial number of cases, agoraphobia is "a clinically significant disorder that exists independently of panic attacks and panic disorders" (p. 153). In fact, agoraphobia may serve as a predictor for the development of panic disorder (Bienvenu, Onyike, Stein et al., 2006).

Further difficulties include rarity of agoraphobia and panic disorders amongst children (e.g., Kenardy, Oei, & Evans, 1990; Klein, Mannuzza, Chapman, & Fyer, 1992; Rachman, 1990; Rosenbaum, Pollock, Otto et al., 1995; Tearnan et al., 1984). "Why should people begin to experience a fear of public places and travel between the ages of 18 and 25?" (Rachman, 1990, p. 73). One would expect that adults who have had many more exposures to situations such as supermarkets and restaurants would be less vulnerable to developing agoraphobia. This claim is compatible with both the behaviorist notion of habit strength, which states that the learned response is strengthened with reinforced repetition (e.g., Hulse, Egeth, & Deese, 1980 pp. 175, 181–185), and findings that fearless experiences tend to immunize the subject from acquiring conditioned fear (e.g., Davey, 1989a, 1989b; Mineka & Cook, 1986; Rachman, 1990, pp. 181–182). Yet the clinical evidence runs contrary to this expectation. The lower prevalence of bizarre fears amongst children is also surprising because children are more prone to develop fears (e.g., fear of animals, darkness, and water) (e.g., Fredrikson, Annas, Fischer, & Wik, 1996; Graham & Gaffan, 1997; King, Eleonora, & Ollendick, 1998; Lautch, 1971; Marks, 1987a, p. 372; McNally & Steketee, 1985; Menzies & Clarke, 1993a;

Milgrom, Mancl, King, & Weinstein, 1995; Moore, Brodsgaard, & Birn, 1991; Rachman, 1990, p. 73; Spence & McCathie, 1993).

Additional problems concern the inability of both behavior and cognitive theories to integrate each others' findings. This problem is also applicable medical and psychodynamic models which are unable to integrate research and clinical data on panic disorder and agoraphobia. For example, none of these theories can explain the high prevalence of panic disorder among people with pulmonary diseases (e.g., Brenes, 2003; Mikkelsen, Middelboe, Pisinger, & Stage, 2004; Nascimento et al., 2002; Roy-Byrne, Craske, & Stein, 2006; Shavitt, Gentil, & Mandetta, 1992; Valença et al., 2006) and mitral valve prolapse which are characterized by nonangina chest pain, palpitations, dyspnea, light-headedness, and anxiety (e.g., Gorman et al., 1988; Hamada, Koshino, Misawa, Isaki, & Geyjo, 1998). Similarly, it is difficult to understand from the perspective of behavioral-cognitive theories why psychoanalytic therapy will yield a positive therapeutic effect with patients who suffer from agoraphobia (see Wolitzky & Eagle, 1999), as will be specified in Part III.

PBT's Integrative Theoretical Model: PBT agrees with both conditioning and cognitive theories regarding the critical importance of bodily sensations in the development of panic disorder and agoraphobia. However, contrary to these theories, PBT claims that these sensations are not necessary condition for the development of these disorders, as seen in the case study of Leonard (1927) which was discussed above. Furthermore, as was elaborated on above when discussing the development of self-deception of illness, according to PBT the misinterpretation of the bodily sensations is a deliberate rational maneuver which enables patients both to facilitate the production of panic attack and to develop the self-explanation of illness, rather than the result of irrational thinking.

This new understanding of panic disorder and agoraphobia enables PBT to integrate the above findings that bodily sensations trigger panic attacks into its theoretical framework. While conditioning theory attribute this effect to conditioning and cognitive theory to misinterpretation of these stimuli, PBT attributes it to belief-challenging conditions. Patients must exhibit panic attack since otherwise they may lose their self-deceptive belief. PBT also resolves aforementioned problems that challenge the validity of behavioral-cognitive theories. These include:

1) Resistance to extinction, as explained by PBT's deceptive cycle;
2) The high prevalence of panic disorder among individuals with pulmonary diseases and mitral valve prolapse, which are accounted for by PBT's principle of availability, as specified above;
3) The development of agoraphobia in the absence of a preceding panic attack to the extent that it serves the individual's coping needs (see Part III the case study by Wolitzky & Eagle, 1999);
4) The rarity of agoraphobia and panic disorder among children, which can be explained by the cost-benefit principle. Children instead prefer to employ other types of fear as coping mechanisms, primarily school phobia (e.g., Last & Francis, 1988; Phelps, Cox, & Bajorek, 1992), which meet PBT's five criteria of bizarreness (see Rofé, 2000). School phobia better suits children's coping demands and imposes fewer restrictions on their daily functioning than agoraphobia and panic disorders.

   Case studies show that school phobia is associated with, or may evolve into, agoraphobia. Deltito and Hahn (1993) have studied a three-generation family presentation of anxiety disorder. The disorder manifested itself as school phobia in childhood, evolved into panic disorder with agoraphobia in young adulthood and developed into diffuse anxiety with hypochondriac features in later life. Similarly, Lepola, Leinonen, and Koponen (1996) reported three case studies of school phobia that were associated with panic and agoraphobic symptoms. Thus, when children are in need of an agoraphobic type of symptom, they will choose one that provides the most desired benefit at the least cost. Later, after their school years, when their cost-benefit considerations have changed, the school phobia might develop into agoraphobia if the need for a bizarre coping strategy persists (for further discussion see see Rofé, 2000, pp. 201–202);

5) The explanation of bizarre phobias, such as Leonard's (1927) train phobia, chocolate phobias (Rachman & Seligman, 1976) and rat germ phobia (Brandt & Mackenzie, 1987), as specified above;
6) The integration of the therapeutic achievements of CBT (cognitive-behavior therapy) in the treatment of panic disorder and agoraphobia, as will be specified in Part III.

One issue which remains unresolved concerns the extreme level of anxiety that panic disorder and agoraphobic patients may experience. How do such attacks of genuine discofort occur if these disorders are indeed voluntary, as claimed by PBT? This seems to be the result of two factors. One factor is the belief, developed by patients following the creation of unawareness, that certain stimuli (e.g., train, rat germs, or bodily sensations) or situations (e.g., public places) are dangerous. In this regard, it is worth mentioning the disastrous effects of belief in non-Western societies. For example, Richter's (1957) anthropological study noted that

> a Brazilian Indian condemned and sentenced by a so-called medicine man, is helpless against his own emotional response to this pronouncement — and dies within hours. In Africa, a young Negro unknowingly eats the inviolably banned wild hen. On discovery of his "crime" he trembles, is overcome by fear and dies in 24 hours. In New Zealand, a Maori woman eats fruit that she only later learns has come

> from a tabooed place. Her chief has been profaned. By noon of the next day she is dead. In Australia, a witch doctor points a bone at a man. Believing that nothing can save him, the man rapidly sinks in spirits and prepares to die (p. 281; see also evidence reviewed by Pruitt, 1974).

Another factor which contributes to the physical experience of panic attack is the stressor which triggers the individual's decision to adopt a panic disorder and agoraphobia, such as in Leonard's case, his wife's suicide. Although bizarre behaviors enable patients to repress their stressors, it seems likely that patients intuitively recall their stressors whenever they are confronted with belief-challenging conditions, such as the increase of bodily sensations. Consequently, these unconscious memories and the fear of losing their pathological coping mechanisms, cause a strong experience of anxiety, and hence genuine experience of panic attack.

Rival Models of Self-Deception

Sackeim and Gur (1978; see also Gur & Sackeim, 1979) have developed a psychoanalytic model of self-deception stating that under certain motivational conditions, individuals can maintain two contradictory beliefs, one of which remains outside the consciousness. In support of this theory, they found that subjects who had experienced failure were unable to identify their own voices heard from a recording device, while simultaneously displaying elevated levels of galvanic skin response (GSR). This theoretical model was then applied by Sackeim, Nordlie, and Gur (1979) to account for a case study of a hysterically blind girl (Grosz & Zimmerman, 1970), who supposedly held two contradictory cognitions (1) the patient consciously believed herself to be blind; and (2) she "unconsciously knew" that she was not blind, because she accurately identified visual objects in 480 experimental trials. In other words, from the standpoint of Sackeim et al. (1979), hysterically blind patients can display accurate visual performance without actually being aware they can see.

However, Sackheim et al.'s position is complicated by the fact that the girl never claimed to be totally blind. "Her behavior showed no signs of any visual deficits except when asked to read small or large print ... [and] she scored 100% loss of vision for reading in both eyes" (Grosz & Zimmerman, 1970, pp. 118–121). This evidence suggests that the girl suffered from selective hysterical blindness similar to the air force patients in World War II who complained of selective ocular hysteria (Ironside & Batchelor, 1945). The authors reported 40 cases of aircrew members who exhibited visual disturbances (e.g., blurred vision or defective night vision) that prevented them from fulfilling flight-related tasks. According to Ironside and Batchelor (1945), these patients suffered from problems related to "looking" rather than from disturbances in "seeing." In looking, "the interference is with the will of the patient, and such functions as perception, appreciation, attention and response are involved; in other words, it is the patient who is at fault, and not his visual mechanism" (p. 89). Thus, it appears that the aforementioned girl deliberately failed to read by consciously disrupting the focus of her eyes. The patient could simultaneously eliminate KSI/TR from her consciousness and reinforce her self-deceptive belief of physical illness based on seemingly objective evidence of blurred vision and the sense of introspective evidence of lack of control of the physical "defect," as specified in Figure 1. This coping strategy enabled the girl to compel her parents, who "appeared to be very busy pursuing their own activities and seemed always to be in a rush to go somewhere or work on some project" (Grosz & Zimmerman, 1970, p. 117), to fulfill their parental duties (e.g., helping with homework).

Von Hippel and Trivers (2011) have developed a more systematic theoretical approach to the issue of self-deception among the general population in everyday life. It is difficult to see how their self-deception model, which constitutes an important contribution to the understanding of everyday life, can promote the understanding of neurotic and psychotic disorders. One of the challenging problems of this model is that "one cannot deceive oneself into believing something while simultaneously knowing it to be false" (Bandura, 2011, p. 16). PBT resolves this issue by stating that patients initially forget (i.e., become unaware of) their KSI/TR and then, immediately afterward, validate a self-deceptive belief based on an extrospective observation that their behavior is maladaptive and an introspective experience of loss of control.

Conclusions

PBT's model of patients' unawareness claims that this cognitive state is a join production of unconscious and conscious processes. This theoretical assumption is suggested due to evidence that challenges the validity of the Freudian unconscious and clinical data indicating the coexistence of awareness and unawareness among patients displaying bizarre behaviors. According to this model, the choice of a specific madness is intuitive and made with little or no conscious awareness. The consciousness is the mechanism that executes the unconscious choice and redisplays it when the patient is confronted with stress, belief challenging conditions, demand characteristics, or when searching for "proofs" to validate their seemingly senseless behaviors. Patients become unaware of KSI/TR through a variety of memory-inhibiting mechanisms and self-deceptive beliefs, which block the accessibility of this information. This model of unawareness has four important advantages upon rival theories:

1. It resolves the clinical evidence of coexisting awareness — unawareness.
2. It explains in rational terms why some patients have a belief that they are ill, that is, that they have no control over their behaviors, whereas others deny that their behavior is deviant;

3. It integrates a vast amount of research and clinical evidence associated with all schools of thoughts. Thus, while PBT acknowledges the critical importance of unawareness in the understanding bizarre behaviors, as does psychoanalysis, it explains this effect by self-deceptive belief rather than the unconscious.

   Similar to non-western societies, who often attribute their unawareness of the underlying causes of their behaviors to spirit possession, those of Western countries deceive themselves that their mad behaviors are controlled by the unconscious and attribute the cause to childhood traumas. Likewise, while medical models attribute the phenomena of JTC to neurological deficits (e.g., Garety et al., 2013; Lunt et al., 2012), PBT views these behaviors as cognitive efforts by which patients rationalize their delusions. In the same way, while behavior–cognitive theories attribute the experience of panic attack, agoraphobia, and OCD, following exposure to the object of their anxiety (e.g., bodily situations, public places, or dirt), to conditioning and irrational thinking, PBT attributes this effect to belief-challenging conditions.
4. It resolves several cardinal theoretical disagreements regarding conversion disorder, DID, panic disorder, agoraphobia, and bizarre phobias.
5. It integrates therapeutic methods pertaining to mad behaviors, such as psychoanalysis, cognitive behavioral therapy (CBT), and religious therapy, in one theoretical framework, as will be demonstrated in Part III.

Based on Karl Popper's (1959) claim that new data is necessary for the acceptance of a new theory, one may undermine the scientific value of PBT's model of unawareness. However, the new trend in the philosophy of science argues, based on empirical data of theories that initially did not have data of their own yet became the dominant theories in their field, that the ability of a theory to explain existing data is more important than its ability to present new supportive evidence (e.g., see Proctor & Capaldi, 2001). For example,

Tyron (2005) noted that "Darwin's evolutionary theory remained on the margins of biology for approximately 75 years until population genetics provided the missing causal explanatory mechanisms." Accordingly, Brush (1989) noted that

> a successful explanation of a fact that other theories have already failed to explain satisfactorily … is more convincing than the prediction of a new fact, at least until the competing theories have had their chance (and failed) to explain it (p. 112; see also Brush, 1989, 1990, 1992, 1993, 2005).

Part III

PBT's Integrative Therapeutic Model

Introduction

Given the inability of traditional theories of psychopathology to incorporate research and clinical findings on the development of psychological disorders into a coherent theoretical system, it is not surprising that they have also failed in their attempts to integrate the relevant therapeutic techniques into one theoretical framework (e.g., see reviews by Feixas & Botella, 2004; Lampropoulos, 2000, 2001). Consequently, researchers have ceased their efforts to find the mechanisms of therapeutic change and have focused instead on empirical evaluations of therapeutic techniques. Based on meta-analysis, some investigators have concluded that all therapies have similar efficacies, and suggest that a number of common factors, such as therapeutic alliance, empathy, support, and emotional catharsis are responsible for therapeutic changes (e.g., see Feixas & Botella, 2004; Lampropoulos, 2000; Luborsky et al., 2002; Reisner, 2005). Others listed a number of empirically supported therapies (ESTs), claiming that they have been found more effective than other techniques in the treatment of specific disorders (see, e.g., Chambless, 2002; Reisner, 2005).

However, while empirical examination of therapies is an important goal, revealing the mechanisms that control therapeutic change is no less important. Rosen and Davison (2003) noted that psychotherapy "should work toward the identification of empirically supported principles of change" (p. 303), rather than focusing on empirical evaluations of effective therapies. Similarly, Tryon (2005) commented, "[the] effectiveness of efforts to persuade clinicians to adopt ESTs may depend substantially on the extent to which science can explain why ESTs work and thereby provide clinicians with an empirically supported explanatory context in addition to effective interventions" (p. 68). Likewise, Power and Brewin (1997) noted that some clinicians

> simply bury their heads in the sand and continue with their favorite techniques. Others, like ourselves, are puzzled and

> are asking if there are common mechanisms that apply across different therapies that might explain both their effectiveness and their (sometimes) lack of effectiveness?" (p. xi).

The historical effort to understand the underlying causes of behavioral disorders was made not for this purpose per se, but mainly because such an understanding would hold the key to the mechanisms of therapeutic change. As noted by Willick (2001)

> we might ask whether it matters what theories of etiology we believe. Do they really influence our clinical work with patients? Of course, it matters to those of us interested in knowing what influences normal and pathological development. For those of us who believe that an understanding of those influences can inform our treatment, it certainly matters. We teach analytic courses on psychopathology ... in the hope that understanding how mental illness develops will guide us in treatment (p. 50).

Accordingly, a genuine therapeutic intervention must not only alleviate the individual's emotional state or symptoms. Rather, the therapy must identify the underlying causes of the behavioral change and take the proper actions to remove these motivating factors.

Part III aims to show that all therapeutic methods pertaining to neuroses and schizophrenia can be integrated within the theoretical framework of psycho-bizarreness theory (PBT). They all obtain their efficacy by affecting one or more components that according to PBT maintains the symptom. The specific therapies include cognitive behavioral therapy (CBT), punishment-reinforcement therapy, religious therapy, psychoanalysis, and drug treatment. Although these methods developed from theories that are conceptually different from PBT (with the exception of religious therapy, which lacks theoretical explanation), they can all be integrated within PBT's theoretical framework, which provides a more economic explanation of their efficacy.

From PBT's perspective, these therapies do not address the underlying causes of mad behaviors. Rather, they are all symptomatic interventions, including psychoanalysis, which itself accused rival approaches of merely treating symptoms rather than the causes that motivate and sustain them (Kazdin, 1982; Tryon, 2008). As will be demonstrated later, these therapies obtain their effects through one or more of the following techniques: (1) sabotaging the self-deceptive belief, and thus preventing the maintenance of unawareness of knowledge of self-involvement (KSI)/true reason (TR). As a result, the symptom becomes costly, losing its repressive value, and increasing the patient's tendency to abandon it; (2) decreasing the controllability value of the symptom by punishment-reinforcement procedures, which again increases the cost of the symptom; (3) diminishing the repressive value of the symptom by increasing the patient's awareness of KSI/TR; (4) relieving the emotional distress by artificial means, such as medications, and thus increasing the likelihood that patients will either adjust to the stress or resolve it.

Part III also suggests a new therapeutic method, Rational-Insight Therapy, which aims to increase patients' awareness of their current stressors and the faulty behavioral methods they use in addressing their problems. Simultaneously, it increases the patient's coping ability through training in coping skills. It should be noted that drug therapy will not be discussed in this part of the book, as it has been already addressed in Part I.

Neurosis

This section presents the original explanations of therapeutic methods pertaining to neurotic disorders and then suggests PBT's alternative explanation for each therapy. Thereby, it demonstrates that research and clinical data relating to each therapy can be integrated within PBT's theoretical framework. The therapies discussed here include CBT, punishment-reinforcement therapy, religious therapy, psychoanalysis, and placebo.

Cognitive Behavioral Therapy

Sabotaging the Self-Deceptive Belief: As elaborated on previously, behavior and cognitive theories attribute the cause of panic disorder and agoraphobia to conditioning and irrational thinking, respectively. The same theoretical approaches have been applied to the explanation of obsessive-compulsive disorder (OCD; Emmelkamp, 1987; Rachman & Hodgson, 1980). As with animals (e.g., Bouton & Swartzentruber, 1991), exposure therapy has been applied to extinguish fears associated with these behavioral disorders. While behavior researchers attribute this therapeutic effect to conditioning, in which patients learn new non-fearful reactions to the fear-arousing stimuli, cognitivists claim that exposure therapy educate patients to think rationally through confrontation with evidence incompatible with their belief (e.g., Beck, 1988; Hoffart, 1993). CBT is a combination of both exposure and cognitive therapy, in which patients are exposed to the fearful stimuli and at the same time are "educated" to think rationally by increasing their awareness about harmless nature of these stimuli (see Aaronson et al., 2008; Taylor, 2000).

As was indicated in the discussion section of Part II, both conditioning and cognitive theories of panic disorder and agoraphobia are confronted with serious challenges to their validity. In contrast, PBT can resolve these difficulties and integrate the findings of both theories into its theoretical framework. This is true also with regard to the therapeutic effects of these therapies. Accordingly, exposure therapy is seen as a therapeutic technique through which patients with bizarre anxiety or fears, including panic disorder, agoraphobia, and OCD, are confronted with incompatible evidence that challenges their self-deceptive beliefs. In this therapeutic method, patients are allowed to produce the first component of the symptom (i.e., fearful experience) but are not permitted to execute the second component of the symptom, that is, the maladaptive behavior (e.g., escape or washing hands). Since the fear has no basis in reality and is merely role-playing adopted as a distractive coping tool, it will subside. Consequently, patients are confronted with extrospective evidence of non-fearful behavior and introspective experience of a sense of control that are incompatible with the self-deceptive belief. These observations sabotage the self-deceptive cycle (Figure 1), which in turn threatens the validity of patients' self-deceptive belief. As a result, unless patients are able to rationalize the challenging evidence, they have to abandon the belief, and in turn the symptoms, as both lose their repressive benefits. This means that exposure does not extinguish the stimulus–response bond, which supposedly was established through conditioning, nor does it educate patients to think rationally. Instead, exposure merely sabotages the self-deceptive belief, counteracts the repressive value of both the belief and the symptom, and thereby, motivates patients to abandon them.

However, when the symptom is still needed for coping purposes, patients will invent self-deceptive excuses in order to resolve the cognitive dissonance caused by exposure therapy and thereby preserve the self-deceptive belief. For example, agoraphobic patients may attribute the incompatible evidence of not being afraid in public to the presence of supportive figures (e.g., therapist or relatives). Therefore, therapy often includes unaccompanied exposure as well. While this is usually part of the formal therapy (see Hafner, 1983; Hoffart, 1993; see also Al-Kubaisy et al., 1992), it can also be performed after the therapy is formally concluded, during therapists' systematic follow-up (e.g., Ollendick, 1995).

Similarly, exposure therapy in OCD is conducted not only in the presence of therapists, but it usually includes self-controlled exposure homework as well (e.g., Abramovitz, 1998; Emmelkamp, 1987; O'Kearney, 1993). The importance of unaccompanied exposure was particularly emphasized with checking rituals (e.g., Emmelkamp,

1982, 1987). Patients suffering from this disorder believe that they "possess pivotal power to provoke or prevent crucial negative outcomes" (Ladouceur, Leger, Rheaume, & Dube, 1996). "For this reason, exposure in the presence of the therapist is often not a genuine exposure, for the patient can easily transfer the responsibility for the action to the therapist" (Emmelkamp, 1987, p. 319).

The elimination of other self-deceptive excuses unique to each patient may also be essential in invalidating the deceptive self-diagnosis of illness. As noted by Salkovskis and Clark (1991), "it is often necessary to identify the factors which are currently preventing a disconfirmation of their beliefs, and then modify these factors" (p. 221). For example, if patients excuse their ability to control panic attacks by performing certain rituals (e.g., tensing muscles, or holding objects; Salkovskis & Clark, 1991), it is essential that exposure nullify these excuses. However, patients sometimes choose a self-deceptive excuse that is more difficult to challenge. For example, Hoffart (1993) described an agoraphobic patient who successfully exposed himself to various parts of the city without experiencing anxiety, yet maintained his deceptive diagnosis of illness by attributing the contradictory evidence to chance. Hoffart concluded, "in the future, he would be just as likely as before to experience over-whelming panic attacks in similar situations" (p. 85). Thus, therapists may not always succeed in disarming patients of their coping mechanism by exposure to incompatible evidence since sophisticated patients can employ self-deceptive excuses in order to nullify the threatening information.

PBT's claim that the therapeutic effect of exposure is because this intervention sabotages the patient's self-deceptive belief can also be applied to explain the therapeutic effect of cognitive therapy. A stated earlier, treatment based on the cognitive theoretical model increases patients' awareness of the catastrophic interpretation of bodily sensations and "educates" them to think rationally by challenging the logical basis of their fears. Thus, from PBT's standpoint, this therapeutic technique sabotages the patient's ability to rationalize their self-deceptive belief through deliberate misinterpretation of their bodily sensations. One application of this treatment strategy is "behavioral experiments" (Salkovskis & Clark, 1991). In this procedure, bodily sensations and panic symptoms are experimentally produced through a number of techniques, such as voluntary hyperventilation (e.g., Clark, Salkovskis, & Chalkley, 1985; Salkovskis & Clark, 1986; Salkovskis, Warwick, Clark, & Wessels, 1986), or reading and dwelling on words representing the catastrophic misinterpretation (e.g., palpitation-dying, breathless suffocation; Clark et al., 1988). This procedure is utilized both to increase patients' awareness of the sequence of bodily sensations and their catastrophic misinterpretation, and also for motivating them to replace the thoughts with non-catastrophic interpretations. Additionally, patients are trained in controlled breathing in order to cope with the hyperventilation sensations and thus facilitate the non-catastrophic interpretation of these sensations. Thus, once the patient's catastrophic misinterpretation is challenged, he or she cannot maintain the self-deceptive belief, and thereby, the manifestation of their bizarre behavior.

An important component of cognitive therapy is the arrangement of experimental or behavioral tests that could debase patients' defensive maneuvers inhibiting the effect of the therapy (e.g., see Hoffart, 1993, 1996; Salkovskis & Clark, 1991). For example, an agoraphobic patient who experienced frequent panic attacks at home, reported that she was unable to enter a room unless the windows or doors were left open (Salkovskis & Clark, 1991). The patient believed that with the windows and doors closed, no air could penetrate the room and that she might rapidly use up whatever existing air there was. In order to challenge this belief, the therapist sprayed air freshener in the corridor outside of room where the patient was sitting. Even though the door was closed, the patient detected the smell of the air freshener and realized that air could penetrate from the outside. Consequently, she was able to enter the room of her house with very little distress.

However, cognitivists have raised the possibility that the aforementioned results do not necessarily prove reeducation, for they can also be attributed to extinction techniques of exposure to bodily sensations or to respiratory control skills that reduce the inconvenient hyperventilation. Therefore, cognitive investigators have conducted research that demonstrates the obtaining of therapeutic gains solely by verbal means, in the absence of the behavioral components. For example, Salkovskis, Clark, and Hackmann (1991) have conducted an experiment aimed at examining the effect of "cognitive therapy without exposure or breathing retraining" (p. 161). Results showed that patients who were given "focal treatment" (i.e., therapy that helps to identify the maladaptive sequence of bodily sensations and their catastrophic misinterpretation, and challenges the patient's belief by providing evidence supporting a non-catastrophic interpretation) displayed a marked reduction in both catastrophic misinterpretation and panic attacks. In contrast, patients who were given "nonfocal treatment" (i.e., therapeutic discussions overlooked bodily sensations and focused instead on negative thoughts regarding life problems), showed no therapeutic benefit.

Given PBT's assumption that madness is aimed to ward off intolerable levels of stress, it is not surprising that a significant number of patients are reluctant to abandon their symptoms, so long as the stress persists. Accordingly, evidence shows that therapy dropout rates among panic disorder and agoraphobia patients may reach 20%–38% (e.g., Arthus, Cottraux, Mollard, Guerin, & Bouvard, 1997; Barlow, Gorman, Shear, & Woods, 2000; Clum, 1989; Haug et al., 2016; Keijsers, Kampman, & Hoogduin, 2001). Similar rates were found with OCD patients (e.g., Abramowitz, 2006; O'Conner, 2005; Schruers, Koning, Luermans, Haack, & Griez, 2005; Stanley & Turner, 1995; Tundo, Salvati, Busto, Di-Spigno, & Falcini, 2007). Although patients attributed their dropout to financial difficulties, time commitments, and schedule constraints (see Taylor, 2002, pp. 187–188), the possibility remains that these are mere excuses to rationalize the termination of the therapy.

Although CBT is an effective therapeutic intervention, its efficacy is limited. Many patients fail to respond to therapy, seek further therapy, develop problems unrelated to the symptom, or undergo relapse (e.g., Brown & Barlow, 1995; Hafner, 1976; Hoffart, 1993; O'Kearney, 1993; O'Sullivan & Marks, 1991; Westen & Morrison, 2001). Moreover, only a small percentage (21%–27%) of those who completed therapy demonstrated high end-state functioning, defined as a clinical cure or functioning within a normative range (e.g., Fisher & Wells, 2005; Jacobson, Wilson, & Tupper, 1988). This limited efficacy may be much lower when considering Westen, Novotny, and Thompson-Brenner's (2004; see also Westen & Morrison, 2001) critique, especially their claim that subjects in EST studies were not randomly assigned to different experimental groups. Instead, patients were "screened to maximize homogeneity of diagnosis and minimize co-occurring conditions that could increase variability of treatment response" (p. 632). From PBT's standpoint, the limited efficacy of CBT stems from the therapy's failure to address the underlying stressor of the neurotic symptom. Indeed, studies have shown that coping skills training, which increase the patient's ability to deal with the initial stressor, enhances the efficacy of CBT (e.g., Biran, 1990; Chambless, Goldstein, Gallagher, & Bright, 1986; Chernen & Friedman, 1993; Craske, Burton, & Barlow, 1989; Hiss, Foa, & Kozak, 1994; O'Kearney, 1993; Richards, Klein, & Austin, 2006).

In conclusion, in line with cognitive theory, PBT views patients' belief as a crucial factor in maintaining neurotic symptoms, such as panic disorder and OCD. However, contrary to the cognitive model, the belief does not reflect irrational thinking. Rather, it constitutes part of patients' cognitive maneuvers in maintaining the unawareness of KSI. Accordingly, while cognitive theory maintains that CBT reeducates patients to think rationally, PBT claims that this intervention merely sabotages patients' self-deceptive beliefs. The advantage of PBT is that it not only integrates the therapeutic findings of CBT, but that it also resolves fundamental problems that challenge the validity of both cognitive and behavior theories of panic disorder and agoraphobia, as specified in the discussion section of Part II.

Religious Therapy

When the symptom is appearing to be activated by a specific stimulus in reality (e.g., dirt in OCD), the best therapeutic intervention for disconfirming the self-deceptive belief is CBT. However, when patients attribute their symptoms to supernatural forces, as is more prevalent in non-Western countries, the most effective therapeutic intervention is religious therapy (e.g., see Alonso & Jeffrey, 1988; Endrawes, O'Brien, & Wilkes, 2007; Hoffman, Laub, & Zim, 1990; Kua, Sim, & Chee, 1986; Razali, 1999; Seltzer, 1983; Wijesinghe, Dissanayake, & Mendis, 1976; Witztum, Grisaru, & Budowski, 1996). The efficiency of this treatment results from the psychological power of the religious figure (e.g., a rabbi, priest, or shaman) to neutralize the evil forces to which patients attribute their symptoms, and thus sabotage the patients' self-deceptive belief. As noted by Kua et al. (1986)

> the healer establishes himself as someone who has extraordinary power and can communicate with supernatural forces. During therapy the healer goes into a trance, and this usually fills the audience with awe and reinforces his status (p. 363).

Resistance to the religious figure's suggestion would be considered heresy. Consequently, once the deceptive function of the self-deceptive belief is sabotaged, it becomes difficult for patients to prolong the symptom and thus increases their tendency to abandon it.

For example, Pattison and Wintrob (1981) reported a case of a young Mexican woman who complained of nightmares and nightly visitations from her fiancée following his death, and believed she was possessed. In the treatment session with the woman, the therapist invited the fiancée's ghost into the house and explained to it that it was now dead, must leave the patient alone, and find an appropriate place for the dead. The ghost was then dismissed out the door and the patient's symptoms subsided rapidly. Similarly, Wijesinghe et al. (1976) described the successful treatment of a spirit possession in which, "the shaman trapped the spirit in the bottle and threw it into the sea, and the subject remained well since" (p. 137). Likewize, Csordas (1987), describing a number of successful religious therapy cases, mentioned a case of a university professor who suddenly developed dissociative fugue, claiming spiritual possession, following a conflict with her husband. Although she had spent 2 years in psychoanalysis prior to the symptom, she refused psychiatric treatment and demanded religious therapy. The psychiatrist, at a loss, advised her to seek a prominent member of a certain cult in Brazil, and, upon filling the cult's religious obligations, she completely recovered.

In another example, Hoffman et al. (1990) described three case studies in which therapists enlisted the services of a rabbi, resulting in a successful therapeutic outcome for religiously observant patients. In one particular case, a 14-year-old Orthodox Jewish boy had suffered the loss of a friend and was subsequently preoccupied with thoughts of her spirit coming to harm him. The rabbi successfully relieved the patient's emotional difficulties by denying the existence of spirits in the Holy Land and by encouraging the patient to say a special prayer every day, "in order to thwart unwanted and frightening thoughts and imaginings" (p. 181).

Razali (1999) described a case of a 38-year-old female Malaysian Muslim, who suddenly developed hysterical paralysis after her husband took a second wife. A number of traditional healers and medical practitioners unsuccessfully treated her, before agreeing to participate in a popular Malaysian spirit-raising séance (*Main Puteri*), which lasted 3 days. The patient's symptom was completely removed on the third day of the "performance," which was attributed to the departure of the "evil spirits" from her body. Thus, since the patient deceived herself that evil forces controlled her symptoms and believed that the "therapist's" rituals "cured" her from these forces, she could no longer rationalize the maintenance of her deviant behavior and therefore she was obliged to abandon it. Kok (1975) describes three additional case studies of conversion disorder in which religious rituals, including the recitation of passages from the Qur'an and offerings of a goat's head or a number of eggs had a curative effect.

Religious authoritative figures can be employed to facilitate the therapy when patients deny deviancy on the grounds of religious belief. For example, Meyer (in Rachman & Hodgson, 1980) described a case study of a religious middle-aged Jewish woman who performed multiple eating and checking rituals. The patient denied that her behavior was deviant, claiming that it had a rational foundation. After unsuccessful attempts to modify the patient's behavior, Meyer arranged for a distinguished rabbi to visit the patient and confirm that she had taken her, "ritual activities to irrational extremes" (p. 19).

Psychodynamic Therapy

According to psychoanalysis, a true recovery from neurosis necessitates the lifting of repression, that is, gaining insight into the underlying causes of deviant behaviors (e.g., see Bachrach, 1996; Barber & Lane, 1995; Bloom, 2003; Charman, 2003; Eagle, 2000; Rofé, 2008). However, studies challenge the existence of both Freudian repression (e.g., McNally, 2003; Piper, Pope, & Borowiecki, 2000; Rofé, 2008) and the unconscious (e.g., Greenwald, 1992; Kihlstrom, 1989, 2000, 2002, 2004; Kihlstrom, Barnhardt, & Tataryn, 1992; O'Brien & Jureidini, 2002; Rofé, 2008). Hence, although psychodynamic therapy has been found effective for neurotic disorders, including eating disorders (e.g., see review by Fonagy, Roth, & Higgitt, 2005), panic disorder (Milrod et al., 2007), and **dissociative identity disorder** (**DID**; e.g., Kihlstrom,

2005; Kluft, 1995), researchers have attributed this efficacy to other factors, such as placebo (e.g., Grünbaum, 1984, 1986, 2007; Jopling, 2001).

One alternative explanation is that the therapeutic success of psychoanalysis, similar to religious therapy, results from the therapist's ability to sabotage the patient's self-deceptive belief. This seems especially applicable to DID, where psychodynamic therapy, in combination with hypnosis, appears to be the therapy of choice (e.g., Adams, 1990; Berman, 1981; Bliss, 1980; Boyd, 1997; Coons, 1994; Dell & Eisenhower, 1990; Kluft, 1987, 1995; Putnam & Loewenstein, 1993; Waiess, 2006; Wilbur, 1984b). Considering claims that DID patients implicitly conceptualize their symptoms as a reflection of unconscious forces (Spanos, Weekes, & Bertrand, 1985; see also Spanos, Weekes, Menary, & Bertrand, 1986), it seems that just like religious therapy, psychodynamic interventions are successful with these patients (e.g., Boyd, 1997; Coons, 1994; Kluft, 1995; Putnam & Loewenstein, 1993; Waiess, 2006) mainly because they succeed in sabotaging patients' self-deceptive beliefs. Since patients deceive themselves that they are "possessed" by evil forces of the unconscious (see Leonard, 1927), the psychoanalytic ritual conducted by a prestigious therapist, produces a new belief that they have been cured of the noxious components of this system. Consequently, since patients can no longer rationalize the symptom by attributing it to forces beyond their conscious control, this should motivate them to abandon it. This claim is consistent with Sampson's (1992) statement that analysts' attitudes are important to the therapeutic process, to the extent that they disconfirm patients' pathogenic beliefs. "If the patient unconsciously perceives the analyst's behavior and attitudes as disconfirming the belief he is testing, the patient will make progress. In this way, direct experiences with the analyst may sometimes lead to significant analytic progress even without interpretation" (pp. 519–520; see also Spanos, 1996; Spanos et al., 1985).

A second explanation of the therapeutic effect of psychoanalysis is lifting of repression. As was indicated in Part I and II, patients become unaware of the underlying causes of their behaviors through the repressive/distractive effects of the symptoms and self-deceptive processes. Accordingly, despite the lack of empirical support for the psychoanalytic concept of lifting of repression, this concept can still be useful in explaining the positive therapeutic effects of psychodynamic therapy to the extent that the therapist increases patients' insight to the current stressor rather than to childhood trauma. Once a patient becomes aware of the underlying motivational factors of thcir symptoms, this behavior loses its repressive effect and increases the patient's willingness to abandon it. The abandonment of the symptom may aggravate patients' depression and result in relapse if the original stressor remains at the same level of intensity. A genuine recovery should occur when the stressor is removed or when the patient is capable of coping with the stressor with the therapist's support and encouragement.

A clinical example demonstrating this theoretical position can be found in a successful psychoanalytic intervention with a 28-year-old married woman suffering from agoraphobia (Wolitzky & Eagle, 1999). The patient's husband had taken a new job about 50 miles from the city where the couple and her parents lived. Planning to move to another city, the couple sold their old apartment, and temporarily moved with their 3-month-old baby into the patient's parents' house. The patient's mother suffered from kidney disease, and from an early age, it had been the patient's job to change the filters for her mother's dialysis machine. According to the authors, "the anticipated move to the new city appeared to precipitate the outbreak of agoraphobic symptoms" (p. 209). At the initial stage of therapy, the husband agreed to change his plan, and seek a job in the city where they lived. Although this caused some emotional relief, it did not affect the patient's agoraphobic symptoms, which persisted at the same level of intensity. The symptoms gradually disappeared when the patient became aware of her conflict pertaining to separation from her sick mother. Soon afterward, the patient moved with her husband and their baby into a new apartment across the street from her parent's house. A follow-up to 5 years showed that the patient remained symptom-free.

From PBT's standpoint, the patient's agoraphobic symptoms played two psychological functions: (1) the husband's decision to move to a new city exacerbated the patient's emotional distress. The symptoms, therefore, constituted a rational counter reaction that compelled him to reconsider his decision; (2) the symptoms intensively preoccupied the patient's attention, thus enabling her to become unaware of her intrapsychic conflict surrounding the separation from her mother. Once the therapy succeeded in generating insight into this conflict, the symptom lost its repressive value and motivated the patient eventually to abandon it. Awareness, however, did not change the patient's apprehension that separation might endanger her mother's life. Nevertheless, this did not aggravate the patient's emotional distress, and a relapse did not occur, because she resolved this problem in an optimal way by separating from her mother, while staying within the close vicinity.

Temple (2001) treated a hospitalized 15-year-old girl suffering from hysterical limb paralysis, using the psychodynamic interpretative method. The patient was in a conflict with her mother concerning her sexual autonomy. The conversion symptoms allowed her to distract her attention from the source of her conflict (i.e., the autonomy over her sexuality), distance herself from her mother (i.e., the stressor), and manipulate her parents to provide sympathy and attention through hospitalization. The psychodynamic interpretive therapy focused on the patient's current stressor and thus increased her awareness of the underlying causes of her behavior. Consequently, the symptom lost its distractive value and "enabled her to find more appropriate ways of recognizing her feelings and the necessity for her to be paralyzed gradually reduced" (p. 292).

However, since the patient did not have sufficient coping abilities, she redisplayed her pathological coping mechanism, "when she was under stress or when a discussion about her return home took place" (p. 292).

In another case study (Viederman, 1995), a 68-year-old Jewish orthodox man was excluded from the local synagogue by the Rabbi who was persuaded to do so by the man's son-in-law. Knowing the father-in-law's aggressive temperament and fearing that he might do "something destructive to his reputation," the family decided to send him on a trip to Florida. Upon his return when he learned of the family's "conspiracy," he developed conversion symptoms expressed by rigidity of the legs and weakness in the neck muscles. From PBT's standpoint, the symptoms improved the patient's emotional condition as they enabled him to: (a) repress his angry feelings resulting from his perception of his family's "subversive" behavior and their "loss of confidence in him"; (b) rationalize his absence in the prayer services at the synagogue; and (c) receive sympathy and support from his wife, children, and perhaps even from the community members.

The brief psychodynamic interpretative method, consisting of 6 weekly meetings, was aimed to increase the patient's awareness of his *current stressor*. For example, the therapist told the patient "you have been unable to walk, because you are afraid to walk into the synagogue. You are afraid of how angry you are. Your confidence has been undermined … I think your symptom will go away with this knowledge. Now get up, and walk around the room comfortably and *without* the cane" (p. 406). The increased awareness of the stressor decreased the repressive value of the symptoms, and thus increased the patient's tendency to abandon these behaviors. Additional contributing factors were the therapist's suggestions, encouragement, and sympathy as well as the participation of his wife in therapy, where the couple "spoke openly and freely to one another of their affections and their dissatisfactions" (p. 405).

Punishment-Reinforcement Therapy

Given PBT's assumption that cost-benefit considerations guide the adoption and maintenance of mad behaviors, it is expected that punishment procedures that reduce the controllability value of the symptom, as well as reinforcement measures that encourage more adaptive behaviors, will increase patients' tendency to abandon this behavior. Indeed, research on ***conversion disorder*** (e.g., Blanchard & Hersen, 1976; Donohue, Thevenin, & Runyon, 1997; Goldblatt & Munitz, 1976; Gooch, Wolcott, & Speed, 1997; Mizes, 1985; Teasell & Shapiro, 1994), OCD (e.g., Brooker, 1982; Emmelkamp, 1987; Kenny, Mowbray, & Lalani, 1978; Kenny, Solyom, & Solyom, 1973; McGuire & Vallance, 1964), and ***anorexia nervosa*** (e.g., Bemis, 1987; Blue, 1979; Okamoto et al., 2002; Touyz, Beumont, Glaun, Phillips, & Cowie, 1984) shows that behavioral therapy that decreases the utility of the symptom (e.g., withdrawal of attention, monetary rewards, and hospital privileges) or increases its cost through punishments (i.e., electric shock and bed confinement), facilitates positive therapeutic outcome.

For example, Tucher and Long (1985) described the case of a 22-year-old soldier who developed hysterical blindness in one eye after experiencing difficulty in adjusting to military stress. The behavioral treatment consisted of verbal reinforcements for the patient's reports of visual improvement, and aversive consequences that included withholding hospital privileges (e.g., time off ward, use of civilian clothes) until the subject's vision improved. The patient was also given a rationale for improvement when instructed to wear an eyepatch over his good left eye in order to "exercise and train" his defective right eye. The subject was told that most people with visual problems improve within 3 days when wearing an eye patch, with complete recovery by the fifth day. The patient reported almost normal vision on the fifth day of treatment and remained so at the 3-day follow-up.

Tucher and Long claimed that, due to the multiple factors employed (reinforcement, punishment, suggestion, and hospitalization), it is difficult to determine the exact cause for the behavioral change. However, taking into consideration studies demonstrating the controllability function of conversion symptoms in military settings (e.g., Ironside & Batchelor, 1945; Mucha & Reinhart, 1970), it seems likely that reinforcement-punishment procedures played a major role in the recovery process. Nevertheless, it is possible that the therapy counteracted the distractibility value of the symptom as well. Prior to therapy, the patient was able to deceive himself that his vision was mediated through the good eye. However, when the patch was put on his good eye, the patient's "bad eye" was constantly bombarded with evidence incompatible with his self-deceptive belief. Consequently, the patient's self-deceptive belief was sabotaged, and thereby the symptom lost its distractibility value. Thus, while it is not possible to determine the exact causes of the therapeutic outcome, both these explanations are consistent with PBT's theoretical assumption.

However, while the punishment-reinforcement therapeutic strategy decreases the controllability value of the symptom and thus facilitates its abandonment, it may result in an adverse therapeutic impact if the stress is high and patients truly lack adequate coping skills. In such cases, patients are likely to exhibit signs of depression and anxiety, suffer aggravated symptoms, or display symptom substitution (e.g., Blanchard & Hersen, 1976; Rachman & Hodgson, 1980, p. 121; Thorpe, Schmidt, Brown, & Castell, 1964; Wilson, 1999). Moreover, punishment techniques that increase the aversive nature (i.e., cost) of the symptom may encourage patients to adopt more extreme coping measures. For example, Kenny et al. (1973) reported that out of five obsessive-compulsive patients that were subjected to aversive therapy, three greatly improved, one improved only moderately (she subsequently developed nightmares), and one became psychotic. Kenny et al. (1973) noted that, "it seems that, as therapy progresses, the faradic disruption technique [shock treatment] increases anxiety and may even 'push' some susceptible patients into psychosis" (p. 455). Similarly, Bevan (1960) reported that electroconvulsive therapy (ECT), which is conceived by some investigators as an aversive stimulus (e.g., Berke, 1981; Fitzgerald, 1973; Furlong, 1972; Ganesan, 1986), was only temporarily effective in the treatment of a woman who suffered from obsessive ruminations. Relapse of the obsessional thoughts was observed and several additional ECTs were ineffective in completely suppressing the thoughts.

It appears that the behaviorists method of punishment-reinforcement may be helpful when the stress is relatively low and patients have the ability to cope if the escape to bizarreness becomes too costly. However, amongst those with poor coping skills, successful outcomes might necessitate coping skills training. For example, Blanchard and Hersen (1976) employed behavioral extinction procedures to treat several case studies of conversion disorder, which included removing the reinforcement (i.e., controllability value) of the symptom, known as secondary gains (e.g., sympathy and attention). However, this symptomatic intervention was insufficient, as symptom substitution occurred when subjects encountered new stressful situations. Effective and long-lasting therapy occurred only when the extinction procedure was accompanied by coping skills training as well. The authors note that

> it would appear that because of a faulty learning history this type of patient has not developed the requisite social skills needed to cope with both the usual and more unusual stresses encountered in life. Therefore, training or retraining in social skills becomes a needed ingredient in a comprehensive therapeutic regime. (p. 127)

Placebo

Occasionally, mere participation in a therapeutic intervention results in a positive outcome. For example, Carl Gustav Jung (1963) informed a middle-aged female patient, who had been suffering from a painful paralyzed leg for 17 years, that he was going to hypnotize her.

Without any hypnotic manipulation, the patient immediately fell into a deep trance and talked without pause for over a half hour, resisting Jung's attempts to awaken her. Soon afterward, she declared herself cured, threw away her crutches, and proceeded to walk. Jung, whose theoretical framework could not account for this unexpected result, announced to his students, "now you've seen what can be done with hypnosis" (p. 120). However, he noted, "in fact I had not the slightest idea what had happened" (p. 120). From PBT's standpoint, it seems likely that the patient unconsciously desired to abandon her symptom even before she sought treatment. However, she felt uncomfortable doing so after so many years of paralysis, and resolved this problem through a pseudo-treatment intervention by a prestigious therapist. This provided her with a rationale (i.e., a self-deceptive excuse), which justified the behavioral change and prevented the aversive feelings of cognitive dissonance and social embarrassment that she might have experienced by spontaneous remission. As noted by Ullmann and Krasner (1975)

> Once the person has made the act, and performed the new role, he cannot shift back into his prior role … The person may continue to play the role because not doing so would cast doubt on his prior behavior in that role. *This is one reason why a placebo may be effective: It gives the person an "out," saves face and avoids many of the aversive consequences in "giving up" the "sick" behavior*. [Italics added] (p. 256; see also Mooney & Gurrister, 2004).

Schizophrenia

The three major therapeutic methods for schizophrenia are drug therapy, psychoanalysis, and CBT. The former two were already discussed in Part I. The third therapy is addressed in the following.

Cognitive Behavioral Therapy

Explanation and Theoretical Weaknesses: Similar to neurosis, cognitive theory attributes the etiology of schizophrenia to irrational thinking. Researchers strengthen this argument through studies demonstrating that patients suffer from neurological, cognitive impairments (e.g., Moritz, Vitzthum, Randjbar, Veckernstedt, & Woodward, 2010; Nuechterlein et al., 2015; Sarin & Wallin, 2014; Skodlar, Henriksen, Sass, Nelson, & Parnas, 2013; Tai & Turkington, 2009). Accordingly, numerous studies demonstrate that educating patients to think rationally through CBT alleviates patients' symptoms (e.g., Morrison, 2009; Sarin & Wallin, 2014; Sarin, Wallin, & Widerlov, 2011; Turkington, Kingdon, & Weiden, 2006; Turkington et al., 2008; Wykes, Steel, Everitt, & Tarrier, 2008). These findings appeared so impressive that both the National Institute for Clinical Excellence in the United Kingdom (NISE, 2003, 2009) and the National Board of Health and Welfare (NBH, 2006) in Sweden, recommended this therapy for schizophrenic patients. Before suggesting PBT's integrative model of these findings, the following comments need to be taken into consideration:

1. Cognitive theory does not seem able to explain the complexity of schizophrenia. For example, it is difficult to see how cognitivists' concept of irrationality can explain the large heterogeneity of schizophrenic symptoms, such as those of Nash, Unabomber, Percy King, and Jennifer, discussed in Part I. How can they accommodate cases of patients suffering from neurological damages alongside data indicating that most patients have no brain abnormality (e.g., Williams, 2012)? Additionally, the concept of irrationality is inconsistent with evidence reviewed in Part I indicating that schizophrenia improves the individual's quality of life.

2. Several anomalies used by cognitivists to support the assumption of irrationality can be explained in rational terms. One example is jumping to conclusions (JTC). Cognitivists interpret this cognitive bias as a reflection of irrational thinking, which supposedly causes the formation and the maintenance of the schizophrenic delusions (e.g., Moritz et al., 2010; Sarin & Wallin, 2014). In contrast, as previously specified, PBT views JTC as a rational maneuver enabling patients to rationalize their self-belief and thus preserve their unawareness. Schizophrenics also display "confirmation bias," in which patients look for evidence consistent with their belief (Bronstein & Cannon, 2017; Freeman, Garety, Kuipers, Fowler, & Bebbingtom, 2002; Sarin & Wallin, 2014), and "attributional bias," in which the blame for negative events is assigned to external factors (e.g., Janssen et al., 2006; Kuipers et al., 2006; Moritz et al., 2010; Moritz & Woodward, 2007). Here too, as elaborated on before, from PBT's point of view, the confirmation bias is a rational maneuver by which patients validate their self-deceptive beliefs.

3. The therapeutic efficacy of CBT is not yet firmly established. Although numerous studies strongly support the efficacy of CBT in schizophrenia, Lynch, Laws, and McKenna (2010) argued that these studies did not consider the potential influence of blindness or the use of control interventions. Accordingly, a meta-analysis in which these factors were taken into account showed that CBT is no better at reducing schizophrenic symptoms or in preventing relapse than usual therapy (Lynch et al., 2010). Similar results were found by Kennedy and Xyrichis (2017). Lynch et al.'s study was criticized on methodological grounds (Hutton, 2013) and a meta-analysis study performed by Sarin, Wallin, and Widerlöv (2011) showed that CBT yielded better outcomes a few months after treatment. However, a more recent meta-analysis, which only included studies in which assessments were carried out by interviewers masked to treatment assignment, found that CBT has a therapeutic effect only in a small range (Jauhar et al., 2014). The authors noted

> given that we, and others including NICE [National Institute for Health and Care Excellence], have found evidence for only small effects on overall symptoms, plus the fact that a large, methodologically rigorous 2008 trail

> failed to demonstrate any effective against relapse, the UK government's continued vigorous advocacy of this form of treatment ... might be considered puzzling" (p. 27).

4. Even if CBT is better therapy than rival interventions, cognitive theory cannot explain why other therapies may also be successful, as demonstrated earlier in the psychoanalytic therapy of Mr. X. (Karon, 2008). Wood and Joseph (2010), in criticizing investigators' effort to demonstrate the superior efficacy of CBT with schizophrenia, argued that, "the research focus should now move from establishing the effectiveness of any one technique, toward studying what common mechanisms underlie all therapeutic contact" (p. 1055).

Mechanisms Affecting the Therapeutic Change: CBT in schizophrenia is a heterogeneous therapy (e.g., see Jones, Hacker, Cormac, Meaden, & Irving, 2012; Tai & Turkington, 2009), which can be classified from PBT's standpoint into techniques that sabotage patients' self-deceptive belief and stress management procedures.

1. Sabotaging the Self-Deceptive Belief: CBT's basic assumption is that the information processing of external and internal stimuli of schizophrenic patients is biased, thereby, "causing systematic distortions of the individual's construction of experience" (Skodlar et al., 2013, p. 252). "Examples of such inappropriate processing of stimuli are 'jumping to conclusion,' 'confirmation biases and externalization, which are specific to positive symptoms" (Sarin & Wallin, 2014, p. 146). "The aim of CBT is thus to change the cognitive errors, dysfunctional beliefs and negative schemas ... that generate the symptoms" (Skodlar et al., 2013, p. 252). Accordingly, the main component of CBT's conventional technique is to challenge the rational and realistic basis of the patient's self-deceptive belief. As noted by Alford and Correia (1994), "the belief in itself was not the focus of discussion; instead, emphasis was placed on evaluating the evidence on which the belief was based ... the subjects themselves were encouraged to articulate arguments against their own beliefs" (p. 19).

One commonly used technique is Socratic questioning aimed "to encourage the probing of the evidence, reason, and rational" of the belief (Tai & Turkington, 2009, p. 866). Another technique is to ask a series of peripheral questions about the person's belief, and thereby to question the rational basis of the belief. For example, a patient was asked, "how could others control your thoughts? What mechanism would they use? … Can microchips really be inserted without your knowledge when you are asleep? … Shall we find out — perhaps on the Internet — what we can about the use of microchips in operations? Also we could check about regulations concerning such operations" (Turkington et al., 2006, p. 368). An additional challenging procedure is to discuss the details of patients' experiences. For example, the clinician can ask the patient "is it like somebody talking to you? Or shouting? … Do other people hear their voices? If not, why not?" (Turkington et al., 2006, p. 368; see also Sarin & Wallin, 2014). CBT also uses a technique called normalization, where the therapist informs patients that their positive symptoms are experienced by normal people as a result of stress, anxiety, sleep deprivation, or other factors (e.g., Sarin & Wallin, 2014; Tai & Turkington, 2009).

Contrary to CBT's assumption that the schizophrenic biased information processing is irrational, PBT claims that the schizophrenic cognitive errors are deliberate and an integral part of the patient's deceptive maneuvers to alleviate their intolerable level of stress. Accordingly, CBT's challenging techniques are viewed as systematic efforts to disarm patients' self-deceptive conviction that their delusions and hallucinations are based on solid evidence. Similarly, the normalization technique sterilizes the coping value of the schizophrenic symptoms and thus increases the patient's tendency to abandon these behaviors. In other words, when therapy leads patients to interpret their hallucinations as a normal phenomenon, it aims to diminish the controllability and distractive values of the symptom. Consequently, since the symptom becomes useless in combating stress-related thoughts, especially when "normalization" is combined with systematic efforts to demolish patients' self-deceptive belief, the patient is motivated to abandon it. In effect, CBT needs to be seen as a cognitive struggle between the therapists equipped with better ammunition to sabotage patients' self-deceptive belief, and the patient who has usually no choice but to obey the therapist's implicit demands to abandon his pathological coping mechanism.

However, the effect of this therapy is highly limited both because (1) sometimes "the patient's delusions are fixed and are not able to be changed" (Sarin & Wallin, 2014, p. 149); (2) it does not address the motivational stressor and therefore cannot yield a real recovery. A case study demonstrating the latter claim is reported by Kinderman and Benn (2002).

2. Stress Management Techniques: The Case of Carol (Bradshaw, 1998): The cognitivists' basic assumption that schizophrenic positive symptoms stem from flawed information processing and that patients should be educated to think rationally is challenged by the fact that stress management techniques alone, used by cognitive therapists, might be effective, as illustrated in case study by Bradshaw (1998).

Carol, a 26-year single white female, was raised in a family where academic success was highly important. She was shy but had a few friends with whom she went out occasionally. After graduation from high school, Carol went to college, where she developed an undifferentiated type of schizophrenia and as a result was hospitalized a number of times. She dropped out college, could not work, and remained supported by the Supplemental Security Income and her family. Carol did not have a family history of mental illness and showed no evidence of brain damage. CBT intervention in this case was highly successful since it enabled Carol to restore the normal functioning that she displayed before going to college.

Unlike the conventional CBT method, in Carol's case, "hallucinations and delusions were not directly challenged, but were interpreted as reactions to stress, personal or interpersonal concerns. The focus was on the context triggering these symptoms rather than on their content" (pp. 19–20). Recovery was obtained by series of therapeutic actions that enhanced Carol's coping skills and removed the stressors maintaining the schizophrenic symptoms. The main components of therapy were as follow:

a. Increasing the patient's awareness to her maladaptive reactions and encouraging productive activities: Carol was instructed to record her activities during the morning, afternoon, and evening in order to manage stress and anxiety and reinforce her coping skills. Both the patient and therapist reviewed this record to identify behaviors that exacerbated or improved her condition. Consequently, Carol became aware of her reactions to different events and their effects on her emotional state. Additionally, she was encouraged to increase her productive activities, initially by focusing on "daily living activities," such as self-care, cooking, cleaning, and time management. Subsequently, after exploring her previous interests and using an interest inventory, she expanded her activities to a wider range. For example, Carol had been previously interested in arts and crafts; thus, she was encouraged to paint and learned macramé (a form of textile making). Further, Carol learned stress management skills, which included relaxation method (meditation) which she practiced for short periods each session, and then daily for 15 minutes. She learned to identify personal signs of stress and symptoms of relapse. These experiences were organized on a "stress thermometer" as low, medium, and high. As soon as she became aware of these incidences, she would meditate briefly as a coping response.

b. Enhancement of social skills: Since Carol's major source of stress was social situations, as is typical in schizophrenia, a special effort was made to enhance her social skills. One problem concerned misreading and misinterpretation of social cues. In order to address this issue, "she was trained to 'check it out' by identifying automatic thoughts, evaluating evidence, exploring alternative explanations and generating new coping self-statements to replace the automatic thoughts" (p. 19). Specific stressful situations were identified and plans were made for adequate coping responses. "Cognitive coping skills were developed by collaborative empiricism, guided discovery, cognitive modeling, rehearsal, role-play and homework assignments" (p. 20).

c. Preventative measures for preventing relapse: As Carol made major progress in various areas of her life (e.g., taking a class at the community college, going out with friends, worked 10 hours a week as a volunteer at a food store), she experienced anxiety, fatigue, or depression within normal limits, which she interpreted as "I'm going crazy." These fears of relapse were addressed by educating her to interpret them as normal reactions to stress, and by taking preventative actions, which included a review of her "stress thermometer, schedule of activities, sleep pattern, exercise, diet and level of stimulation" (p. 20). Additionally, her fears were challenged using "Socratic questioning, examining evidence and alternative explanations" (p. 20).

d. Enhancement of self-concept: Other therapeutic activities included specific programs aimed to strengthen Carol's self-concept (e.g., she was asked to identify three positive events in her life each day) and several techniques, which helped her preserve the therapeutic changes.

Six months and 1-year follow-ups showed that Carol almost completely recovered as she displayed major improvements in work, independent living, social, and family relationships. "There were few symptoms present and little distress reported by her. Interpersonal functioning was relatively unimpaired and affect and cognition were within normal limits" (p. 22).

This case study strengthens PBT's claim that stress, rather than irrational thinking, is the underlying cause of schizophrenia. This evidence sharply contrasts the disease model of schizophrenia. In accordance with this claim, recent study shows that enhancing stress regulation and lowering the distress due to psychotic symptoms by CBT, reduces the pituitary volume, which plays a key role in physiological stress regulation (Premkumar et al., 2018).

Conclusions

Cognitive theory is too simple to account for the complex phenomena of schizophrenia. The implicit claim that patients, both neurotics and psychotics, are in effect "stupid" and need to be educated to think rationally fails to consider the intolerable level of stress with which they are confronted. CBT is a heterogeneous therapy composed of two major interventions: belief challenging techniques and stress management. While both interventions can be accounted for by PBT, it seems that cognitive theory would have difficulty explaining why the later intervention yields better therapeutic results.

Discussion: Mechanisms of Therapeutic Change

As demonstrated earlier, all therapies pertaining to neuroses and schizophrenia obtain their therapeutic effects of abandoning the symptom by affecting one of the mechanisms which according to PBT maintain this behavior. This therapeutic goal is obtained by one of the following methods:

1. Sabotaging Self-Deceptive Belief: Some therapies nullify the patient's self-deceptive belief and thereby pose cognitive difficulty in redisplaying the symptom. One example is **CBT** which either increases patients' awareness of the illogical basis of their beliefs or confronts them with inconsistent evidence. A second example is **religious therapy**, where a prestigious religious figure of the same faith performs some ritual that supposedly neutralizes the harmful effects of supernatural forces. A third example is **psychoanalysis**, where a prestigious psychoanalyst deceives patients through psychoanalytic rituals (e.g., hypnosis or free association) that they have been freed from the evil effects of "repressed trauma," which supposedly controlled their behavior.

2. Changing the Cost-Benefit Equilibrium: This behavioral method, which is effective especially with conversion disorder and anorexia nervosa, motivates patients to abandon their symptoms by increasing the cost of these behaviors.

3. Lifting of Repression: This method, originally suggested by psychoanalysis, increases the patient's insight regarding the current stressor. Thereby, it nullifies the repressive value of the symptom and thus diminishes the utility of this behavior. The efficacy of this intervention was demonstrated with a number of disorders, such as conversion disorder and agoraphobia.

4. Stress Management: Although traditional theories do not view current stressors as the central cause of psychological disorders, categorized by PBT as madness, therapies promoted by these theories incorporate coping skills training as central components of a genuine recovery.

5. Alleviation of Depression: Drug therapy, which was discussed in Part I, does not have curative effects as in physical diseases. Apparently, both antidepressants and antipsychotics alleviate patients' emotional distress and consequently some may temporarily renounce the symptoms. Sometimes, drugs have an indirect curative effect either because patients are given time-out from depression, which allows them to search for more adaptive solutions to their stressors, or because of positive events that occur during this period.

6. Placebo: Placebo may be effective when patients search for excuses to abandon their symptoms, either because the stress has already been removed or because they have become habituated to it.

In sum, despite tremendous research efforts, researchers have arrived at the conclusion that it is impossible to integrate the various therapeutic methods into one theoretical framework (e.g., see reviews by Feixas & Botella, 2004; Lampropoulos, 2000, 2001). PBT succeeds in implementing this goal for two major reasons: First, the five criteria of madness enable us to classify neurosis and schizophrenia under one theoretical roof. Second, contrary to the axiomatic assumption of traditional theories, clinical and research data show that these behaviors are rational coping mechanisms that individuals intuitively adopt when confronted with an extreme level of stress. This new insight of the underlying mechanisms that control the adoption and maintenance of madness enable us to integrate all therapeutic methods pertaining to these behaviors under one theoretical umbrella.

Efficacy of Traditional Therapies

Throughout the last century, the issue of symptom substitution was at the core of a bitter theoretical dispute between psychoanalysts and behaviorists. According to psychoanalysis, a necessary condition for successful therapy is the removal of the underlying causes of the symptom. Failing to do so would lead to symptom substitution. In contrast, behaviorists, based on learning theories, disregard the etiology of the symptom, believing that the goal of therapy is the attainment of positive behavioral change. This controversy seemingly ended with the victory of the behaviorists as researchers arrived at the conclusion that the "clinical concerns regarding the danger of symptom substitution were greatly exaggerated and are essentially baseless in fact" (Tryon, 2008, p. 967). However, this conclusion is premature since, as demonstrated earlier, from PBT's perspective, all these therapies, including psychoanalysis, are in fact symptomatic interventions. The rarity of symptom substitution (e.g., Nurnberger & Hingtgen, 1973) is due to reasons other than those suggested by behaviorists (e.g., Kazdin, 1982). First, patients may be unwilling to replace the symptom with other deviant behaviors either because they are unfamiliar with these behaviors or because of the cost involved. Second, therapists often enhance patients' ability to remove the stressors through coping skills training before or after the occurrence of the symptom substitution (e.g., Blanchard & Hersen, 1976).

In the introduction to Part III, it was stated that some investigators claim that all therapies have similar efficacies and attribute the effect of therapy to therapeutic alliance, empathy, support, and emotional catharsis. Others list a number of ESTs, claiming they have been found to be more effective than other techniques in the treatment of specific disorders. PBT demonstrates that both approaches are right. On the one hand, as was demonstrated earlier with regards to conversion disorder, different methods which stemmed from different theories, such as psychoanalysis, behavior therapy, and religious therapy, may yield positive therapeutic outcomes. On the other hand, although the emotional components of therapy are highly important, each of these therapies obtain their positive effects not because of these components but rather because of their unique ability to nullify different factors that according to PBT maintains the symptom.

For these reasons, psychoanalysis is the most successful in the treatment of DID, because patients attribute their symptoms to evil unconscious forces, which can be nullified especially by this therapy. Religious therapy is effective particularly in non-Western countries and certain sections in Western society where patients attribute their symptoms to supernatural forces. In the Western countries, punishment-reinforcement procedure is the most useful intervention for conversion disorder because it nullifies the controllability value of the symptom. Similarly, CBT is effective for anxiety disorders, such as panic disorder, agoraphobia, and OCD, especially because of its ability to sabotage the patient's self-deceptive belief.

Thus, PBT denies the statement that "techniques do not do anything to the client" (Feixas & Botella, 2004, p. 197) and that therapeutic effects are the consequence of common factors associated with patient–therapist relationships. This theory provides a theoretical framework for both EST's findings that certain therapies are more effective for specific disorders, and to some extent for the rival approach that all therapies yield similar outcomes.

PBT's Therapeutic Contributions

In addition to its theoretical value, PBT also has three main practical contributions: diagnostic criteria, theoretical eclecticism, and insight-rational therapy.

Diagnostic Criteria

PBT's set of diagnostic criteria, specified in Part I, is an important contribution to therapy because it is based on empirical data, rather than on the consensus of biased experts as seen in the *Diagnostic Statistical Manual (DSM)*, and because it is derived from a theory that provides insight into the etiology of a specific disorder.

Theoretical Eclecticism

Given the theoretical confusion in psychotherapy, many therapists employ an eclectic approach, termed "*technical eclecticism*" (e.g., Carter, 2006; Duncan, Parks, & Rusk, 1990a, 1990b; Lazarus, 1989, 1995, 2008), that "permits one to select techniques from any discipline without necessarily endorsing any of the theories that spawned them" (Lazarus, 1995, p. 31). Under these circumstances, the selection of a given therapy is made in darkness and upon a purely intuitive basis. In contrast, PBT provides an improved eclectic approach, which can be termed "*theoretical eclecticism,*" whereby a therapeutic intervention is selected based on a theoretical framework, which matches the patient's specific symptoms and needs to a given therapeutic approach. It equips clinicians with a set of principles that can guide them to wise decisions, and thus facilitate and enhance the therapeutic outcome.

Insight-Therapy

Medical models, psychoanalysis, and PBT each views "insight" as an important part of any treatment. Yet each theory uses the concept differently and taken a different stance as to whether or not such insight may be a necessary condition for recovery.

Medical models Insight: Given medical models' premise that schizophrenia is a brain disease, psychiatrists make every effort to convince patients that they are mentally ill in order to motivate them to take drugs, believing that doing so is necessary for genuine recovery (e.g., Siebert, 2000). In one example, Tony, a 20-year-old unemployment factory worker, was admitted to a mental hospital for a court-ordered examination after having beaten up his father in a first fight. The psychiatric said to the patient:

> Tony, your behavior is sick. We can treat you here as an outpatient, but you must understand you are mentally ill before we can make any progress". Tony shouted, "No, I'm not! You doctors are crazy if you think I'm mentally ill!" The psychiatrist raised his voice: "We've argued about this before. You must believe you are mentally ill or we can't help you!" Tony's face got red. His nostrils flared. He yelled, "I'm not mentally ill!" Tony's wife reached over and put her hand on his arm. The resident yelled, 'Yes, you are!' (Siebert, 2000, p. 36).

As noted by Hoffer and Osmond (1966) in their book How to Live with Schizophrenia, schizophrenic patients are commonly told:

> You have a grave responsibility to yourself and to your family to get well. You will have no problem if you are convinced

> that you are ill. But no matter what you think, you must do all you can to accept the statement of your doctor that you are ill (p. 153).

"When a patient disagrees, this is diagnosed as resistance or 'lack of insight' and viewed as another sign of 'mental illness'" (Siebert, 2000, p. 38).

Psychoanalytic Insight: Psychoanalytic theory attributes the underlying causes of madness to repressed childhood trauma. Accordingly, Breuer and Freud's (1895) claim that lifting repression is a necessary condition for therapeutic success. This idea is a central component of classic psychoanalysis (e.g., see Bergmann, 1992; Blum, 2003; Fenichel, 1946, Grünbaum, 2002; Kluft, 1995), and as noted by Eagle (2000), "The therapeutic value of lifting of repressions remains as one of the core theoretical assumptions underlying psychoanalytic, as well as other, related treatments" (p. 168). However, as indicated earlier, numerous studies refute the existence of Freudian repression, and report that this intervention is an ineffective therapy (e.g., see review by Rofé, 2008).

PBT's Rational-Insight: PBT agrees with both psychoanalysis and medical models regarding the critical importance of insight for a genuine recovery. However, "insight" in PBT refers to the patient's awareness that he or she has adopted the mad behavior and is responsible for its continued maintenance. Furthermore, contrary to these theories, it claims that genuine recovery does not necessitate insight. As was demonstrated above, both neurotic (see Blanchard & Hersen, 1976; Wolitzky & Eagle, 1999) and schizophrenic (e.g., See Bradshow, 1998; Karon, 2008) patients can fully recover by traditional symptomatic methods if the therapy successfully sabotages one of the components that according to PBT maintain the symptom and either removes the stress or enhances patients' coping skills. Moreover, insight should be induced only if the therapist is confident that the patient has the ability, with the therapist's assistance, to cope with the stress that motivated the adoption of the mad behavior. Otherwise, insight may aggravate the patient's emotional condition, especially in schizophrenic patients who constitutionally suffer from poor coping abilities due to severe brain impairments. An effective approach for these patients would be overlooking their schizophrenic bizarre behaviors of hallucination and delusions (unless if the patient poses a danger to himself or others) and focusing in improving their general emotional state and quality of life. This can be obtained by enhancing life conditions within a protected environment and encouraging a normal lifestyle through sheltered or supported employment, which was found to be found to be essential for patients' well-being (Cheng, Chen, & Lin, 2016; Davis, Lysaker, Kristeller et al., 2015; Evensen, Wisløff, Lystad et al., 2019).

PBT's insight-therapy approach consists of three types of interventions whose relative efficacy depends on various factors, such as the nature of the symptoms, the complexity of the stress to which the individual is subjected, duration of the disorder and the strength of patients' coping resources. The first intervention is to tell the patient that he or she deliberately adopted the mad behavior and then to encourage him or her to abandon it. Unless the patient's self-deceptive belief is very weak, this intervention is unlikely to be effective and it may be even harmful.

This type of intervention has been proven to be effective by Symonds (see Merskey, 1979) in treatment of dissociative fugue characterized by reversible amnesia for personal identity (e.g., see case study by Masserman, 1946). This is a relatively easy disorder to treat, using insight, since patents have difficulty producing effective self-deceptive beliefs that enable the forgetting of personal details (e.g., names, family ties, etc.). Symonds induced full recovery by telling fugue patients: "I know from experience that your pretended loss of memory is the result of some intolerable emotional situation" (pp. 264–265). The therapist further stated that if the patient would tell the whole story he would respect the patient's confidence, even to the point of telling the patient's doctor and relatives that he or she had been cured by hypnotism. Symonds reported that all of his patients admitted to having faked their symptoms, i.e., they abandoned their pathological coping strategy.

The second PBT method of insight is to use Socratic Questioning (e.g., Tai & Turkington, 2009) to make patients aware that they have adopted their symptoms as a way of alleviating some extreme emotional distress in their lives. This kind of intervention, for example, played a critical role in the rapid recovery of the schizophrenic patient Molly, following a single clinical interview (Siebert, 2000). By calling Molly's attention to the stressful events in her life, Siebert led her to the realization that her symptoms were simply rational strategies she had adopted to soothe herself. She simultaneously realized that her "crazy" behavior was not the result of brain disease, and was in fact within her power to maintain or abandon it.

A.S. (Al Siebert): Molly? (She looks up at me.) I am curious about something. Why are you here in a psychiatric hospital?

Molly: God spoke to me and said I was going to give birth to the second Savior.

A.S.: That may be, but why are you here in this hospital?

Molly: (startled, puzzled) Well, that's crazy talk.

A.S.: According to whom?

Molly: What?

A.S.: Did you decide when God spoke to you that you were crazy?

Molly: Oh. No. They told me I was crazy.

A.S.: Do you believe you are crazy?

Molly: No. But I am, aren't I? (dejected)

A.S.: If you will put that in the form of a question, I'll answer you.

Molly: (slightly puzzled, pauses to think) Do you think I am crazy?

A.S.: No.

Molly: But that couldn't have happened, could it?

A.S.: As far as I am concerned, you are the only person who knows what happens in your mind. Did it seem real at the time?

Molly: Oh yes!

A.S.: Tell me what you did after God spoke to you.

Molly: What do you mean?

A.S.: Did you start knitting booties and sweaters and things?

Molly: (laughs) No, but I did pack my clothes and wait by the door several times.

A.S.: Why?

Molly: I felt like I would be taken someplace.

A.S.: It wasn't where you expected, was it?

Molly: (laughing) No!

A.S.: One thing I'm curious about.

Molly: What?

A.S.: Why is it that of all women in the world, God chose you to be the mother of the second Savior?

Molly: (breaks into a big grin) You know; I've been trying to figure that out myself!

A.S.: So your dad and mom didn't love you, the patients were critical and didn't like you, and your boyfriend just wanted to be friends. That made you feel very sad and lonely.

Molly: (head down, dejected) Yes, there didn't seem to be anyone in the whole world who cared for me at all.

A.S.: And then God spoke to you.

Molly: Yes. (quietly)

A.S.: How did you feel after God gave you the good news?

Molly: (looks up, smiles warmly at me) I felt like the most special person in the whole world.

A.S.: That's a nice feeling, isn't it?

Molly: Yes, it is. (The kitchen crew came into the dining room to set up for lunch.)

A.S.: I must go now.

Molly: Please don't tell them what we've been talking about. No one seems to understand.

A.S.: I know what you mean. I promise not to tell if you won't.

Molly: I promise.

Two days later, upon meeting the "therapist", the patient asked: "I've been thinking about what we talked about. I've been wondering. Do you think I imagined God's voice to make myself feel better?"

Siebert's method of insight may yield a positive outcome under two conditions: (1) The intervention takes place at the very early stages of the disorder, before it crystallizes into a lifestyle as seen, for example, in the case of King (see Part I); (2) The stress is environmental, rather than the result of poor coping skills stemmed from brain impairments.

PBT's third insight intervention, which can be termed informational exposure therapy, calls for exposing the patient over 8–10 sessions to scientific facts that refute the validity of traditional theories of psychopathology. The therapist tells the patient, "I would like to give you a short course on psychology in which you will learn the different hypotheses that have been made over the last 100 years regarding the causes of behavior disorders". During these sessions patients get to know the main ideas of psychoanalysis and medical models mainly by video presentation of patients who fully recovered from disorders, such as DID and schizophrenia. They are then presented with evidence reviewed in the introduction to this book that refutes the validity of the traditional explanations of these cases. They learn PBT's main ideas and are led to understand that the mad behaviors of these patients were quite rational insofar as they enabled them to alleviate their unbearable emotional distress. The therapy then focuses on the patient's specific disorder, using a Socratic Questioning method which, like in CBT, aims to encourage the probing of the evidence, reason, and rationale behind the patient's belief (Tai & Turkington, 2009, p. 866). As specified above in discussing CBT's intervention in treatment of schizophrenia, the patient is led to understand that they are the only person responsible for the quality of their life, and that the therapist has the ability to help them find more adaptive solutions for their problems.

For example, Nash would have been confronted with each of his specific stressors and asked to reevaluate his response to them. One such stressor may have been guilt surrounding his father's death: Nash would have been asked, using Socratic Questioning method, whether his father's demand that he marry Eleanor, who was seven years older than him and much less intelligent, was justified, given the fact, which his father was not aware of, that Alicia, "a beautiful young physics student… adored him" (Nasar, 1998, p. 15). Nash should have considered the possibility that his father's death may have been purely the result of health problems. The same approach should be applied to his other stressors, such as his frustration that he did not get a position at Princeton University. Did his disappointment justify the development of mad behavior? Clinical studies are needed, of course, to examine the efficacy of PBT's insight methods.

Part IV
General Discussion

PBT's Theoretical Advantages

PBT meets five major requirements that are expected of an ideal theory of psychopathology, as opposed to traditional theories that can meet none. These expectations include (1) providing operational criteria for the diagnosis of neuroses, criminal insanity, and **schizophrenia**, which differentiates them from non-bizarre behaviors; (2) explanation of a variety of mad behaviors by one set of theoretical concepts; (3) specifying the factors that cause the variability of mad behaviors **within** each disorder (e.g., blindness, paralysis, and psychogenic movements in conversion disorder; disorganized speech, serial killings, and sophisticated bizarre symptoms in schizophrenia), **between** different types of madness (e.g., conversion disorder, obsessive-compulsive disorder [OCD], agoraphobia, criminal insanity, or schizophrenia), **among different types of social groups** (e.g., females vs. males, western vs. developed countries) and across different period of times; (4) integrating the seemingly incompatible data into one theoretical paradigm, such as evidence indicating that schizophrenia can be developed both in the presence and absence of genetic vulnerability; and (5) providing a unified theory of therapy.

Although PBT differs from all traditional theories of psychopathology, it is closer to psychoanalysis than other theories. Both theories (1) focus on the explanation of bizarre behaviors, which they divide into neuroses and psychoses; (2) are parsimonious approaches, as using the same theoretical concepts for the explanation and treatment of these disorders; (3) view repression and unawareness as keys to the understanding and treatment of these disorders; (4) claim that the patient's insight into the underlying causes of their bizarre behaviors is critically important for genuine recovery.

However, there are profound differences between the two theories. **First**, PBT claims that the current stressors, rather than historical events, are the underlying causes of the individual's bizarre behaviors. **Second**, contrary to psychoanalysis, which shares the same axiomatic assumption of rival theories that psychological disorders are involuntary, PBT claims that madness is a coping mechanism that people intuitively/unconsciously choose when confronted with intolerable levels of stress and consciously implemented by them. **Third**, PBT views mad behaviors as an economic product the selection of which is determined by the same principles that guide a consumer's decision-making process. **Fourth**, while Freud undermined the role of the conscious in the development and treatment of bizarre behaviors, PBT claims that the conscious is a major actor in the development and treatment of these behaviors. **Fifth**, although in both theories repression is perceived as a psychological process that causes the elimination of threatening materials from the consciousness/attention, there are fundamental differences between them in the conception of this notion. While Freudian repression consists of five components, none of which have received empirical confirmation (Rofé, 2008), PBT's repression is nothing more than conscious distraction. Most importantly, contrary to psychoanalysis, in PBT, repression is the consequence rather than the cause of madness.

Sixth, the two theories have completely different conceptions of unawareness. Although PBT acknowledges the existence of the unconscious, it limits its effect to intuitive processes through which a specific symptom is selected. In PBT, unawareness is a creation activity in which the conscious plays a major role. It enables patients to forget knowledge of self-involvement (KSI)/true reason (TR) and results in the development of self-deceptive belief. This new concept of unawareness enables us to integrate data indicating that patients are unaware of the underlying causes of their behaviors and yet control their manifestation. Also, this concept allows us to understand the type of self-deceptive beliefs that patients maintain (illness vs. denial), to resolve fundamental theoretical problems (e.g., etiology and mechanisms that control the development of conversion disorder, DID, panic disorder and agoraphobia; see the Discussion in Part-II), and to gain insight into the mechanism of therapeutic change. Thus, although Freud's theory failed, and even though PBT is radically different from this theory, Freud has made priceless contributions to the understanding of psychological disorders. He has paved the way for PBT's breakthrough into the understanding of madness.

Many scholars raise the question whether Freud is still alive or if he is really dead. In this regard, Kihlstrom (2015), one of the distinguished cognitive researchers, note on his webpage that

> from a scientific point of view, classical Freudian psychoanalysis is dead as both a theory of the mind and a mode of therapy … At best, Freud is a figure of only historical interest for psychologists. He is better studied as a writer, in departments of language and literature, than as a scientist, in departments of psychologists. Psychologists can get along without him.

PBT is a proof that Kihlstrom's portrait of Freud is a complete distortion of the truth. Freud made invaluable scientific contributions to psychology, more than any other figure in the history of psychopathology. His most significant contribution is his vision that a necessary condition for the understanding behavioral disorders is the distinction between bizarre and non-bizarre behaviors, and that bizarre behaviors have to be explained by one set of theoretical concepts. He was also right that the patient's insight into the underlying causes of his symptoms is crucially important for a genuine recovery. Although it is absolutely true that psychoanalysis is dead, it is doubtful whether PBT would have been alive without Freud's spirit.

When considering the bitter historical controversy between psychoanalysis and behaviorism, there seems to be no doubt that the psychoanalytic approach, not psychoanalysis itself, won the contest. Not only does behavior–cognitive theory have difficulty in explaining bizarre phobias (e.g., train phobia, Leonard, 1927; chocolate phobia, Rachman & Seligman, 1976; insect phobia, Jacobs & Nadel, 1985; rat germ phobia, Brandt & Mackenzie, 1987), including panic disorder and agoraphobia, as elaborated on above, but they have significant problems in accounting even for the development of simple phobias (see review by Rofé & Rofé, 2015). PBT resolves the historical controversy between psychoanalysis and behavior–cognitive theories by making a sharp distinction between bizarre and non-bizarre phobia, and revising the Pavlovian explanation of simple phobia (Rofé, 2000; Rofé & Rofé, 2015). It is difficult to imagine, when considering the complex process by which mad behaviors develop, Watson's and his followers' pretention to understand the development of behavioral disorders by investigating rats' behaviors. Although behavioral-cognitive therapies proved their therapeutic efficacy as demonstrated above, their therapeutic methods and findings are more adequately explained by PBT than by behavior–cognitive concepts.

PBT's most revolutionary contribution concerns the universally accepted belief that schizophrenia is a brain disease. Although many researchers have criticized this belief (e.g., Williams, 2012), given the inability of psychological theories to provide more convincing explanation, their critique has not significantly damaged the reputation of medical models. The special merit of this book is not in the critique of the disease models of schizophrenia, to which it contributes a great deal, but rather in providing an alternative theory which is able to incorporate both neurological data and case studies of a variety of bizarre behaviors with lack of such evidence into one theoretical system.

Practical Implications

PBT has four major practical implications. **First**, it provides objective diagnostic criteria for neuroses, criminal insanity, and schizophrenia. As demonstrated in this book, PBT's diagnostic approach received significant empirical support and emerged out of a theory which provides insight into the etiology and mechanisms of therapeutic change, as opposed to the DSM-5, which lacks scientific validation and is supposedly atheoretical. Accordingly, the DSM should be revised in accordance with PBT's diagnostic criteria. The revised edition should distinguish between bizarre and non-bizarre deviant behaviors, categorizing bizarre behaviors into neuroses, psychoses, and criminal insanities

Second, PBT's insight into the processes by which bizarre behaviors develop improves the therapeutic intervention in two ways. One is PBT's "theoretical eclecticism", which equips clinicians with a set of principles which enable them to choose a specific therapeutic method, as opposed to the previous intuitive eclectic approach, termed "technical eclecticism", which "permits one to select arbitrarily techniques from any discipline without necessarily endorsing any of the theories that spawned them" (Lazarus, 1995, p. 31). The second way is via a new therapeutic intervention, termed Rational-Insight Therapy, which makes patients aware of their conscious involvement in the adoption and maintenance of their symptoms, encouraging them to abandon their mad behavior in favor of better coping mechanisms.

Third, following research and clinical data have disproven the disease conception of schizophrenia, the primary therapeutic intervention should be psychological. Such intervention should focus on addressing the patient's stressors and on enhancing their coping abilities. Neverthless while the long-term use of antipsychotics should be prohibited, given their dreadful side-effects, they can be employed on a short-term basis (Haddad & Correll, 2018; Whitaken, 2010), especially when a patient is extremely depressed and suicidal (Kaneda, 2007; Keck, Strakowski, & McElroy, 2000).

Fourth, the courts currently lack objective criteria for diagnosing criminal insanity, and usually base their verdicts on the subjective evaluations of psychiatrists (e.g., Frances, 2013). Additionally, the legal system tends to regard criminally insane individuals as not responsible for their criminal behaviors. Both psychoanalysts and advocates of medical models have arrived at this conclusion mainly due to the fact that, unlike normal criminal acts in which individuals strive for desirable objectives and are aware of the reasons for their actions, criminally insane behaviors appear to be senseless, lack incentives, and leave the individual largely oblivious to the underlying causes of their actions. Contrary to the dominant view in contemporary legal system, PBT maintains that such people commit their crimes both consciously and selfishly. Therefore, these individuals should be viewed as responsible for their actions and punished accordingly, while taking into account their extreme level of depression which often motivate them to commit suicide.

Concluding Remarks

Evidence reviewed in this book indicates that psychopathology is in a serious theoretical crisis that bears no resemblance to difficulties in any other field. There is perhaps no case in the history of science in which theories that prevailed for over a century were proven so utterly misguided, as is the case in modern psychopathology. The inadequacy of Freud's theory was noticed in the initial presentation of his theory when he failed to explain the correlation between schizophrenia and neurological impairments. This theoretical failure paved the way for the neurologically invasive approach of medical models, which legitimized the employment of barbaric treatments, such as lobotomies and shock insulin. Meanwhile, the scientific legitimacy of Freud's theory collapsed with the emergence of studies refuting the existence of repression, the cornerstone of psychoanalysis.

The fall of psychoanalysis increased the pseudo-scientific status of medical models, allowing them to expand their approach to all types of behavioral disorders. Today these models prevail despite the abundance of evidence refuting their most foundational assumptions. Such evidence includes the significant proportion of schizophrenics who display no neurological impairments whatsoever; the significant percentage of patients who have fully recovered without drugs, especially in undeveloped countries; and the low prospects of recovery coupled with the high risk of complications for patients undergoing drug treatments.

Behavior-cognitive theories tell a similar story. Their explanations of fear and phobia encounter serious difficulties when trying to account for the development of agoraphobia, panic disorder, and other types of bizarre phobias such as train, chocolate, and rat germ phobias. Yet thus far these difficulties have not damaged their scientific popularity.

The peculiar situation in which a theory continues to function despite a wealth of contradictory evidence is consistent with recent developments in the philosophy of science which contend that scientific theories are in practice not overthrown by new data, as Karl Popper once understood (1959), but rather by alternative theories that better explain the existing data (e.g., Brush, 1989, 2006).

The idea that madness, which may be displayed in a variety of seemingly irrational behaviors, is a direct result of stress, and that these behaviors are in fact rational is the most plausible explanation of this phenomenon. This explanation simplifies the therapeutic intervention, making it more humanistic and can reduce the likelihood of horrible criminal insanities. Many innocent lives of those who had been murdered by various criminally insane serial killers, could have been saved if therapists to whom these individuals had applied were aware of the potential danger and could have addressed their intolerable levels of stress. Certainly, PBT can help therapists in this matter.

Critique

Two possible critiques which could be used to weaken PBT's position must be considered. One problem concerns the scientific credibility of case studies, which constitutes PBT's major supporting data. As was noted by Wolpert and Fonagy (2009) in their critique of psychoanalysis,

> an analytic case history is essentially subjective and anecdotal, and it also ignores other approaches to mental

> illnesses. No analyst is likely to consider the possibility that the patients' condition may be due to a genetic defect or some other physical illness. For example, there is good evidence that depression has a strong genetic component and so does schizophrenia. It is unlikely that psychoanalysts would even recognize such diagnoses of the patient's condition (p. 483).

In reference to this issue, we need to consider researchers' claim, presented earlier, that the scientific value of case studies is no less than that of other research methods, especially at early stage of formulating a new theory. These studies support PBT's major arguments that mad behaviors have common diagnostic criteria and etiology, are goal-oriented, and that the choice of a specific madness resembles the consumer decision-making processes. Additionally, the case studies used in this book are not subjective as they were originally reported by scholars who were unfamiliar with PBT. Most importantly, none of the existing theories can provide a better explanation of these cases, nor they can integrate other theorists' clinical and research data pertaining to the development and treatment of rival theories into their theoretical framework, as PBT does. These include studies regarding genetic and neurological defects pertaining to schizophrenia, Freud's clinical observations that repression and unawareness are key factors for understanding the development and treatment of madness, behaviorists and cognitive studies concerning the development and treatment of panic disorder, agoraphobia and schizophrenia. Thus, it would be erroneous to attribute PBT's supporting data only to case studies.

Another possible avenue of critique which needs to be addressed concerns the lack of evidence supporting PBT's therapeutic suggestions. In to this regard two concepts must be considered: (1) PBT's major goal in this book is not providing new therapeutic interventions, but rather to uncover the underlying mechanisms that are involved in both the development and treatment of mad behaviors; (2) as specified earlier, especially in Part-III, all traditional therapeutic techniques suggested by rival theories actually support PBT. This means that the therapeutic findings of rival theories strengthen PBT's theoretic approach rather than the theoretical approach which originally developed these techniques. Thus, the critique against PBT should be limited only to its new therapeutic suggestions, an effort which undoubtedly requires intensive clinical research. In this regard, one case study which applied PBT's new therapeutic suggestions (Rofé, 2010), is the first step in this direction.

References

Aaronson, C. J., Shear, M. K., Goetz, R. R., Allen, L. B., Barlow, D. H., White, K. S., ... Gorman, J. M. (2008). Predictors and tie course of response among panic disorder patients treated with cognitive-behavioral therapy. *The Journal of Clinical Psychiatry*, *69*, 418–424.

Abas, M. A., Sahakian, B. J., & Levy, R. (1990). Neuropsychological deficits and CT scan changes in elderly depressives. *Psychological Medicine*, *20*, 507–520.

Abramovitz, J. S. (1997). Effectiveness of psychological and pharmacology treatment for obsessive-compulsive disorder: A quantitative review. *Journal of Consulting and Clinical Psychology*, *65*, 44–52.

Abramovitz, J. S. (1998). Does cognitive-behavioral therapy cure obsessive-compulsive disorder? A meta-analytic evaluation of clinical significance. *Behavior Therapy*, *29*, 339–355.

Abramowitz, J. S. (2006). The psychological treatment of obsessive-compulsive disorder. *Canadian Journal of Psychiatry*, *51*, 407–416.

Abramowitz, J. S., Deacon, B. J., Woods, C. M., & Tolin, D. F. (2004). Association between protestant religiosity and obsessive-compulsive symptoms and cognitions. *Depression and Anxiety*, *20*, 70–76.

Abrams, K., Schruers, K., Cosci, F., & Sawtell, S. (2008). Biological challenge procedures used to study co-occurring nicotine dependence and panic disorder. *Addictive Behaviors*, *33*, 1463–1469.

Abse, D. W. (1959). Hysteria. In S. Arieti (Ed.), *American handbook of psychiatry* (Vol. 1). New York, NY: Basic Books.

Acheson, D. T., Forsyth, J. P., Prenoveau, J. M., & Bouton, M. E. (2007). Interoceptive fear conditioning as a learning model of panic disorder: An experimental evaluation using 20% CO_2-enriched air in a non-clinical sample. *Behaviour Research and Therapy*, *45*, 2280–2294.

Acocella, J. (1999). *Creating hysteria: Women and multiple personality disorder*. San Francisco, CA: Jossey-Bass.

Acosta, F. J., Aguilar, E. J., Cejas, M. R., & Gracia, R. (2013). Beliefs about illness and their relationship with hopelessness, depression, insight and suicide attempts in schizophrenia. *Psychiatria Danubina*, *25*, 49–54.

Adams, M. E. (1990). Some observations on the nature and treatment of multiple personality disorder. *Psychoanalysis and Psychotherapy, 8*, 161–168.

Adityanjee, A., Raju, G. S. P., & Khandelwal, S. K. (1989). Current status of multiple personality disorder in India. *American Journal of Psychiatry, 146*, 1607–1610.

Akdemir, D., & Ünal, F. (2006). Early onset conversion disorder: A case report. *Türk Psikiyatri Dergisi, 17*, 65–71.

Akhtar, S. (1988). Four culture-bound psychiatric syndromes in India. *International Journal of Social Psychiatry, 34*, 70–74.

Alexander, F. (1932). *The medical value of psychoanalysis*. New York, NY: Norton.

Alexander, F. (1950). *Psychosomatic medicine*. New York, NY: Norton.

Alexander, P. E. (1991). Management of panic disorders. *Journal of Psychoactive Drugs, 23*, 329–333.

Alford, B. A., & Correia, C. J. (1994). Cognitive therapy of schizophrenia: Theory and empirical status. *Behavior Therapy, 25*, 17–33.

Al-Kubaisy, T., Marks, I. M., Logsdail, S., Marks, M. P., Lovell, K., Sungur, M., & Araya, R. (1992). Role of exposure homework in phobia reduction: A controlled study. *Behavior Therapy, 23*, 599–621.

Allen, J. J. B., & Movius, H. L., II. (2000). The objective assessment of amnesia in dissociative identity disorder using event-related potentials. *International Journal of Psychophysiology, 38*, 21–41.

Allison, D. J., Sharma, B., & Timmons, B. W. (2019). The efficacy of anti-inflammatory treatment interventions on depression in individuals with major depressive disorder and high levels of inflammation: A systematic review of randomized clinical trials. *Physiology & Behavior, 207*, 104–112.

Allport, G. W. (1929). Scientific method in aesthetics. *Psychological Bulletin, 26*, 711.

Alonso, L., & Jeffrey, D. (1988). Mental illness complicated by the santeria belief in spirit possession. *Hospital and Community Psychiatry, 39*, 1188–1191.

Amador, X. F., & Paul-Odouard, R. (2000). Defending the Unabomber: Anosognosia in schizophrenia. *Psychiatric Quarterly, 71*, 363–371.

American Psychiatric Association (1952). *Diagnostic and statistical manual of mental disorders*, 1st ed. (DSM-I). Washington, DC: American Psychiatric Association.

American Psychiatric Association (1968). *Diagnostic and statistical manual of mental disorders*, 2nd ed. (DSM-II). Washington, DC: American Psychiatric Association.

American Psychiatric Association (1976). *Task force on nomenclature — progress report on the preparation of DSM-III.*

American Psychiatric Association (1980). *Diagnostic and statistical manual of mental disorders* (3rd ed. [*DSM-III*]). Washington, DC: Author.

American Psychiatric Association (1994). *Diagnostic and statistical manual of mental disorders* (4th ed. [*DSM-III-IV*]). Washington, DC: Author.

American Psychiatric Association (2000). *Diagnostic and statistical manual of mental disorders* (4th ed., text revision [*DSM-IV*-TR]). Washington, DC: Author.

American Psychiatric Association (2013). *Diagnostic and statistical manual of mental disorders: DSM-5* (5th ed.). Washington, DC: Author.

Andersen, A. E., & DiDomenico, L. (1992). Diet vs. shape content of popular male and female magazines: A dose-response relationship to the incidence of eating disorders? *International Journal of Eating Disorders, 11*, 283–287.

Anderson, C. A., Shibuya, A., Ihori, N., Swing, E. L., Bushman, B. J., Sakamoto, A., … Saleem, M. (2010). Violent video game effects on aggression, empathy, and prosocial behavior in Eastern and Western countries: A meta-analytic review. *Psychological Bulletin, 136*, 151–173.

Anderson, M. C. (2005). The role of inhibitory control in forgetting unwanted memories: A consideration of three methods. In N. Ohta, C. MacLeod, & B. Uttl (Eds.), *Dynamic cognitive processes* (pp. 159–189). Tokyo: Springer-Verlag.

Anderson, M. C., & Green, C. (2001). Suppressing unwanted memories by executive control. *Nature, 410*, 366–369.

Anderson, M. C., Ochsner, K. N., Kuhl, B., Cooper, J., Robertson, E., Gabrieli, S. W., … Gabrieli, J. D. E. (2004). Neural systems underlying the suppression of unwanted memories. *Science, 303*, 232–235.

Andreasen, N. C. (1985). *The broken brain: The biological revolution in psychiatry*. London: Harper & Row.

Arntz, A. (2002). Cognitive therapy versus interoceptive exposure as treatment of panic disorder without agoraphobia. *Behaviour Research and Therapy, 40*, 325–341.

Artaloytia, J. F., Arango, C., Lahti, A., Sanz, J., Pascual, A., Gubero, P., … Palomo, T. (2006). Negative signs and symptoms secondary to antipsychotics: A double-blind, randomized triangle of a single dose of placebo, haloperidol, and risperidone in healthy volunteers. *The American Journal of Psychiatry, 163*, 488–493.

Artazcoz, L., Benach, J., Borrell, C., & Cortes, I. (2004). Unemployment and mental health: Understanding the interactions among gender, family roles, and social class. *American Journal of Public Health, 94*, 82–88.

Arthus, M., Cottraux, J., Mollard, E., Guerin, J., & Bouvard, M. (1997). Cognitive-behaviour therapy in agoraphobia: A retrospective study of 345 cases. *L'Encéphale: Revue de psychiatrie clinique biologique et thérapeutique, 23*, 300–307.

Aumann, R. J. (2006). War and peace. *PNAS: Proceedings of the National Academy of Sciences of the United States of America, 103*, 17075–17078.

Aumann, R. J. (2016, September 4). *Letter of recommendation to editors: Federmann Center for the Study of Rationality*. Jerusalem: Hebrew University.

Austin, D. W., & Richards, J. C. (2001). The catastrophic misinterpretation model of panic disorder. *Behaviour Research and Therapy, 39*, 1277–1291.

Ayalon, M., & Merom, H. (1985). The teacher interview. *Schizophrenia Bulletin, 11*, 117–120.

Bacaltchuk, J., Hay, P., & Mari, J. (2000). Antidepressants versus placebo for the treatment of bulimia nervosa: A systematic review. *Australian and New Zealand Journal of Psychiatry, 34*, 310–317.

Bachrach, H. M. (1996). On the efficacy of psychotherapy. In *The Hatherleigh guide to psychotherapy*. New York, NY: Hatherleigh Press.

Baker, A. (2007). Occam's Razor in science: A case study from biogeography. *Biology & Philosophy, 22*, 193–215.

Balhara, Y. P. S., & Verma, R. (2012). Schizophrenia and suicide. *East Asian Archives of Psychiatry, 22*, 126–133.

Bandura, A. (1969). *Principles of behavior modification*. New York, NY: Holt, Rinehart & Winston.

Bandura, A. (2011). Self-deception: A paradox revisited. *Behavioral and Brain Sciences, 34*, 16–17.

Baradell, J. G., & Klein, K. (1993). Relationship of life stress and body consciousness to hypervigilant decision making. *Journal of Personality and Social Psychology, 64*, 267–273.

Barber, S., & Lane, R. C. (1995). Efficacy research in psychodynamic therapy: A critical review of the literature. *Psychotherapy in Private Practice, 14*, 43–69.

Bargh, J. A. (2014). The historical origins of priming as the preparation of behavioral responses: Unconscious carryover and contextual influences of real-world importance. In D. C. Molden (Ed.), *Understanding priming effects in social psychology* (pp. 218–233). New York, NY: Guilford Press.

Bargh, J. A., & Morsella, E. (2008). The unconscious mind. *Perspectives on Psychological Science, 3*, 73–79.

Baribeau, D. A., & Anagnostou, E. (2013). A comparison of neuroimaging findings in childhood onset schizophrenia and autism spectrum disorder: A review of the literature. *Frontiers in Psychiatry, 4*, 175–189.

Barlow, D. H. (1988). *Anxiety and its disorders: The nature and treatment of anxiety and panic*. New York, NY: Guilford Press.

Barlow, D. H. (2004). Psychological treatments. *American Psychologist, 59*, 869–878.

Barlow, D. H., Brown, T. A., & Craske, M. G. (1994). Definitions of panic attacks and panic disorder in the *DSM-IV*: Implications for research. *Journal of Abnormal Psychology, 103*, 553–564.

Barlow, D. H., Gorman, J. M., Shear, M. K., & Woods, S. W. (2000). Cognitive-behavioral therapy, imipramine, or their combination for panic disorder: A randomized controlled trial. *Journal of the American Medical Association, 283*, 2529–2536.

Bartoli, F., Dell'Osso, B., Crocamo, C., Fiorillo, A., Ketter, T. A., Suppes, T., . . . Carrà, G. (2017). Benefits and harms of low and high second-generation antipsychotics doses for bipolar depression: A meta-analysis. *Journal of Psychiatric Research, 88*, 38–46.

Bass, C. (2001). Factitious disorders and malingering. In P. W. Halligan, C. Bass, & J. F. Marshall (Eds.), *Contemporary approaches to the study of hysteria* (pp. 126–142). New York, NY: Oxford.

Bayer, R., & Spitzer, R. L. (1985). Neurosis, psychodynamics and *DSM-III*: A history of the controversy. *Archives of General Psychiatry, 42*, 187–196.

Beckfield, D. F. (1985). Interpersonal competence among college men hypothesized to be at risk for schizophrenia. *Journal of Abnormal Psychology, 94*, 397–404.

Beckman, K., & Burns, G. L. (1990). Relation of sexual abuse and bulimia in college women. *International Journal of Eating Disorders, 9*, 487–492.

Behnke, S. H. (1997). Assessing the criminal responsibility of individuals with multiple personality disorder: Legal cases, legal theory. *Journal of the American Academy of Psychiatry and the Law, 25*(3), 391–399.

Beisser, H. R., Glasser, N., & Grant, M. (1967). Psychosocial adjustment of children of schizophrenic mothers. *Journal of Nervous and Mental Diseases, 145*, 429–440.

Beitman, B. D., Lamberti, J. W., Mukerji, V., DeRosear, L., Basha, I., & Schmid, L. (1987). Panic disorder in patients with angiographically normal coronary arteries. *Psychosomatics: Journal of Consultation and Liaison Psychiatry, 28*, 480–484.

Beitman, B. D., Mukerji, V., Russell, J. L., & Grafing, M. (1993). Panic disorder in cardiology patients: A review of the Missouri Panic/Cardiology Project. *Journal of Psychiatric Research, 27*, 35–46.

Bellack, A. S., Morrison, R. L., Wixted, J. T., & Mueser, K. T. (1990). An analysis of social competence in schizophrenia. *The British Journal of Psychiatry, 156*, 809–818.

Bellack, A. S., Schooler, N. R., Marder, S. R., Kane, J. M., Brown, C. H., & Yang, Y. (2004). Do clozapine and risperidone affect social competence and problem solving? *The American Journal of Psychiatry, 161*, 364–367.

Bemis, K. M. (1987). The present status of operant conditioning for the treatment of anorexia nervosa. *Behavior Modification, 11*, 432–463.

Benninghoven, D., Raykowski, L., Solzbacher, S., Kunzendorf, S., & Jantschek, G. (2007). Body images of patients with anorexia nervosa, bulimia nervosa and female control subjects: A comparison with male ideals of female attractiveness. *Body Image, 4*, 51–59.

Benzick, J. M. (2001). Serotonin syndrome preceding pseudoseizures in an adolescent. *Psychosomatics: Journal of Consultation Liaison Psychiatry, 42*, 441–443.

Bergmann, M. V. (1992). An infantile trauma, a trauma during analysis, and their psychic connections. *International Journal of Psychoanalysis, 73*, 447–454.

Berke, J. H. (1981). Psychodynamic appraisal of electroconvulsive therapy (ECT). *Psiquis: Revista de Psiquiatria, Psicologia y Psicosomatica, 2*, 3–5 (in Spanish).

Berkowitz, D. (1993). Work roles and news selection in local TV: Examining the business-journalism dialectic. *Journal of Broadcasting & Electronic Media, 37*, 67–81.

Berkowitz, L. (1988). Frustrations, appraisals, and aversively stimulated aggression. *Aggressive Behavior, 14*, 3–11.

Berkowitz, L. (1989). Frustration and aggression hypothesis: Examination and reformulation. *Psychological Bulletin, 106*, 59–73.

Berkowitz, A. D., & Perkins, H. W. (1987). Recent research on gender differences in collegiate alcohol use. *Journal of American College Health, 36*, 123–129.

Berman, E. (1981). Multiple personality: Psychoanalytic perspectives. *International Journal of Psycho-Analysis, 62*, 283–300.

Bet, P. M., Hugtenburg, J. G., Penninx, B. W., & Hoogendijk, W. J. (2013). Side effects of antidepressants during long-term use in a naturalistic setting. *European Neuropsychopharmacology, 23*, 1443–1451.

Bevan, J. R. (1960). Learning theory applied to the treatment of a patient with obsessional ruminations. In E. J. Eysenck (Ed.), *Behavior therapy and the neuroses: Reading in modern methods of treatment derived from learning theory*. Oxford, England: Pergamon.

Bhadrinath, B. R. (1990). Anorexia nervosa in adolescents of Asian extraction. *British Journal of Psychiatry, 156*, 565–568.

Bienvenu, O. J., Onyike, C. U., Stein, M. B., Chen, L. S., Samuels, J., Nestadt, G., & Eaton, W. W. (2006). Agoraphobia in adults: Incidence and longitudinal relationship with panic. *The British Journal of Psychiatry, 188*, 432–438.

Bijlsma, E. Y., Chan, J. S., Olivier, B., Veening, J. G., Millan, M. J., Waldinger, M. D., & Oosting, R. S. (2014). Sexual side effects of serotonergic antidepressants: Mediated by inhibition of serotonin on central dopamine release? *Pharmacology Biochemistry and Behavior, 121*, 88–101.

Bilge, T., Handan, N., Rumeysa, T., & Alp, U. (2015). Clinical variables associated with suicide attempts in schizophrenia before and after the first episode. *Psychiatry Research, 229*, 252–256.

Biran, M. W. (1990). Resourcefulness and successful treatment of agoraphobia. In M. Rosenbaum (Ed.), *Learned resourcefulness: On coping skills, self-control, and adaptive behavior*. New York, NY: Springer.

Black, D. W., Wesner, R., Bowers, W., & Gabel, J. (1993). A comparison of fluvoxamine, cognitive therapy, and placebo in the treatment of panic disorder. *Archives of General Psychiatry, 50*, 44–50.

Blair, R. J. R. (2010). Psychopathy, frustration, and reactive aggression: The role of ventromedial prefrontal cortex. *British Journal of Psychology, 101*, 383–399.

Blanchard, E. B., & Hersen, M. (1976). Behavioral treatment of hysterical neurosis: Symptom substitution and symptom return reconsidered. *Psychiatry, 39*, 118–129.

Blaney, P. H. (1986). Affect and memory: A review. *Psychological Bulletin, 99*, 229–246.

Blanz, B., Schmidt, M. H., Detzner, U., & Lay, B. (1994). Is there a sex-specific difference in onset age of schizophrenia that started before age 18? *European Child & Adolescent Psychiatry, 3*, 267–276.

Bliss, E. L. (1980). Multiple personalities. *Archives of General Psychiatry, 37*, 1388–1397.

Bliss, E. L. (1983). Multiple personalities, related disorders and hypnosis. *American Journal of Clinical Hypnosis, 26*, 114–123.

Bliss, E. L. (1984). Spontaneous self-hypnosis in multiple personality disorder. *Psychiatric Clinics of North America, 7*, 135–148.

Bloom, H. S. (2003). Using "short" interrupted time-series analysis to measure the impacts of whole-school reforms: With applications to a study of accelerated schools. *Evaluation Review, 27*, 3–49.

Blue, R. (1979). Use of punishment in treatment of anorexia nervosa. *Psychological Reports*, *44*, 743–746.

Blum, H. P. (2003). Psychoanalytic controversies: Repression, transference and reconstruction. *International Journal of Psychoanalysis*, *84*, 497–513.

Boag, S. (2012). *Freudian repression, the unconscious, and the dynamics of inhibition*. London, England: Karnac Books.

Boag, S. (2015). Repression, defence, and the psychology of science. In S. Boag, L. A. W. Brakel, & V. Talvitie (Eds.), *Philosophy, science, and psychoanalysis: A critical meeting* (pp. 247–268). London, England: Karnac Books.

Bonanno, G. A. (2006). The illusion of repressed memory. *Behavioral and Brain Sciences*, *29*, 515–516.

Bonanno, G. A., & Keuler, D. J. (1998). Psychotherapy without repressed memory: A parsimonious alternative based on contemporary memory research. In S. J. Lynn & K. M. McConkey (Eds.), *Truth in memory* (pp. 437–463). New York, NY: Guilford Press.

Bonner, R. L., & Rich, A. R. (1990). Psychosocial vulnerability, life stress, and suicide ideation in a jail population: A cross-validation study. *Suicide and Life Threatening Behavior*, *20*, 213–224.

Bornstein, R. F. (2001). The impending death of psychoanalysis. *Psychoanalytic Psychology*, *16*, 3–20.

Bouton, M. E., Mineka, S., & Barlow, D. H. (2001). A modern learning theory perspective on the etiology of panic disorder. *Psychological Review*, *108*, 4–32.

Bower, G. H. (1981). Mood and memory. *American Psychologist*, *36*, 129–148.

Bowers, K. S., & Farvolden, F. (1996). Revisiting a century-old Freudian slip — from suggestion disavowed to the truth repressed. *Psychological Bulletin*, *119*, 355–380.

Bowers, K. S., & Woody, E. Z. (1996). Hypnotic amnesia and the paradox of intentional forgetting. *Journal of Abnormal Psychology*, *105*, 381–390.

Boyd, J. D. (1997). Clinical hypnosis for rapid recovery from dissociative identity disorder. *American Journal of Clinical Hypnosis*, *40*, 97–110.

Boyle, M. (2002). It's all done with smoke and mirrors. Or, how to create the illusion of a schizophrenic brain disease. *Clinical Psychology*, *12*, 9–16.

Boysen, G. A., & VanBergen, A. (2014). Simulation of multiple personalities: A review of research comparing diagnosed and simulated dissociative identity disorder. *Clinical Psychology Review*, *34*, 14–28.

Bozorgmehr, A., Alizadeh, F., Ofogh, S. N., Hamzekalayi, M. R. A., Herati, S., Moradkhani, A., & Ghadirivasfi, M. (2018). What do the genetic association data say about the high risk of suicide in people with depression? A novel network-based approach to find common molecular basis for depression and suicidal behavior and related therapeutic targets. *Journal of Affective Disorders*, *229*, 463–468.

Bradshaw, W. (1998). Cognitive-behavioral treatment of schizophrenia: A case study. *Journal of Cognitive Psychotherapy*, *12*, 13–25.

Brady, J. P., & Lind, D. L. (1961). Experimental analysis of hysterical blindness. *Archives of General Psychiatry*, *4*, 331–339.

Braginsky, B. M., & Braginsky, D. D. (1967). Schizophrenic patients in the psychiatric interview: An experimental study of their effectiveness at manipulation. *Journal of Consulting Psychology*, *31*, 543–547.

Braginsky, B. M., & Braginsky, D. D. (1971). Schizophrenic patients in the psychiatric interview: An experimental study of their effectiveness at manipulation. *Journal of Consulting Psychology*, *31*, 543–547.

Braginsky, B. M., Brkaginsky, D. D., & Ring, K. (1969). *Methods of madness: The mental hospital as a last resort*. New York, NY: Holt, Rinehart and Winston.

Braginsky, B. M., Grosse, M., & Ring, K. (1966). Controlling outcomes through impression-management: An experimental study of the manipulative tactics of mental patients. *Journal of Consulting Psychology*, *30*, 295–300.

Braithwaite, J. (2007). Occam's Razor: The principle of parsimony, Behavioural Sciences Center, School of Psychology, University of Birmingham, UK.

Branch, H., & Eurman, L. J. (1980). Social attitudes toward patients with anorexia nervosa. *The American Journal of Psychiatry*, *137*, 631–632.

Brandt, K. R., & Mackenzie, T. B. (1987). Obsessive-compulsive disorder exacerbated during pregnancy: A case report. *International Journal of Psychiatry in Medicine*, *17*, 361–366.

Bremner, J. D. (2008). The neurobiology of trauma and memory in children. In M. L. Howe, G. S. Goodman, & D. Cicchetti (Eds.), *Stress, trauma, and children's memory development: Neurobiological, cognitive, clinical, and legal perspectives* (pp. 11–49). New York, NY: Oxford University Press.

Bremner, J. D., Southwick, S. M., Johnson, D. R, Yehuda, R., & Charney, D. S. (1993). Childhood physical abuse and combat-related posttraumatic stress disorder in Vietnam veterans. *The American Journal of Psychiatry*, *150*, 235–239.

Brenes, G. A. (2003). Anxiety and chronic obstructive pulmonary disease: Prevalence, impact, and treatment. *Psychosomatic Medicine*, *65*, 963–970.

Breslow, R., Kocsis, J. H., & Belkin, B. (1980). Memory deficits in depression: Evidence utilizing the Wechsler memory scale. *Perceptual and Motor Skills*, *51*, 541–542.

Breuer, J., & Freud, S. (1895). Studies in hysteria. In J. Strachey (Ed. & Trans.), *The Standard edition of the complete psychological works of Sigmund Freud* (Vol. 2, pp. 1–17). London, England: Hogarth Press.

Brewin, C. R., & Andrews, B. (1997). Reasoning about repression: Inferences from clinical and experimental data. In M. A. Conway (Ed.), *Recovered memories and false memories* (pp. 192–205). New York, NY: Oxford University Press.

Bringager, C. B., Gauer, K., Arnesen, H., Friis, S., & Dammen, T. (2008). Nonfearful panic disorder in chest-pain patients: Status after nine-year follow-up. *Psychosomatics*, *49*, 426–437.

Brody, L. R., & Hall, J. (1993). Gender and emotion. In M. Lewis & J. Haviland (Eds.), *Handbook of emotions* (pp. 447–461). New York, NY: Guilford Press.

Broman, C. L., Hamilton, V. L., Hoffman, W. S., & Mavaddat, R. (1995). Race, gender, and the response to stress: Autoworkers vulnerability to long-term unemployment. *American Journal of Community Psychology*, *23*, 813–842.

Bronstein, M. V., & Cannon, T. D. (2017). Bias against disconfirmatory evidence in a large nonclinical sample: Associations with schizotypy and delusional beliefs. *Journal of Experimental Psychopathology*, *8*, 289–303.

Brooker, A. E. (1982). Behavioral treatment of obsessive-compulsive disorders: Current status. *Psychological Reports*, *50*, 1035–1044.

Brown, S. A. (1987). Alcohol use and type of life events experienced during adolescence. *Psychology of Addictive Behaviors, 1*, 104–107.

Brown, D., Scheflin, A. W., & Whitfield, C. L. (1999). Recovered memories: The current weight of the evidence in science and in the courts. *Journal of Psychiatry and Law, 27*, 5–156.

Brown, R. J., Poliakoff, E., & Kirkman, M. A. (2007). Somatoform dissociation and somatosensory amplification are differentially associated with attention to the tactile modality following exposure to body-related stimuli. *Journal of Psychosomatic Research, 62*, 159–165.

Brown, T. A., & Barlow, D. H. (1995). Long-term outcome in cognitive-behavioral treatment of panic disorder: Clinical predictors and alternative strategies for assessment. *Journal of Consulting and Clinical Psychology, 63*, 754–765.

Brown, T. A., & Deagle, E. A. (1992). Structured interview assessment of nonclinical panic. *Behavior Therapy, 23*, 75–85.

Bruch, H. (1973). *Eating disorders: Obesity, anorexia nervosa, and the person within*. New York, NY: Basic Books.

Bruch, H. (1978). *The golden cage: The enigma of anorexia nervosa.* Cambridge, MA: Harvard University Press.

Brush, S. G. (1989). Prediction and theory evaluation: The case of light bending. *Science, 246*, 1124–1129.

Brush, S. G. (1990). Prediction and theory evaluation: Alfven on space plasma phenomena. *Eos, 71*, 19–33.

Brush, S. G. (1992). How cosmology became a science. *Scientific America, 267*, 62–70.

Brush, S. G. (1993). Prediction and theory evaluation: Cosmic microwaves and the revival of the big bang. *Perspectives on Science, 1*, 565–602.

Brush, S. G. (2005). Testing hypotheses: Prediction and prejudice: Comment. *Science, 308*(5727), 1410–1410.

Buchanan, T. W. (2007). Retrieval of emotional memories. *Psychological Bulletin, 133*, 761–779.

Buller, R., Mair, W., & Benkert, O. (1987). Das Herzangst-Syndrom-ein Subtyp des Pani-Syndroms. In D. O. Nutzinger, D. Pyserman, T. Welan, & H. G. Zapotoczky (Eds.), *Herzphobie*. Stuttgart: Enke.

Burnett, C., & Francisco, J. (2013). Role of intuition in creativity. *Encyclopedia of Creativity, Invention, Innovation and Entrepreneurship*, 1564–1570.

Burrows, G. D., Judd, F. K., & Norman, T. R. (1993). Long-term drug treatment of panic disorder. *Journal of Psychiatric Research, 27*, 111–125.

Burstow, B. (2005). A critique of posttraumatic stress disorder and the DSM. *Journal of Humanistic Psychology, 7*, 429–445.

Bushnell, J. A., Wells, J. E., & Oakley-Browne, M. A. (1992). Long-term effects of interfamilial sexual abuse in childhood. *Acta Psychiatrica Scandinavica, 85*, 136–142.

Byrne, M., Hodges, A., Grant, E., Owens, D. C., & Johnstone, E. E. (1999). Neuropsychological assessment of young people at high genetic risk for developing schizophrenia compared with controls: Preliminary findings of the Edinburgh High Risk Study (EHRS). *Psychological Medicine, 29*, 1161–1173.

Bystritsky, A. (2004). Current pharmacological treatments for obsessive compulsive disorder. *Essential Psychopharmacology, 5*, 251–272.

Calogero, R. M., Davis, W. N., & Thompson, J. K. (2004). The sociocultural attitudes toward appearance questionnaire (SATAQ-3): Reliability and normative comparisons of eating disordered patients. *Body Image, 1*, 193–198.

Campanella, J., & Rovee-Collier, C. (2005). Latent learning and deferred imitation at 3 months. *Infancy, 7*, 243–262.

Cannon, M., Jones, P., Gilvarry, C., Rifkin, L., McKenzie, K., Foerster, A., & Murray, R. M. (1997). Premorbid social function in schizophrenia and bipolar disorder: Similarities and differences. *American Journal of Psychiatry, 154*, 1544–1550.

Capps, D. (2003). John Nash's pre delusional phase: A case of acute identity confusion. *Pastoral Psychology, 51*, 361–386.

Capps, D. (2004). The decades of life: Relocating Erikson's stages. *Pastoral Psychology, 53*, 3–32.

Capps, D. (2005). John Nash: Three phases in the career of a beautiful mind. *Journal of Religion & Health, 44*, 363–376.

Capps, D. (2011). John Nash, game theory, and the schizophrenic brain. *Journal of Religion & Health, 50*, 145–162.

Carden, N. L., & Schramel, D. J. (1966). Observations of conversion reactions seen in troops involved in the Vietnam conflict. *American Journal of Psychiatry, 123*, 21–31.

Carella, M. J. (1974). Psychoanalysis and the mind-body problem. *Psychoanalytic Review, 61*, 53–61.

Carey, G., & Gottesman, I. I. (1981). Twin and family studies of anxiety, phobic, and obsessive disorders. In D. F Klein & J. G. Rabkin (Eds.), *Anxiety: New research and changing concepts*. New York, NY: Raven Press.

Carlat, D. J., Camargo, C. A., & Herzog, D. B. (1997). Eating disorders in males: A report on 135 patients. *American Journal of Psychiatry, 154*, 1127–1132.

Carley, R. (2013). Agile materialisms: Antonio Gramsci, Stuart Hall, racialization, and modernity. *Journal of Historical Sociology, 26*, 413–441.

Carson, R. C., Butcher, J. N., & Coleman, J. C. (1988). *Abnormal psychology and modern life* (8th ed.), New York, NY: Harper Collins.

Carter, J. A. (2006). Theoretical pluralism and technical eclecticism. In C. D. Goodheart, A. E. Kazdin, & R. J. Sternberg (Eds.), *Evidence-based psychotherapy: Where practice and research meet* (pp. 63–79). Washington, DC: American Psychological Association.

Carter, M. M., & Barlow, D. H. (1995). Learned alarms: The origins of panic. In W. O'Donohue & L. Krasner (Eds.), *Theories of behavior therapy: Exploring behavior change* (pp. 209–228). Washington, DC: American Psychological Association.

Casey, D. E., Haupt, D. W., Newcomer, J. W., Henderson, D. C., Sernyak, M. J., Davidson, M., … Hennekens, C. H. (2004). Antipsychotic-induced weight gain and metabolic abnormalities: Implications for increased mortality in patients with schizophrenia. *The Journal of Clinical Psychiatry, 65*, 4–18.

Cassady, J. D., Kirschke, D. L., Jones, T. F., Craig, A. S., Bermudez, O. B., & Schaffner, W. (2005). Case series: Outbreak of conversion disorder among Amish adolescent girls. *Journal of the American Academy of Child and Adolescent Psychiatry, 44*, 291–297.

Ceci, S. J., & Loftus, E. F. (1994). Memory work: A royal road to false memories? *Applied Cognitive Psychology, 8*, 351–364.

Cella, M., Dymond, S., Cooper, A., & Turnbull, O. H. (2012). Cognitive decision modelling of emotion-based learning impairment in schizophrenia: The role of awareness. *Psychiatry Research, 196*, 15–19.

Cha, D. S., Luo, X., Ahmed, J., Becirovic, L., Cha, R. H., & McIntyre, R. S. (2019). Brexpiprazole as an augmentation agent to antidepressants in treatment resistant major depressive disorder. *Expert Review of Neurotherapeutics*. Advance Online Publication.

Chalavi, S., Vissia, E. M., Giesen, M. E., Nijenhuis, E. R. S., Draijer, N., Cole, J. H., … Reinders, A. A. (2015). Abnormal hippocampal morphology in dissociative identity disorder and post-traumatic stress disorder correlates with childhood trauma and dissociative symptoms. *Human Brain Mapping, 36*, 1692–1704.

Chambless, D. L. (2002). Identification of empirically supported counseling psychology interventions: Commentary. *The Counseling Psychologist, 30*, 302–308.

Chambless, D. L., Goldstein, A. J., Gallagher, R., & Bright, P. (1986). Integrating behavior therapy and psychotherapy in the treatment of agoraphobia. *Psychotherapy, 23*, 150–159.

Charman, D. P. (2003). Paradigms in current psychotherapy research: A critique and the case for evidence-based psychodynamic psychotherapy research. *Australian Psychologist, 38*, 39–45.

Cheit, R. E. (1998). Consider this, skeptics of recovered memory. *Ethics and Behavior, 8*, 141–160.

Cheng, K.-Y., Chen, S.-Y., & Lin, C.-Y. (2016). Mortality among patients with schizophrenia and vocational rehabilitation program services under Taiwan's psychiatric care reform. *International Journal of Mental Health Systems, 10*, 10–32.

Chernen, L., & Friedman, S. (1993). Treating the personality disordered agoraphobic patient with individual and marital therapy: A multiple replication study. *Journal of Anxiety Disorders, 7*, 163–177.

Chesler, B. E. (1995). The impact of stress, fear of fatness, and panic disorder with agoraphobia on eating disorder symptomatology: A case study. *International Journal of Eating Disorders, 18*, 195–198.

Chiu, L. P. (1989). Attempted suicide in Hong Kong. *Acta Psychiatrica Scandinavica, 79*, 425–430.

Cho, M., Lee, T. Y., Kwak, Y. B., Yoon, Y. B., Kim, M., & Soo, J. (2019). Adjunctive use of anti-inflammatory drugs for schizophrenia: A meta-analytic investigation of randomized controloed trails. *Australians & New Zealnd Journal of Psychiatry, 53*, 742–759.

Christopher, G., & MacDonald, J. (2005). The impact of clinical depression on working memory. *Cognitive Neuropsychiatry, 10*, 379–399.

Chu, J. A., Frey, L. M., Ganzel, B. L., & Matthews, J. A. (1999). Memories of childhood abuse: Dissociation, amnesia and corroboration. *American Journal of Psychiatry, 156*, 749–755.

Clarizio, H. F. (1991). Obsessive-compulsive disorder: The secretive syndrome. *Psychology in the Schools, 28*, 106–115.

Clark, D. A. (1999). Cognitive behavioral treatment of obsessive-compulsive disorders: A commentary. *Cognitive and Behavioral Practice, 6*, 408–415.

Clark, D. M. (1986). A cognitive approach to panic. *Behaviour Research and Therapy, 24*, 461–470.

Clark, D. M. (1988). A cognitive model of panic attacks. In S. Rachman & J. D. Maser (Eds.), *Panic: Psychological perspectives*. Hillsdale, NJ: Erlbaum.

Clark, D. M. (1999). Anxiety disorders: Why they persist and how to treat them. *Behaviour Research and Therapy, 37*, S5–S27.

Clark, D. M., Salkovskis, P. M., & Chalkley, A. J. (1985). Respiratory control as a treatment for panic attacks. *Journal of Behavior Therapy and Experimental Psychiatry, 16*, 23–30.

Clark, D. M., Salkovskis, P. M., Gelder, M. G., Koehler, C., Martin, M., Anastasiades, P., … Jeavons, A. (1988). Tests of a cognitive theory of panic. In I. Hand & H. U. Wittchen (Eds.), *Panic and Phobia II.* New York, NY: Springer-Verlag.

Clark, M. S., Milberg, S., & Ross, J. (1983). Arousal cues arousal-related material in memory: Implications for understanding effects of mood and memory. *Journal of Verbal Learning and Verbal Behavior, 22*, 633–649.

Clarke, N. A., Hartmann, T., Jones, E. L., Ballard, C. G., & Francis, P. T. (2011). Antipsychotic medication is associated with selective alterations in ventricular cerebrospinal fluid Aβ 40 and tau in patients with intractable unipolar depression. *International Journal of Geriatric Psychiatry, 26*, 1283–1291.

Claus, P. J. (1979). Spirit possession and spirit mediumship from the perspective of Tulu oral traditions. *Culture Medicine and Psychiatry, 3*, 29–52.

Clum, G. A. (1989). Psychological interventions vs. drugs in the treatment of panic. *Behavior Therapy, 20*, 429–457.

Clum, G. A., Luscomb, R. L., & Patsiokas, A. T. (1991). On the stress/parasuicide or parasuicide/stress relationship. *Psychological Reports, 68*, 1317–1318.

Cohen, C. I. (1993). Poverty and the course of schizophrenia: Implications for research and policy. *Hospital and Community Psychiatry, 44*, 951–958.

Coleman, J. C. (1984). *Abnormal psychology and modern life* (3rd ed.). Chicago, IL: Scott Foresman.

Coleman, J. C., Butcher, J. N., & Carson, R. C. (1984). *Abnormal Psychology and Modern Life* (7th ed.). Glenview, IL: Scott, Foresman.

Conrad, N. (1992). Stress and knowledge of suicidal others as factors in suicidal behavior of high school adolescents. *Issues in Mental Health Nursing, 13*, 95–104.

Coons, P. M. (1994). Confirmation of childhood abuse in child and adolescent cases of multiple personality disorder and dissociative disorder not otherwise specified. *Journal of Nervous and Mental Diseases, 182*, 461–464.

Cornblatt, B. A., Carrion, R. E., Addington, J., Seidman, L., Walker, E. F., Cannon, T. D., … Lencz, T. (2012). Risk factors for psychosis: Impaired social and role functioning. *Schizophrenia Bulletin, 38*, 1247–1257.

Cornblatt, B. A., Dworkin, R. H., Wolf, L. E., & Erlenmeyer-Kimling, L. (1996). Markers, developmental processes, and schizophrenia. In M. F. Lenzenweger & J. J. Haugaard (Eds.), *Frontiers of developmental psychopathology* (pp. 125–147). New York, NY: Oxford University Press.

Cornblatt, B. A., Obuchowski, M., Roberts, S., Pollack, S., & Erlenmeyer-Kimling, L. (1999). Cognitive and behavioral precursors of schizophrenia. *Development and Psychopathology, 11*, 487–508.

Cosway, R., Byrne, M., Clafferty, R., Hodges, A., Grant, E., Morris, J., … Johnstone, E. C. (2000). Sustained attention in young people at high risk for schizophrenia. *Psychological Medicine, 32*, 277–286.

Cottraux, J., Bouvard, M. A., & Maud, M. (2005). Combining pharmacotherapy with cognitive-behavioral interventions for obsessive compulsive disorder. *Cognitive Behavioral Therapy*, *34*, 185–192.

Cramer, P. (2001). The unconscious status of defense mechanisms. *American Psychologist*, *56*, 762–763.

Craske, M. G., & Barlow, D. H. (1989). Nocturnal panic. *Journal of Nervous and Mental Disease*, *177*, 160–167.

Craske, M. G., Burton, T., & Barlow, D. H. (1989). Relationships among measures of communication, marital satisfaction and exposure during couple's treatment of agoraphobia. *Behaviour Research and Therapy*, *21*, 131–140.

Craske, M. G., & Rowe, M. K. (1997). Nocturnal panic. *Clinical Psychology: Science and Practice*, *4*, 153–174.

Crews, F. (2006). What Erdelyi has repressed. *Behavioral and Brain Sciences*, *29*, 516–517.

Crnic, K. A., Neece, C. L., McIntyre, L. L., Blacher, J., & Baker, B. L. (2017). Intellectual disability and developmental risk: Promoting intervention to improve child and family well-being. *Child Development*, *88*, 436–445.

Crumlish, N., Whitty, K. P., Kamali, M., Clarke, M., Browne, S., McTigue, O., … O'Callaghan, E. (2005). Early insight predicts depression and attempted suicide after 4 years in first-episode schizophrenia and schizophreniform disorder. *Acta Psychiatrica Scandinavica*, *112*, 449–455.

Csordas, T. (1987). Health and holy in African and Afro-American spirit possession. *Social Science and Medicine*, *24*, 1–11.

Culberg, J., & Engström-Lindberg, M. (1988). Prevalence and incidence of eating disorders in a suburban area. *Acta Psychiatric Scandinavica*, *78*, 314–319.

Culler, E. (1930). A phobic case. *British Journal of Medical Psychology*, *10*, 46–69.

Cybulska, E. M. (1997). Globus hystericus — a somatic symptom of depression? The role of electroconvulsive therapy and antidepressants. *Psychosomatic Medicine*, *59*, 67–69.

Dagnan, D., & Sandhu, S. (1999). Social comparison, self-esteem and depression in people with intellectual disability. *Journal of Intellectual Disability Research*, *43*, 372–379.

Dalenberg, C. J., Brand, B. L., Gleaves, D. H., Dorahy, M. J., Loewenstein, R. J., Cardena, E., … Spiegel, D. (2012). Evaluation of the evidence for the trauma and fantasy models of dissociation. *Psychological Bulletin, 138*, 550–588.

Dane, E., Baer, M., Pratt, M., & Oldham, G. (2011). Rational versus intuitive problem solving: How thinking "off the beaten path" can stimulate creativity. *Psychology of Aesthetics, Creativity, and the Arts, 5*, 3–12.

Davey, G. C. L. (1989a). UCS revaluation and conditioning models for acquired fears. *Behaviour Research and Therapy, 27*, 521–528.

Davey, G. C. L. (1989b). Dental phobias and anxieties. *Behaviour Research and Therapy, 27*, 51–58.

Davidson, M., Reichenberg, A., Rabinowitz, J., Weiser, M., Kaplan, Z., & Mark, M. (1999). Behavioral and intellectual markers for schizophrenia in apparently healthy male adolescents. *American Journal of Psychiatry, 156*, 1328–1335.

Davis, L. W., Lysaker, P. H., Kristeller, J. L., Salyers, M. P., Kovach, A. C., & Woller, S. (2015). Effect of mindfulness on vocational rehabilitation outcomes in stable phase schizophrenia. *Psychological Services, 12*, 303–312.

Davison, G. C., & Neale, J. M. (1986). *Abnormal psychology. An experimental clinical approach* (4th ed.). New York, NY: Wiley.

De Lange, F. P., Roelofs, K., & Toni, I. (2007). Increased self-monitoring during imagined movements in conversion paralysis. *Neuropsychologia, 45*, 2051–2058.

De Mille, R. (1962). Intellect after lobotomy in schizophrenia: A factor analytic study. *Psychological Monographs: General and Applied, 76*, 1–18.

De Poderoso, C. M., Julian, C., & Linezky, L. (2005). Panic disorder and agoraphobia: A psychodynamic approach. In C. M. Velotis (Ed.), *Anxiety disorder research* (pp. 165–187). Hauppauge, NY: Nova Science.

De Silva, P., & Marks, M. (1999). The role of traumatic experiences in the genesis of obsessive-compulsive disorder. *Behaviour Research and Therapy, 37*, 941–951.

De Vignemont, F. (2009). Hysterical conversion: A mirror image of anosognosia? In T. Bayne & J. Fernandez (Eds.), *Delusion and self-deception: Affective and motivational influences on belief formation* (pp. 243–261). New York, NY: Psychology Press.

DeBattista, C., & Hawkins, J. (2009). Utility of atypical antipsychotics in the treatment of resistant unipolar depression. *CNS Drugs*, *23*, 369–377.

Deeley, Q., Oakley, D., Toone, B., Bell, V., Walsh, E., Marquand, A. F., … Halligan, P. W. (2013). The functional anatomy of suggested limb paralysis. *Cortex*, *49*, 411–422.

Delis, D. C., & Wetter, S. R. (2007). Cogniform disorder and cogniform condition: Proposed diagnoses for excessive cognitive symptoms. *Archives of Clinical Neuropsychology*, *22*, 589–604.

Dell, P. F., & Eisenhower, J. W. (1990). Adolescent multiple personality disorder: A preliminary study of eleven cases. *Journal of the American Academy of Child and Adolescent Psychiatry*, *29*, 359–366.

Dell'Osso, B., Nestadt, G., Allen, A., & Hollander, E. (2006). Serotonin-norepinephrine reuptake inhibitors in the treatment of obsessive-compulsive disorder: A critical review. *Journal of Clinical Psychiatry*, *67*, 600–610.

Deltito, J. A., & Hahn, R. (1993). A three-generational presentation of separation anxiety in childhood with agoraphobia in adulthood. *Psychopharmacology Bulletin*, *29*, 189–193.

Demal, U., Zitterl, W., Lenz, G., Zapotoczky, H. G., & Zitterl-Eglseer, K. (1996). Obsessive compulsive disorder and depression: First results of a prospective study on 74 patients. *Progress in Neuro-Psychopharmacology and Biological Psychiatry*, *20*, 801–813.

Denys, D., de Geus, F., van Megen, H., & Westenberg, H. G. M. (2004). Symptom dimensions in obsessive-compulsive disorder: Factor analysis on a clinician-rated scale and a self-report measure. *Psychopathology*, *37*, 181–189.

Derossett, J. E. (2013). *Every parent's nightmare: Adam Lanza & Sandy Hook elementary*. USA: CreateSpace Independent Publishing Platform.

Dill, J. C., & Anderson, C. A. (1995). Effects of frustration and justification on hostile aggression. *Aggressive Behavior*, *21*, 359–369.

DiNardo, L., & Rainey, D. (1991). The effects of illumination level and exposure time on facial recognition. *Psychological Records*, *41*, 329–334.

Ding J. M., & Kanaan, R. A. (2016). What should we say to patients with unexplained neurological symptoms? How explanation affects offence. *Journal of Psychosomatic Research*, *91*, 55–60.

Dinwiddie, S. H., North, C. S., & Yutzy, S. H. (1993). Multiple personality disorder: Scientific and medicolegal issues. *Bulletin of the American Academy of Psychiatry & the Law*, *21*, 69–79.

Dohrenwend, B. P., & Dohrenwend, B. S. (1969). *Social status and psychological disorder*. New York, NY: Wiley.

Dold, M., Aigner, M., Lanzenberger, R., & Kasper, S. (2013). Antipsychotic augmentation of serotonin reuptake inhibitors in treatment-resistant obsessive-compulsive disorder: A meta-analysis of double-blind, randomized, placebo-controlled trials. *The International Journal of Neuropsychopharmacology*, *16*, 557–574.

Dold, M., Bartova, L., Kautzky, A., Serretti, A., Porcelli, S., Souery, D., . . . Kasper, S. (2018). Clinical factors associated with augmentation treatment with second-generation antipsychotics and lithium in major depression — Results from a European multicenter study. *European Neuropsychopharmacology*, *28*, 1305–1313.

Dollard, J., & Miller, N. E. (1950). *Personality and psychotherapy: An analysis in terms of learning, thinking, and culture*. New York, NY: McGraw-Hill.

Donoghue, K., Doody, G. A., Murray, R. M., Jones, P. B., Morgan, C., Dazzan, P., … MacCabe, J. H. (2014). Cannabis use, gender and age of onset of schizophrenia: Data from the ÆSOP study. *Psychiatry Research*, *215*, 528–532.

Donohue, B., Thevenin, D. M., & Runyon, M. K. (1997). Behavioral treatment of conversion disorder in adolescence. *Behavior Modification*, *21*, 231–251.

Dörfler, V., & Ackermann, F. (2012). Understanding intuition: The case for two forms of intuition. *Management Learning*, *43*, 545–564.

Doroshow, D. B. (2006). Performing a cure for schizophrenia: Insulin coma therapy on the wards. *Journal of the History of Medicine and Allied Sciences*, *62*, 213–243.

Dougherty, D. D., Rauch, S. L., & Jenike, M. A. (2004). Pharmacotherapy for obsessive compulsive disorder. *Journal of Clinical Psychology*, *60*, 1195–1202.

Doyle, A., & Pollack, M. H. (2004). Long term management of panic disorder. *Journal of Clinical Psychiatry*, *65*, 24–28.

Dudley, R., Daley, K., Nicholson, M., Shaftoe, D., Spencer, H., Cavanagh, K., & Freeston, M. (2013). "Jumping to conclusions" in first-episode psychosis: A longitudinal study. *British Journal of Clinical Psychology, 52*, 380–393.

Dudley, R., John, C. H., Young, A. W., & Over, D. E. (1997). The effect of self-referent material on the reasoning of people with delusions. *British Journal of Clinical Psychology, 36*, 575–584.

Dudley, R., Taylor, P., Wickham, S., & Hutton, P. (2016). Psychosis, delusions and the "jumping to conclusions" reasoning bias: A systematic review and meta-analysis. *Schizophrenia Bulletin, 42*, 652–665.

Dudley, R. E., & Over, D. E. (2003). People with delusions jump to conclusions: A theoretical account of research findings on the reasoning of people with delusions. *Clinical Psychology & Psychotherapy, 10*, 263–274.

Duncan, B. L., Parks, M. B., & Rusk, G. S. (1990a). Eclectic strategic practice: A process constructive perspective. *Journal of Marital and Family Therapy, 16*, 165–178.

Duncan, B. L., Parks, M. B., & Rusk, G. S. (1990b). Strategic eclecticism: A technical alternative for eclectic psychotherapy. *Psychotherapy, 27*, 568–577.

Dutton, D. G., & Karakanta, C. (2013). Depression as a risk marker for aggression: A critical review. *Aggression and Violent Behavior, 18*, 310–319.

Dworkin, R. H., Lewis, J. A., Cornblatt, B., & Erlenmeyer-Kimling, L. (1994a). Social competence deficits in adolescents at risk for schizophrenia. *Journal of Nervous and Mental Disease, 182*, 103–108.

Dworkin, R. H., Lewis, J. A., Cornblatt, B., & Erlenmeyer-Kimling, L. (1994b). "Social competence deficits in adolescents at risk for schizophrenia": Correction. *Journal of Nervous and Mental Disease, 182*, 301.

Eagle, M. (2000). Repression: Part II of II. *Psychoanalytic Review, 87*, 161–187.

Eagly, A. H., & Wood, W. (1991). Explaining sex differences in social behavior: A meta-analytic perspective. *Personality and Social Psychology Bulletin, 17*, 306–315.

Ebert, A., & Bar, K.-J. (2010). Emil Kraepelin: A pioneer of scientific understanding of psychiatry and psychopharmacology. *Indian Journal of Psychiatry, 52*, 191–192.

Edelstein, E. L. (1989). *Anorexia nervosa and other dyscontrol syndromes*. Berlin: Springer.

Eich, E. (1995). Mood as a mediator of place dependent memory. *Journal of Experimental Psychology: General, 124*, 293–308.

Eich, E., Macaulay, D., & Ryan, L. (1994). Mood dependent memory for events of the personal past. *Journal of Experimental Psychology: General, 123*, 201–215.

Eifert, G. H. (1992). Cardiophobia: A paradigmatic behavioral model of heart-focused anxiety and non-anginal chest pain. *Behaviour Research and Therapy, 30*, 329–345.

Einfeld, S. L., Piccinin, A. M., Mackinnon, A., Hofer, S. M., Taffe, J., Gray, K. M., ... Tonge, B. J. (2006). Psychopathology in young people with intellectual disability. *Journal of the American Medical Association, 296*, 1981–1989.

Eisler, R. M., & Blalock, J. A. (1991). Masculine gender role stress: Implications for the assessment of men. *Clinical Psychology Review, 11*, 45–60.

Ekinci, O., Ugurlu, G. K., Albayrak, Y., Arslan, M., & Caykoylu, A. (2012). The relationship between cognitive insight, clinical insight, and depression in patients with schizophrenia. *Comprehensive Psychiatry, 53*, 195–200.

Elal, G. (2003). Abnormal eating attitudes and disorders in Turkey: Feminine attractiveness or liberal modernity? In G. M. Ruggiero (Ed.), *Eating disorders in the Mediterranean area: An exploration in transcultural psychology* (pp. 57–78). Hauppauge, NY: Nova Science.

Elie, D., Poirier, M., Chianetta, J. M., Durand, M., Gregoire, C. A., & Grignon, S. (2010). Cognitive effects of antipsychotic dosage and polypharmacy: A study with the BACS in patients with schizophrenia and schizoaffective disorder. *Journal of Psychopharmacology, 24*, 1037–1044.

Emmelkamp, P. M. G. (1982). *Phobic and obsessive-compulsive disorders: Theory, research and practice*. New York, NY: Plenum.

Emmelkamp, P. M. G. (1987). Obsessive-compulsive disorders. In L. Michelson & L. M. Ascher (Eds.), *Anxiety and stress disorders: Cognitive-behavioral assessment and treatment*. New York, NY: Guilford.

Emmerson, P. G. (1986). Effects of environmental context on recognition memory in an unusual environment. *Perceptual and Motor Skills, 63,* 1047–1050.

Emsseley, R. (2018). Antipsychotic maintenance treatment in schizophrenia and the importance of preventing relapse. *World Psychiatry, 17,* 168–169.

Endrawes, G., O'Brien, L., & Wilkes, L. (2007). Mental illness and Egyptian families. *International Journal of Mental Health Nursing, 16,* 178–187.

Engs, R. C., & Hanson, D. J. (1990). Gender differences in drinking patterns and problems among college students: A review of the literature. *Journal of Alcoholism and Drug Abuse, 35,* 36–47.

Epstein, R. (1984). The principle of parsimony and some applications in psychology. *Journal of Mind and Behavior, 5,* 119–130.

Erdelyi, M. H. (1985). *Psychoanalysis: Freud's cognitive psychology.* New York, NY: Freeman.

Erdelyi, M. H. (2006). The unified theory of repression. *Behavioral and Brain Sciences, 29,* 499–551.

Erdelyi, M. H., & Goldberg, B. (1979). Let's not sweep repression under the rug: Toward a cognitive psychology of repression. In J. F. Kihlstrom & F. J. Evans (Eds.), *Functional disorder of memory.* Hillsdale, NJ: Erlbaum.

Erickson, K., Drevets, W. C., Clark, L., Cannon, D. M., Bain, E., Zarate, C. A., Jr., … Sahakian, B. J. (2005). Mood-congruent bias in affective go/no-go performance of unmedicated patients with major depressive disorder. *The American Journal of Psychiatry, 162,* 2171–2173.

Evans, J. S. B. T. (2008). Dual-processing accounts of reasoning, judgment, and social cognition. *Annual Review of Psychology, 59,* 255–278.

Evensen, S., Wisløff, T., Lystad, J. U., Bull, H., Martinsen, E. W., Ueland, T., & Falkum, E. (2019). Exploring the potential cost-effectiveness of a vocational rehabilitation program for individuals with schizophrenia in a high-income welfare society. *BMC Psychiatry, 19,* Article ID 140.

Erwin, E. (1980). Psychoanalytic therapy. The Eysenck argument. *American Psychologist, 35,* 435–443.

Eysenck, H. J. (1976). The learning theory model of neurosis: A new approach. *Behaviour Research and Therapy*, *14*, 251–267.

Eysenck, H. J., & Rachman, S. J. (1965). *The causes and cures of neurosis*. San Diego, CA: Robert R. Knapp.

Faatehi, M., Basiri, M., Nezhadi, A., Shabni, M., Masoumi-Ardakani, Y., Soltani, Z., & Nozari, M. (2019). Early enriched environment prevenrs cognitive impairment in an animal model of schizophrenia induced by MK-801: Role of hippocampal BDNF. *Brain Research*, *1711*, 115–119.

Fahy, T. A. (1988). The diagnosis of multiple personality disorder: A critical review. *British Journal of Psychiatry*, *153*, 597–606.

Fakhoury, W. K. H., Wright, D., & Wallace, M. (2001). Prevalence and extent of distress of adverse effects of antipsychotics among callers to a United Kingdom National Mental Health Helpline. *International Clinical Psychopharmacology*, *16*, 153–162.

Falcone, M. A., Murray, R. M., O'Connor, J. A., Hockey, L. N., Gardner-Sood, P., Di Forti, M., … Jolley, S. (2015). Jumping to conclusions and the persistence of delusional beliefs in first episode psychosis. *Schizophrenia Research*, *165*, 243–246.

Falkai, P., Rossner, M. J., Schulze, T. G., Hasan, A., Brzózka, M. M., Malchow, B., … Schmitt, A. (2015). Kraepelin revisited: Schizophrenia from degeneration to failed regeneration. *Molecular Psychiatry*, *20*, 671–676.

Faraone, S. V., Ghirardi, L., Kuja-Halkola, R., Lichtenstein, P., & Larsson, H. (2017). The familial co-aggregation of attention-deficit/hyperactivity disorder and intellectual disability: A register-based family study. *Journal of the American Academy of Child & Adolescent Psychiatry*, *56*, 167–174.

Faries, D., Ascher-Svanum, H., Zhu, B., Correll, C., & Kane, J. (2005). Antipsychotic monotherapy and polypharmacy in the naturalistic treatment of schizophrenia with atypical antipsychotics. *BMC Psychiatry*, *5*, 1–11.

Fava, G. A., Rafanelli, C., Tossani, E., & Grandi, S. (2008). Agoraphobia is a disease: A tribute to Sir Martin Roth. *Psychotherapy and Psychosomatics*, *77*, 133–138.

Favaro, A., & Santonastaso, P. (2000). Self-injurious behavior in anorexia nervosa. *Journal of Nervous and Mental Disease*, *188*, 537–542.

Fayek, A. (2005). The centrality of the system UCS in the theory of psychoanalysis: The nonrepressed unconscious. *Psychoanalytic Psychology*, *22*, 524–543.

Feixas, G., & Botella, L. (2004). Psychotherapy integration: Reflections and contributions from a constructivist epistemology. *Journal of Psychotherapy Integration*, *14*, 192–222.

Fenichel, O. (1934). *Outline of clinical psychoanalysis*. New York, NY: Psychoanalytic Quarterly & Norton Press.

Fenichel, O. (1946). *Psychoanalytic theory of neurosis*. London, England: Routledge & Kegan.

Ferguson, C. P., & Pigott, T. A. (2000). Anorexia and bulimia nervosa: Neurobiology and pharmacotherapy. *Behavior Therapy*, *31*, 237–263.

Fernández, L. B., & Cano, T. R. (2005). Uso de antipsicóticos en el tratamiento de pacientes con trastorno de la conducta alimentaria: Estudio con risperidona [Antipsychotics in treatment of patients with eating disorders: A study with risperidone]. *Actas Españolas de Psiquiatría*, *33*, 33–40.

Fervaha, G., Agid, O., Takeuchi, H., Foussias, G., & Remington, G. (2014). Effect of antipsychotic medication on overall life satisfaction among individuals with chronic schizophrenia: Findings from the NIMH CATIE study. *European Neuropsychopharmacology*, *24*, 1078–1085.

Fineberg, N. A., Pampaloni, I, Pallanti, S., Ipser, J., & Stein, D. J. (2007). Sustained response versus relapse: The pharmacotherapeutic goal for obsessive compulsive disorder. *International Clinical Psychopharmacology*, *22*, 313–322.

Fink, G. R., Halligan, P. W., & Marshall, J. C. (2006). Neuroimaging of hysteria. In M. Hallett, S. Fahn, J. Jankovic, A. E. Lang et al. (Eds.), *Psychogenic movement disorders: Neurology and neuropsychiatry* (pp. 230–237). Philadelphia, PA: Lippincott Williams & Wilkins.

Fischer, A. H. (1993). Sex differences in emotionality: Factor stereotype? *Feminism and Psychology*, *3*, 303–318.

Fisher, P. L., & Wells, A. (2005). How effective are cognitive and behavioral treatments for obsessive-compulsive disorder? A clinical significance analysis. *Behaviour Research and Therapy*, *43*, 1543–1558.

Fisher, S., & Greenberg, R. P. (1977). Stomach symptoms and up-down metaphors and gradients. *Psychosomatic Medicine*, *39*, 93–101.

Fitzgerald, T. J. (1973). The use of electroconvulsive therapy as an aversive stimulus: A single subject design. *Newsletter for Research in Mental Health and Behavioral Sciences*, *15*, 24–26.

Fleet, R. P., Martel, J. P., Lavoie, K. L., Dupuis, G., & Beitman, B. D. (2000). Non-fearful panic disorder: A variant of panic in medical patients? *Psychosomatics: Journal of Consultation and Liaison Psychiatry*, *41*, 311–320.

Flyvbjerg, B. (2006). Five misunderstandings about case-study research. *Qualitative Inquiry*, *12*, 219–245.

Foa, E. B. (1979). Failure in treating obsessive-compulsives. *Behaviour and Research Therapy*, *17*, 169–176.

Folks, D. G., Ford, C. V., & Regan, W. M. (1984). Conversion symptoms in a general hospital. *Psychosomatics*, *25*, 285–295.

Follette, W. C., & Houts, A. C. (1996). Models of scientific progress and the role of theory in taxonomy development: A case study of the *DSM*. *Journal of Consulting and Clinical Psychology*, *64*, 1120–1132.

Fonagy, P., Roth, A., & Higgit, A. (2005). Psychodynamic psychotherapies: Evidence-based practice and clinical wisdom. *Bulletin of the Menninger Clinic*, *69*, 1–58.

Forney, M. A., Forney, P. D., Sheets, K., Sitorius, M., Rixey, S., McGinty, D., Smith, S., & Yates, M. L. (1990). The relationship between stress and substance used among first year medical students: An exploratory investigation. *Journal of Alcohol and Drug Education*, *35*, 54–65.

Frances, A. (2013). The new crisis in confidence in psychiatric diagnosis. *Annnals in Internal Medicine*, *159*, 221–222.

Frankel, F. H. (1974). Trance capacity and genesis of phobic behavior. *Archives of General Psychiatry*, *31*, 261–263.

Fredrikson, M., Annas, P., Fischer, H., & Wik, G. (1996). Gender and age differences in the prevalence of specific fears and phobias. *Behaviour Research and Therapy*, *34*, 33–39.

Freedman, L. R., Rock, D., Roberts, S. A., Cornblatt, B. A., & Erlenmeyer-Kimling, K. L. (1998). The New York high-risk project: Attention, anhedonia and social outcome. *Schizophrenia Research*, *30*, 1–9.

Freeman, D., Garety, P., Kuipers, E., Fowler, D., & Bebbingtom, P. E. (2002). A cognitive model of persecutory delusions. *British Journal of Clinical Psychology*, *41*, 331–347.

Freeston, M. H., Ladouceur, R., Gagnon, F., Thibodeau, N., Rhéaume, J., Letarte, H., & Bujold, A. (1997). Cognitive-behavioral treatment of obsessive thoughts: A controlled study. *Journal of Consulting and Clinical Psychology*, *65*, 405–413.

Freud, A. (1936). *The ego and the mechanisms of defense*. New York, NY: International Universities Press.

Freud, S. (1894/1962). The neuro-psychoses of defense. In J. Strachey (Ed. & Trans.), *The standard edition of the complete psychological works of Sigmund Freud* (Vol. 3). London, England: Hogarth Press.

Freud, S. (1905/1964). Three essays on the theory of sexuality. In J. Strachey (Ed. & Trans.), *The standard edition of the complete psychological works of Sigmund Freud* (Vol. 7, pp. 125–245). London, England: Hogarth Press.

Freud, S. (1909/1964). Analysis of a phobia in a five-year-old boy. In J. Strachey (Ed. & Trans.), *The standard edition of the completed psychological works of Sigmund Freud* (Vol. 10, pp. 5–149). London, England: Hogarth Press.

Freud, S. (1913). The disposition to obsessional neurosis: A contribution to the problem of choice of neurosis. *The Standard Edition of the Complete Psychological Works of Sigmund Freud* (Vol. 12, pp. 311–326). London: Hogarth Press.

Freud, S. (1914). On the history of the psychoanalytic movement. In J. Strachey (Ed. & Trans.), *The standard edition of the complete psychological works of Sigmund Freud* (Vol. 14, pp. 7–66). London, England: Hogarth Press.

Freud, S. (1915a). Instincts and their vicissitudes. In J. Strachey (Ed. & Trans.), *The standard edition of the complete psychological works of Sigmund Freud* (Vol. 14, pp. 117–140). London, England: Hogarth Press.

Freud, S. (1915b). Repression. In J. Strachey (Ed. & Trans.), *The standard edition of the complete psychological works of Sigmund Freud* (Vol. 14, pp. 141–158). London, England: Hogarth Press.

Freud, S. (1915c). The unconscious. In J. Strachey (Ed. & Trans.), *The standard edition of the complete psychological works of Sigmund Freud* (Vol. 14, pp . 166–204). London, England: Hogarth Press.

Freud, S. (1926/1964). Inhibition, symptoms and anxiety. In J. Strachey (Ed. & Trans.), *The standard edition of the complete psychological works of Sigmund Freud* (Vol. 20, pp. 77–175). London, England: Hogarth Press.

Freud, S. (1936/1963). *The problem of anxiety* (H. A. Bunker, Trans.). New York, NY: Norton.

Friedman, S., Smith, L., Fogel, D., Paradis, C., Viswanathan, R., Ackerman, R., & Trappler, B. (2002). The incidence and influence of early traumatic life events in patients with panic disorder: A comparison with other psychiatric outpatients. *Journal of Anxiety Disorder*, *16*, 259–272.

Fiedorowicz, J. G., Cyranowski, J. M., Liu, Z., & Swartz, H. A. (2019). Changes in inflammation with treatment for bipolar II depression: Pilot trial data on differential effects of psychotherapy and medication. *Neurology, Psychiatry and Brain Research*, *33*, 112–118.

Fukunishi, I., Sugawara, Y., Takayama, T., Makuuchi, M., Kawarasaki, H., & Surman, O. S. (2001). Psychiatric disorders before and after living-related transplantation. *Psychosomatics: Journal of Consultation and Liaison Psychiatry*, *42*, 337–343.

Furlong, F. W. (1972). The mythology of electroconvulsive therapy. *Comprehensive Psychiatry*, *13*, 235–239.

Furukawa, T., Watanabe, N., & Churchill, R. (2006). Psychotherapy plus antidepressant for panic disorder with or without agoraphobia. *British Journal of Psychiatry*, *188*, 305–312.

Fusar-Poli, P., Papanastasiou, E., Stahl, D., Rocchetti, M., Carpenter, W., Shergill, S., & McGuire, P. (2015). Treatments of negative symptoms in schizophrenia: Meta-analysis of 168 randomized placebo-controlled trials. *Schizophrenia Bulletin*, *41*, 892–899.

Fusar-Poli, P., Smieskova, R., Kempton, M. J., Ho, B. C., Andreasen, N. C., & Borgwart, S. (2013). Progressive brain changes in schizophrenia related to antipsychotic treatment? A meta-analysis of longitudinal MRI studies. *Neuroscience and Biobehavioral Reviews*, *37*, 1680–1691.

Gallagher, I., & Hall, I. (2015). Lubitz "only had 30% vision": Killer co-pilot concerned he was losing eyesight "due to detached retina." Mail Online, 30 March.

Ganaway, G. K. (1995). Hypnosis, childhood trauma, and dissociative identity disorder: Toward an integrative theory. *International Journal of Clinical and Experimental Hypnosis*, *43*, 127–144.

Ganesan, V. (1986). Electroconvulsive therapy under fire. *Indian Journal of Clinical Psychology*, *13*, 145–147.

Garaigordobil, M., & Pérez, J. I. (2007). Self-concept, self-esteem and psychopathological symptoms in persons with intellectual disability. *The Spanish Journal of Psychology*, *10*, 141–150.

Garety, P., Joyce, E., Jolley, S., Emsley, R., Waller, H., Kuipers, E., … Freeman, D. (2013). Neuropsychological functioning and jumping to conclusions in delusions. *Schizophrenia Research*, *150*, 570–574.

Garfinkel, P. E., & Kaplan, A. S. (1986). Anorexia nervosa: Diagnostic conceptualizations. In K. D. Brownell & J. P. Foryet, (Eds.), *Handbook of eating disorders: Physiology, psychology, and treatment of anorexia and bulimia.* New York, NY: Basic Books.

Garner, D. M. (1986). Cognitive therapy for anorexia nervosa. In K. D. Brownell & J. P. Foryet, (Eds.), *Handbook of eating disorders: Physiology, psychology, and treatment of anorexia and bulimia.* New York, NY: Basic Books.

Garner, D. M., Vitousek, K. M., & Pike, K. M. (1997). Cognitive-behavioral therapy for anorexia nervosa. In D. M. Garner & P. E. Garfinkel (Eds.), *Handbook of treatment for eating disorders* (pp. 94–144). New York, NY: Guilford Press.

Gaweda, L., Staszkiewich, M., & Balzan, R. P. (2017). The relationship between cognitive biases and psychological dimensions of delusions: The importance of jumping to conclusions. *Journal of Behavior and Experimental Psychiatry*, *56*, 51–56.

Gelder, M. G. (1992). Treatment of neuroses. *International Journal of Mental Health*, *21*, 3–42.

Gerretsen, P., Chakravarty, M. M., Mamo, D., Menon, M., Pollock, B. G., Rajji, T. K., & Graff-Guerrero, A. (2013). Frontotemporoparietal asymmetry and lack of illness awareness in schizophrenia. *Human Brain Mapping*, *34*, 1035–1043.

Gerlsma, C., Emmelkamp, P. M., & Arrindell, W. A. (1990). Anxiety, depression, and perception of early parenting: A meta-analysis. *Clinical Psychology Review*, *10*, 251–277.

Gerretsen, P., Chakravarty, M. M., Mamo, D., Menon, M., Pollock, B. G., Rajji, T. K., & Graff-Guerrero, A. (2013). Frontotemporoparietal asymmetry and lack of illness awareness in schizophrenia. *Human Brain Mapping, 34*, 1035–1043.

Gershuny, B. S., Baer, L., Radomsky, A. S., Wilson, K. A., & Jenike, M. A. (2003). Connections among symptoms of obsessive-compulsive disorder and posttraumatic stress disorder: A case series. *Behaviour Research and Therapy, 41*, 1029–1041.

Gibbert, M., Ruigrok, W., & Wicki, B. (2008). What passes as a rigorous case study? *Strategic Management Journal, 29*, 1465–1474.

Giesbrecht, T., Lynn, S. J., Lilienfeld, S. O., & Merckelbach, H. (2008). Cognitive processes in dissociation: An analysis of core theoretical assumptions. *Psychological Bulletin, 134*, 617–647.

Giesbrecht, T., Lynn, S. J., Lilienfeld, S. O., & Merckelbach, H. (2010). Cognitive processes, trauma, and dissociation — misconceptions and misrepresentations: Reply to Bremner (2010). *Psychological Bulletin, 136*, 7–11.

Gigerenzer, G. (2007). *Gut feelings: The intelligence of the unconscious.* New York, NY: Viking.

Gilmore, L., & Cuskelly, M. (2014). Vulnerability to loneliness in people with intellectual disability: An explanatory model. *Journal of Policy and Practice in Intellectual Disabilities, 11*, 192–199.

Gleaves, D. H. (1996). The sociocognitive model of dissociative identity disorder: A reexamination of the evidence. *Psychological Bulletin, 120*, 42–59.

Glenn, P. (2015). Andreas: Ascent into madness. *The Telegraph*, 2 April.

Glisky, E. L., Ryan, L., Reminger, S., Hardt, O., Hayes, S. M., & Hupbach, A. (2004). A case of psychogenic fugue: I understand, aber ich verstehe nichts. *Neuropsychologia, 42*, 1132–1147.

Glöckner, A., & Witteman, C. (2010). Beyond dual-process models: A categorization of processes underlying intuitive judgment and decision making. *Thinking & Reasoning, 16*, 1–25.

Goldblatt, M., & Munitz, H. (1976). Behavioral treatment of hysterical leg paralysis. *Journal of Behavior Therapy and Experimental Psychiatry, 7*, 259–263.

Golding, J. M. (2005). Directed forgetting tasks in cognitive research. In A. Wenzel & D. C. Rubin (Eds.), *Cognitive methods and their application to clinical research* (pp. 177–196). Washington, DC: American Psychological Association.

Goldney, R. D. (1989). Suicide: The role of the media. *Australian and New Zealand Journal of Psychiatry, 23*, 30–34.

Gooch, J. L., Wolcott, R., & Speed, J. (1997). Behavioral management of conversion disorder in children. *Archives of Physical Medicine and Rehabilitation, 78*, 264–268.

Good, G. E., Sherrod, N. B., & Dillon, M. G. (2000). Masculine gender role stressors and men's health. In R. M. Eisler & M. Hersen (Eds.), *Handbook of gender, culture, and health* (pp. 63–81). Mahwah, NJ: Lawrence Erlbaum Associates.

Goodwin, R. D., Faravelli, C., Rosi, S., Cosci, F., Truglia, E., de-Graaf, R., & Wittchen, H. U. (2005). The epidemiology of panic disorder and agoraphobia in Europe. *European Neuropsychopharmacology, 15*, 435–443.

Gorman, J. M., Goetz, R. R., Fyer, M., King, D. L., Fyer, A. J., Liebowitz, M. R., & Klein, D. F. (1988). The mitral valve prolapse-panic disorder connection. *Psychosomatic Medicine, 50*, 114–122.

Gottheil, E., Backup, C. E., & Cornelison, F. S. (1969). Denial and self-image confrontation in a case of anorexia nervosa. *Journal of Nervous and Mental Disease, 148*, 238–250.

Gottlob, L. R., Golding, J. M., & Hauselt, W. J. (2006). Directed forgetting of a single item. *Journal of General Psychology, 133*, 67–80.

Gøtzsche, P. (2014). Benzodiazepines and the risk for Alzheimer's disease. *BMJ: British Medical Journal, 349*, g5312.

Graeber, C. (2013). *The good nurse: A true story of medicine, madness and murder*. New York, NY: Hachette Book.

Graham, J., & Gaffan, E. A. (1997). Fear of water in children and adults: Etiology and familial effects. *Behaviour Research and Therapy, 35*, 91–108.

Graysmith, R. (1996). *Unabomber: A desire to kill mass*. New York, NY: Amazon.

Green, C., Garety, P. A., Freeman, D., Fowler, D., Bebbington, P., Dunn, G., & Kuipers, E. (2006). Content and affect in persecutory delusions. *British Journal of Clinical Psychology, 45*, 561–577.

Green, M. (2016). Impact of cognitive and social cognitive impairment on functional outcomes in patients with schizophrenia. *Journal of Clinical Psychiatry*, *77*, 8–11.

Greenberg, D., & Witztum, E. (1994). The influence of cultural factors on obsessive compulsive disorder: Religious symptoms in a religious society. *Israel Journal of Psychiatry and Related Sciences*, *31*, 211–220.

Greenfeld, D. G., Anyan, W. R., Hobart, M., Quinlan, D. M., & Plantes, M. (1991). Insight into illness and outcome in anorexia nervosa. *International Journal of Eating Disorders*, *10*, 101–109.

Greenwald, A. G. (1992). Unconscious cognition reclaimed. *American Psychologist*, *47*, 766–779.

Greenwood, C. M., Husted, J., Bomba, M. D., Hodgkinson, K. A., & Bassett, A. S. (2004). Elevated rates of schizophrenia in a familial sample with mental illness and intellectual disability. *Journal of Intellectual Disability Research*, *48*, 531–539.

Griffiths, R. F., & Ellis, P. M. (2007). Visual conversion disorder in a harbor pilot leading to sudden loss of control of a large vessel. *Aviation, Space, and Environmental Medicine*, *78*, 59–62.

Grinker, R. R. (2010). The five lives of the psychiatry manual. *Nature*, *468*, 168–170.

Grisaru, N., & Witztum, E. (1995). The "Zar" phenomena amongst Ethiopian new immigrants to Israel: Cultural and clinical aspects. *Sichot*, *9*, 209–219.

Gross, M. L. (1978). *The psychological society: A critical analysis of psychiatry, psychotherapy, psychoanalysis, and the psychological revolution*. New York, NY: Random House.

Grosz, H. J., & Zimmerman, J. (1965). Experimental analysis of hysterical blindness: A follow-up report and new experimental data. *Archives of General Psychiatry*, *13*, 255–260.

Grosz, H. J., & Zimmerman, J. (1970). A second detailed case study of functional blindness: Further demonstration of the contribution of objective psychological laboratory data. *Behavior Therapy*, *1*, 115–123.

Grubb, T., & Watt, N. F. (1979). *Longitudinal approaches to promoting social adjustment through public school programs*. Paper presented at the meeting of the Society for Research in Child Development, San Francisco, CA.

Grünbaum, A. (1984). *The foundations of psychoanalysis: A philosophical critique*. Berkeley, CA: University of California Press.

Grünbaum, A. (1986). Précis of the foundations of psychoanalysis: A philosophical critique. *Behavioral and Brain Sciences*, *9*, 217–228.

Grünbaum, A. (2002). Critique of psychoanalysis. In E. Erwin (Ed.), *The Freud encyclopedia: Theory, therapy and culture*. New York, NY: Routledge.

Grünbaum, A. (2007). The reception of my Freud-critique in the psychoanalytic literature. *Psychoanalytic Psychology*, *24*, 545–576.

Guntrip, H. (1969). The schizoid personality and the external world. In H. Guntrip (Ed.), *Schizoid phenomena, object relations and the self.* New York, NY: International University Press.

Guo, S., Palaniyappan, L., Liddle, P. F., & Feng, J. (2016). Dynamic cerebral reorganization in the pathophysiology of schizophrenia: An MRI-derived cortical thickness study. *Psychological Medicine*, *46*, 2201–2214.

Gupta, A., & Kumar, D. (2005). Multiple personality disorder: A case report from northern India. *German Journal of Psychiatry*, *8*, 98–100.

Gur, R. C., & Sackeim, H. A. (1979). Self-deception: A concept in search of a phenomenon. *Personality and Social Psychology*, *37*, 147–169.

Gureje, O., Aderibigbe, Y. A., Olley, O., & Bamidele, R. W. (1994). Premorbid functioning in schizophrenia: A controlled study of Nigerian patients. *Comprehensive Psychiatry*, *35*, 437–440.

Gustafson, R. (1989). Frustration and successful vs. unsuccessful aggression: A test of Berkowitz's completion hypothesis. *Aggressive Behavior*, *15*, 5–12.

Gutheil, T. G. (1993). True or false members of sexual abuse? A forensic psychiatric view. *Psychiatric Annals*, *23*, 527–531.

Haddad, P. M., & Correll, C. U. (2018). The acute efficacy of antipsychotics in schizophrenia: A review of recent meta-analyses. *Therapeutic Advances in Psychopharmacology*, *8*, 303–318.

Hafner, R. J. (1976). Fresh symptoms emergence after intensive behavior therapy. *British Journal of Psychiatry*, *129*, 378–383.

Hafner, R. J. (1983). Behavior therapy for agoraphobic men. *Behaviour Research and Therapy*, *21*, 51–56.

Haggerty, K. D. (2009). Modern serial killers. *Crime, Media, Culture: An International Journal*, *5*, 168–187.

Hakola, H., Puranen, M., Repo, L., & Tiihonen, J. (1993). Long-term effects of bilateral frontal lobe lesions from neuropsychiatric and neuroradiological aspects. *Dementia and Geriatric Cognitive Disorders*, *4*, 109–112.

Halligan, P. W., & Oakley, D. A. (2013). Hypnosis and cognitive neuroscience: Bridging the gap. *Cortex*, *49*, 359–364.

Hamada, T., Koshino, Y., Misawa, T., Isaki, K., & Gejyo, F. (1998). Mitral valve prolapse and autonomic function in panic disorder. *Acta Psychiatrica Scandinavica*, *97*, 139–143.

Hammarstrom, A., & Janlert, U. (2002). Early unemployment can contribute to adult health problems: Results from a longitudinal study of school leavers. *Journal of Epidemiology and Community Health*, *56*, 624–630.

Han, C., Pae, C., Wang, S., Lee, S., Patkar, A. A., Masand, P. S., & Serretti, A. (2014). The potential role of atypical antipsychotics for the treatment of posttraumatic stress disorder. *Journal of Psychiatric Research*, *56*, 72–81.

Hans, S. L., Auerbach, J. G., Asarnow, J. R., Styr, B., & Marcus, J. (2000). Social adjustment of adolescents at risk for schizophrenia: The Jerusalem Infant Development Study. *Journal of the American Academy of Child & Adolescent Psychiatry*, *39*, 1406–1414.

Hans, S. L., Marcus, J., Henson, L., Auerbach, J. G., & Mirsky, A. F. (1992). Interpersonal behavior of children at risk for schizophrenia. *Psychiatry*, *55*, 314–335.

Harrington, P. J., Schmidt, N. B., & Telch, M. J. (1996). Prospective evaluation of panic potentiation following 35% CO_2 challenge in nonclinical subjects. *The American Journal of Psychiatry*, *153*, 823–825.

Harrow, M., & Jobe, T. H. (2013). Does long-term treatment of schizophrenia with antipsychotic medications facilitate recovery? *Schizophrenia Bulletin*, *39*, 962–965.

Harrow, M., Jobe, T. H., & Faull, R. N. (2012). Do all schizophrenia patients need antipsychotic treatment continuously throughout their lifetime? A 20-year longitudinal study. *Psychological Medicine, 42*, 2145–2155.

Haug, T., Nordgreen, T., Öst, L. G., Tangen, T., Kvale, G., Hovland, O. J., … Havik, O. E. (2016). Working alliance and competence as predictors of outcome in cognitive behavioral therapy for social anxiety and panic disorder in adults. *Behaviour Research and Therapy, 77*, 40–51.

Hauri, P. J., Friedman, M., & Ravaris, C. L. (1989). Sleep in patients with spontaneous panic attacks. *Sleep: Journal of Sleep Research & Sleep Medicine, 12*, 323–337.

Hawkins, J. D., Lishner, D. M., Catalano, R. F., & Howard, M. O. (1985). Childhood predictors of adolescent substance abuse: Toward an empirically grounded theory. *Journal of Children in Contemporary Society, 18*, 11–48.

Hayward, C., & Wilson, K. A. (2007). Anxiety sensitivity: A missing piece to the agoraphobia-without-panic puzzle. *Behavior Modification, 31*, 162–173.

Hecker, T., Bamewitz, E., Stenmark, H., & Iversen, V. (2016). Pathological spirit possession as a cultural interpretation of trauma-related symptoms. *Psychological Trauma: Theory, Research, Practice, and Policy, 8*, 468–476.

Heine, R. W. (1953). A comparison of patients' reports on psychotherapeutic experience with psychoanalytic, nondirective, and Adlerian therapists. *American Journal of Psychotherapy, 7*, 16–23.

Heinrich, L. M., & Gullone, E. (2006). The clinical significance of loneliness: A literature review. *Clinical Psychology Review, 26*, 695–718.

Henriken, M. G., & Parnas, J. (2016). The self in schizophrenia. La traduzione italiana di questo testo (curata da Valeria Bizzari) è apparsa su La Società degli Individui 57, 2016/3, Franco Angeli.

Hiss, H., Foa, E. B., & Kozak, M. J. (1994). Relapse prevention program for treatment of obsessive-compulsive disorder. *Journal of Consulting and Clinical Psychology, 62*, 801–808.

Ho, B., Andreasen, N. C., Ziebell, S., Pierson, R., & Magnotta, V. (2011). Long-term antipsychotic treatment and brain volumes. A longitudinal study of first-episode. *Archives of General Psychiatry, 68*, 128–137.

Hoek, H. W. (1993). Review of the epidemiological studies of eating disorders. *International Review of Psychiatry*, *5*, 61–74.

Hoek, H. W., Van Harten, P. N., Hermans, K. M. E., Katzman, M. A., Matroos, G. E., & Susser, E. S. (2005). The incidence of anorexia nervosa on Curacao. *American Journal of Psychiatry*, *162*, 748–752.

Hoek, H. W., & Van Hoeken, D. (2003). Review of the prevalence and incidence of eating disorders. *International Journal of Eating Disorders*, *34*, 383–396.

Hoffart, A. (1993). Cognitive treatments of agoraphobia: A critical evaluation of theoretical basis and outcome evidence. *Journal of Anxiety Disorders*, *7*, 75–91.

Hoffart, A. (1996). In vivo cognitive therapy of panic attacks. *Journal of Cognitive Psychotherapy: An International Quarterly*, *10*, 281–289.

Hoffer, A., & Osmond, H. (1966). *How to live with schizophrenia.* New York: University Press.

Hoffman, L., & Halmi, K. (1993). Psychopharmacology in the treatment of anorexia nervosa and bulimia nervosa. *Psychiatric Clinics of North America*, *16*, 767–778.

Hoffman, R. E., & Hampson, M. (2012). Functional connectivity studies of patients with auditory verbal hallucinations. *Frontiers in Human Neuroscience*, *6*, 1–7.

Hoffman, S. G., Laub, B., & Zim, S. (1990). Collaboration of clergy and psychotherapists in treating psychiatric patients. *Israel Journal of Psychiatry and Related Sciences*, *27*, 180–185.

Hoffnung, R., Aizenberg, D., Hermesh, H., & Munitz, H. (1989). Religious compulsions and the spectrum concept of psychopathology. *Psychopathology*, *22*, 141–144.

Hogarth, R. M. (2001). *Educating intuition*. Chicago, IL: University Chicago Press.

Hogarth, R. M. (2010). Intuition: A challenge for psychological research on decision making. *Psychological Inquiry*, *21*, 338–353.

Hogarty, G. E., Goldberg, S. C., & Collaborative Study Group (1973). Drug and sociotherapy in the aftercare of schizophrenic patients: One year relapse rates. *Archives of General Psychiatry*, *28*, 54–64.

Hollander, E. (1999a). Managing aggressive behavior in patients with obsessive-compulsive disorder and borderline personality disorder. *The Journal of Clinical Psychiatry, 60*, 38–44.

Hollander, E. (1999b). Managing aggressive behavior in patients with obsessive-compulsive disorder and borderline personality disorder. *The Journal of Clinical Psychiatry Monograph Series, 17*, 28–31.

Holmes, D. S. (1974). Investigations of repression: Differential recall of material experimentally or naturally associated with ego threat. *Psychological Bulletin, 81*, 632–653.

Holmes, D. S. (1990). The evidence for repression: An examination of sixty years of research. In J. L. Singer (Ed.), *Repression and dissociation: Implications for personality theory, psychopathology, and health.* Chicago, IL: University of Chicago Press.

Hoover, C. F., & Insel, T. R. (1984). Families of origin in obsessive-compulsive disorder. *Journal of Nervous and Mental Disease, 172*, 207–215.

Hopper, A., Ciorciari, J., Johnson, G., Spensley, J., Sergejew, A., & Stough, C. (2002). EEG coherence and dissociative identity disorder: Comparing EEG coherence in DID hosts, alters, controls, and acted alters. *Journal of Trauma & Dissociation, 3*, 75–88.

Horowitz, L. M. (2004). *Interpersonal foundations of psychopathology.* Washington, DC: American Psychological Association.

Horwitz, B. N., Luong, G., & Charles, S. T. (2008). Neuroticism and extraversion share genetic and environmental effects with negative and positive mood spillover in a nationally representative sample. *Personality and Individual Differences, 45*, 636–642.

Hourihan, K. L., & Taylor, T. L. (2006). Cease remembering: Control processes in directed forgetting. *Journal of Experimental Psychology: Human Perception and Performance, 32*, 1354–1365.

Houston, J. P. (1991). *Fundamentals of learning and memory* (4th ed.). New York, NY: Harcourt Brace Jovanovich.

Huebner, H. F. (1993). *Endorphins, eating disorders, and other addictive behaviors.* New York, NY: W. W. Norton.

Huesmann, L. R. (2010). *The psychology of reactions to policy oriented mass media research about aggression.* XIX International Society for Research on Aggression World Conference.

Huggler, J. (2015a). Germanwings pilot Andreas Lubitz kept diary that shows his descent into depression. *The Telegraph*, 21 September.

Huggler, J. (2015b). Germanwings pilot's doctor suggested he seek treatment in a psychiatric hospital two weeks before Alps crash. *The Telegraph*.

Hulse, S. H., Egeth, H., & Deese, J. (1980). *The psychology of learning*. New York, NY: McGraw Hill.

Husa, A. P., Rannikko, I., Moilanen, J., Haapea, M., Murray, G. K., Barnett, J., … Jaaskelainen, E. (2014). Lifetime use of antipsychotic medication and its relation to change of verbal learning and memory in midlife schizophrenia — an observational 9-year follow-up study. *Schizophrenia Research, 158*, 134–141.

Hutton, P. (2013). Cognitive-behavioral therapy for schizophrenia: A critical commentary on the Howes and Wood meta-analysis. *Psychology and Psychotherapy: Theory, Research and Practice, 86*, 139–145.

Inouye, E. (1972). Genetic aspects of neurosis: A review. *International Journal of Mental Health, 1*, 176–189.

Ironside, R., & Batchelor, I. R. C. (1945). The ocular manifestations of hysteria in relation to flying. *British Journal of Ophthalmology, 29*, 88–98.

Ishikura, R., & Tashiro, N. (2002). Frustration and fulfillment of needs in dissociative and conversion disorders. *Psychiatry and Clinical Neurosciences, 56*, 381–390.

Ishii, K. (1991). Measuring mutual causation: Effects of suicide news on suicides in Japan. *Social Science Research, 20*, 188–195.

Ismail, K. (2005). Correspodence. *British Journal of Psychiatry, 186*, 76–80.

Jacobs, W. J., & Nadel, L. (1985). Stress induced recovery of fears and phobias. *Psychological Review, 92*, 512–531.

Jacobson, N. S., Wilson, L., & Tupper, C. (1988). The clinical significance of treatment gains resulting from exposure-based interventions for agoraphobia: A reanalysis of outcome data. *Behavior Therapy, 19*, 539–554.

Jafari-Sabet, M., & Jannat-Dastjerdi, I. (2009). Muscimol state-dependent memory: Involvement of dorsal hippocampal μ-opioid receptors. *Behavioural Brain Research, 202*, 5–10.

James, D. (1998). Multiple personality disorder in the courts: A review of the North American experience. *Journal of Forensic Psychiatry, 9*, 339–361.

Janis, I. L., & Mann, L. (1977). *Decision making: A psychological analysis of conflict, choice, and commitment*. New York: Free Press.

Janssen, I., Versmissen, D., Campo, J. A., Myin-Germeys, I., Van Os, J., & Krabbendam, L. (2006). Attribution style and psychosis: Evidence for an externalizing bias in patients but not in individuals at high risk. *Psychological Medicine, 36*, 771–778.

Jaroff, L. (1993). Lies of the mind. *Time, 142*, 56–61.

Jauhar, S., McKenna, P. J., Radua, J., Fung, E., Salvador, R., & Laws, K. R. (2014). Cognitive-behavioral therapy for the symptoms of schizophrenia: Systematic review and meta-analysis with examination of potential bias. *The British Journal of Psychiatry, 204*, 20–29.

Jones, C., Hacker, D., Cormac, I., Meaden, A., & Irving, C. B. (2012). Cognitive behavior therapy versus other psychosocial treatments for schizophrenia. *Schizophrenia Bulletin, 38*, 908–910.

Jones, K. (2000). Insulin coma therapy in schizophrenia. *Journal of the Royal Society of Medicine, 93*,147–149.

Jones, M. M. (1980). Conversion reaction: Anachronism or evolutionary form? A review of neurologic, behavioral and psychoanalytic literature. *Psychological Bulletin, 87*, 427–441.

Jones, S. R. (2010). Do we need multiple models of auditory verbal hallucinations? Examining the phenomenological fit of cognitive and neurological models. *Schizophrenia Bulletin, 36*, 566–575.

Jones-Webb, R., Toomey, T. L., Short, B., Murray, D. M, Wagenaar, A., & Wolfson, M. (1997). Relationships among alcohol vulnerability, drinking location, alcohol consumption and drinking problems in adolescents. *Substance Use and Misuse, 32*, 1261–1285.

Jopling, D. A. (2001). Placebo insight: The rationality of insight-oriented psychotherapy. *Journal of Clinical Psychology, 57*, 19–36.

Jung, C. G. (1963). *Memories, dreams, reflections*. New York, NY: Crown Publishing Group/Random House.

Kaczynski, T. (1995). The Unabomber manifesto: The industrial society and its future. *The Washington Post*.

Kaczynski, T. (1999, June). Interview with Ted Kaczynski, Administrative Maximum Facility Prison Florence, Colorado, USA. *Earth First! Journal*.

Kaffman, M., & Sadeh, T. (1989). Anorexia nervosa in the kibbutz: Factors influencing the development of a monoideistic fixation. *International Journal of Eating Disorders*, *8*, 33–53.

Kahneman, D. (2003). A perspective on judgment and choice: Mapping bounded rationality. *American Psychologist*, *58*, 697–720.

Kanaan, R. A., Carson, A., Wessely, S. C., Nicholson, T. R., Aybek, S., & David, A. S. (2010). What's so special about conversion disorder? A problem and a proposal for diagnostic classification. *The British Journal of Psychiatry*, *196*, 427–428.

Kandler, C., Gottschling, J., & Spinath, F. M. (2016). Genetic and environmental parent–child transmission of value orientations: An extended twin family study. *Child Development*, *87*, 270–284.

Kane, J. M., Fleischhacker, W. W., Hansen, L., Perlis, R., Pikalov, A., & Assunção-Talbott, S. (2009). Akathisia: An updated review focusing on second-generation antipsychotics. *Journal of Clinical Psychiatry*, *70*, 627–643.

Kaneda, Y. (2007). Depression and suicide risk in patients with schizophrenia during the treatment by second generation antipsychotic agents: A mini-review. *Clinical Psychopharmacology and Neuroscience*, *5*, 14–18.

Kant, G. L., D'Zurilla, T. J., & Maydeu-Olivares, A. (1997). Social problem solving as a mediator of stress-related depression and anxiety in middle-aged and elderly community residents. *Cognitive Therapy and Research*, *21*, 73–96.

Kao, Y., & Liu, Y. (2011). Suicidal behavior and insight into illness among patients with schizophrenia spectrum disorders. *Psychiatric Quarterly*, *82*, 207–220.

Karbasi, A. L. (2010). Enhanced cognitive-behavioral therapy (CBT-E) for eating disorders: Case study of a client with anorexia nervosa. *Clinical Case Studies*, *9*, 225–240.

Karon, B. P. (2008). Psychotherapy of schizophrenia works. *Pragmatic Case Studies in Psychotherapy*, *4*, 55–61.

Kasper, S., & Akimova, E. (2013). The role of atypical antipsychotics in inadequate-response and treatment-resistant depression. In S. Kasper & S. Montgomery (Eds.), *Treatment-resistant depression* (pp. 107–128).

Kato, M., & Chang, C. (2013). Augmentation treatments with second-generation antipsychotics to antidepressants in treatment-resistant depression. *CNS Drugs*, *27*, 11–19.

Kaye, W. H., Strober, M., & Klump, K. L. (2002). Serotonin neuronal function in anorexia nervosa and bulimia nervosa. In F. Lewis-Hall, T. S. Williams, J. A. Panetta, & J. M. Herrera (Eds.), *Psychiatric illness in women: Emerging treatments and research* (pp. 557–575). Washington, DC: American Psychiatric Publishing.

Kazdin, A. E. (1982). Symptom substitution, generalization, and response covariation: Implications for psychotherapy outcome. *Psychological Bulletin*, *91*, 349–365.

Keck, P., Strakowski, S., & McElroy, S. (2000). The efficacy of atypical antipsychotics in the treatment of depressive symptoms, hostility, and suicidality in patients with schizophrenia. *Journal of Clinical Psychiatry 61*, 4–9.

Keedy, S. K., Reilly, J. L., Bishop, J. R., Weiden, P. J., & Sweeney, J. A. (2015). Impact of antipsychotic treatment on attention and motor learning systems in first-episode schizophrenia. *Schizophrenia Bulletin*, *41*, 355–365.

Keel, P. K., & Klump, K. L. (2003). Are eating disorders culture-bound syndromes? Implications for conceptualizing their etiology. *Psychological Bulletin*, *129*, 747–769.

Keijsers, P. J., Kampman, M., & Hoogduin. A. L. (2001). Dropout prediction in cognitive behavior therapy for panic disorder. *Behavior Therapy*, *32*, 739–749.

Kemp, A. H., Pe Benito, L., Quintana, D. S., Clark, C., McFarlane, A., Mayur, P., … Williams, L. M. (2010). Impact of depression heterogeneity on attention: An auditory oddball event related potential study. *Journal of Affective Disorders*, *123*, 202–207.

Kenardy, J., Fried, L., Kraemer, H. C., & Taylor, C. B. (1992). Psychological precursors of panic attacks. *British Journal of Psychiatry*, *160*, 668–673.

Kenardy, J., Oei, T. P., & Evans, L. (1990). Neuroticism and age of onset for agoraphobia with panic attacks. *Journal of Behavior Therapy and Experimental Psychiatry, 21*, 193–197.

Kenardy, J., & Taylor, C. B. (1999). Expected versus unexpected panic attacks: A naturalistic prospective study. *Journal of Anxiety Disorders, 13*, 435–445.

Kendall-Tackett, K. A., Williams, L. M., & Finkelhor, D. (1993). Impact of sexual abuse on children: A review and synthesis of recent empirical studies. *Psychological Bulletin, 113*, 164–180.

Kennedy, L., & Xyrichis, A. (2017). Cognitive behavioral therapy compared with non-specialized therapy for alleviating the effect of auditory hallucinations in people with reoccurring schizophrenia: A systematic review and meta-analysis. *Community Mental Health Journal, 53*, 127–133.

Kenny, F. T., Mowbray, R. M., & Lalani, S. (1978). Faradic disruption of obsessive ideation in the treatment of obsessive neurosis: A controlled study. *Behavior Therapy, 9*, 209–221.

Kenny, F. T., Solyom, L., & Solyom, C. (1973). Faradic disruption of obsessive ideation in the treatment of obsessive neurosis. *Behavior Therapy, 4*, 448–457.

Keshavan, M. S., Diwadkar, V. A., Montrose, D. M., Rajarethinam, R., & Sweeney, J. A. (2005). Premorbid indicators and risk for schizophrenia: A selective review and update. *Schizophrenia Research, 79*, 45–57.

Keshavan, M. S., Nasrallah, H. A., & Tandon, R. (2011). Schizophrenia, "Just the Facts" 6. Moving ahead with the schizophrenia concept: From the elephant to the mouse. *Schizophrenia Research, 127*, 3–13.

Keynejad, R. C., Carson, A. J., David, A. S., & Nicholson, T. R. (2017). Functional neurological disorder: Psychiatry's blind spot. *The Lancet Psychiatry, 4*, e2–e3.

Khanna, S., & Channabasavanna, S. (1988). Phenomenology of obsessions in obsessive-compulsive neurosis. *Psychopathology, 21*, 12–18.

Kihlstrom, J. F. (1987). The cognitive unconscious. *Science, 237*, 1445–1452.

Kihlstrom, J. F. (1989). Hypnosis and memory — and much, much more. *Contemporary Psychology: A Journal of Reviews, 34*, 985–986.

Kihlstrom, J. F. (1994). One hundred years of hysteria. In J. W. Rhue & S. J. Lynn (Eds.), *Dissociation: Clinical and theoretical perspectives* (pp. 365–394). New York, NY: Guilford.

Kihlstrom, J. F. (2000). Not taking the evidence into account. *Contemporary Psychology, 45*, 235–236.

Kihlstrom, J. F. (2002). No need for repression. *Trends in Cognitive Sciences, 6*, 502.

Kihlstrom, J. F. (2004). Availability, accessibility, and subliminal perception. *Consciousness and Cognition, 13*, 92–100.

Kihlstrom, J. F. (2005). Dissociative disorders. *Annual Review of Clinical Psychology, 1*, 227–253.

Kihlstrom, J. F. (2006). Repression: A unified theory of a will-o'-the-wisp. *Behavioral and Brain Sciences, 29*, 523.

Kihlstrom, J. F. (2015). *Is Freud still alive? No not really*. Retrieved from https://www.ocf.berkeley.edu/~jfkihlstrom/freuddead.htm

Kihlstrom, J. F., Barnhardt, T. M., & Tataryn, D. J. (1992). The psychological unconscious: Found, lost, and regained. *American Psychologist, 47*, 788–791.

Kinderman, P., & Benn, A. (2002). Attributional therapy: A case of paranoia and hallucinations. In A. P. Morrison (Ed.), *A casebook of cognitive therapy for psychosis* (pp. 197–216). New York, NY: Brunner-Routledge.

King, M. B. (1993). Cultural aspects of eating disorders. *International Review of Psychiatry, 5*, 205–216.

King, N. J., Eleonora, G., & Ollendick, T. H. (1998). Etiology of childhood phobias: Current status of Rachman's three pathways theory. *Behaviour Research and Therapy, 36*, 297–309.

Kiviniemi, M., Suvisaari, J., Koivumaa-Honkanen, H., Hakkinen, U., Isohanni, M., & Hakko, H. (2013). Antipsychotics and mortality in first-onset schizophrenia: Prospective Finnish register study with a 5-year follow-up. *Schizophrenia Research, 150*, 274–280.

Klein, D. F. (1993). Panic disorder with agoraphobia. *The British Journal of Psychiatry, 163*, 835–837.

Klein, D. F., Mannuzza, S., Chapman, T., & Fyer, A. J. (1992). Child panic revisited. *Journal of the American Academy of Child & Adolescent Psychiatry, 31*, 112–114.

Klerman, G. L. (1992). Treatments for panic disorder. *Journal of Clinical Psychiatry, 53*, 14–19.

Kluft, R. P. (1987). An update on multiple personality disorder. *Hospital and Community Psychiatry, 38*, 363–373.

Kluft, R. P. (1995). Psychodynamic psychotherapy of multiple personality disorder and allied forms of dissociative disorder not otherwise specified. In J. P. Barber & P. Crits-Christoph (Eds.), *Dynamic therapies for psychiatric disorders* (Axis I). New York, NY: Basic Books.

Kok, L. P. (1975). Epidemic hysteria (a psychiatric investigation). *Singapore Medical Journal, 16*, 35–38.

Konopaske, G. T., Dorph-Petersen, K., Pierri, J. N., Wu, Q., Sampson, A. R., Lewis, D. A. (2007). Effect of chronic exposure to antipsychotic medication on cell numbers in the parietal cortex of macaque monkeys. *Neuropsychopharmacology, 32*, 1216–1223.

Konopaske, G. T., Dorph-Petersen, K., Sweet, R. A., Pierri, J. N., Zhang, W., Sampson, A. R., & Lewis, D. A. (2008). Effect of chronic antipsychotic exposure on astrocyte and oligodendrocyte numbers in macaque monkeys. *Biological Psychiatry, 63*, 759–765.

Konsztowicz, S., & Lepage, M. (2019). The role of illness engulfment in the association between insight and depressive symptomatology in schizophrenia. *Journal of Psychiatric Research, 111*, 1–7.

Koon, R. E. (1983). Conversion dysphagia in children. *Psychosomatics: Journal of Consultation Liaison Psychiatry, 24*, 182–184.

Koran, L. M., Bullock, K. D., Hartston, H. J., Elliot, M. A., & D'Andrea, V. (2002). Citalopram treatment of compulsive shopping: An open-label study. *Journal of Clinical Psychiatry, 63*, 704–708.

Kosten, T. R., Rounsaville, B. J., Kosten, T. A., & Merikangas, K. (1991). Gender differences in the specificity of alcoholism transmission among the relatives of opioid addicts. *Journal of Nervous and Mental Disease, 179*, 392–400.

Kotler, L. A., & Walsh, B. T. (2000). Eating disorders in children and adolescents: Pharmacological therapies. *European Child and Adolescent Psychiatry, 9*, I108–I116.

Kozak, M. J., & Foa, E. B. (1994). Obsessions, overvalued ideas, and delusions in obsessive-compulsive disorder. *Behaviour Research and Therapy, 32*, 345–353.

Krahn, L. E., Bostwick, J. M., & Stonnington, C. M. (2008). Looking toward *DSM-V*: Should factitious disorder become a subtype of somatoform disorder? *Psychosomatics*, *49*, 277–282.

Kraines, S. H. (1948). *The therapy of the neurosis and psychoses* (3rd ed.). Philadelphia, PA: Lea & Febiger.

Krames, L., & MacDonald, M. R. (1985). Distraction and depressive cognitions. *Cognitive Therapy and Research*, *9*, 561–573.

Kroft, S. (2013). First serial killer on 60 minutes in 45 years. *CBS News.*

Kua, E. H., Sim, L. P., & Chee, T. C. (1986). A cross-cultural study of the possession-trance in Singapore. *Australian and New Zealand Journal of Psychiatry*, *20*, 361–364.

Kucharska-Pietura, K., & Mortimer, A. (2013). Can antipsychotics improve social cognition in patients with schizophrenia? *CNS Drugs*, *27*, 335–343.

Kuipers, E., Garety, P., Fowler, D., Freeman, D., Dunn, G., & Bebbington, P. (2006). Cognitive emotional, and social processes in psychosis: Refining cognitive behavioral therapy for persistent positive symptoms. *Schizophrenia Bulletin*, *32*, S24–S31.

Kuloglu, M., Atmaca, M., Tezcan, E., Gecici, O., & Bulut, S. (2003). Sociodemographic and clinical characteristics of patients with conversion disorder in eastern Turkey. *Social Psychiatry and Psychiatric Epidemiology*, *38*, 88–93.

Kunzendorf, R. G., & Wigner, L. (1985). Smoking and memory: State-specific effects. *Perceptual and Motor Skills*, *61*, 558.

Kushner, M. G., & Beitman, B. D. (1990). Panic attacks without fear: An overview. *Behaviour Research and Therapy*, *28*, 469–479.

La Via, M. C., & Brewerton, T. D. (1996). Cataplexy and the switch process of multiple personality disorder. *Psychiatry Research*, *63*, 231–232.

Lacasse, J. R. (2014). After DSM-5: A critical mental health research agenda for the 21st century. *Research on Social Work Practice*, *24*, 5–10.

Ladouceur, R., Leger, E., Rheaume, J., & Dube, D. (1996). Correction of inflated responsibility in the treatment of obsessive-compulsive disorder. *Behaviour Research and Therapy*, *34*, 767–774.

Laing, R. D. (1964). Is schizophrenia a disease? *International Journal of Social Psychiatry*, *10*, 184–193.

Lampropoulos, G. K. (2000). Evolving psychotherapy integration: Eclectic selection and prescriptive applications of common factors in therapy. *Psychotherapy*, *37*, 285–297.

Lampropoulos, G. K. (2001). Bridging technical eclecticism and theoretical integration: Assimilative integration. *Journal of Psychotherapy Integration*, *11*, 5–19.

Landau, S. F., & Rahav, G. (1989). Suicide and attempted suicide: Their relation to subjective social stress indicators. *Genetic, Social, and General Psychology Monographs*, *115*, 273–294.

Langdon, R., & Ward, P. (2009). Taking the perspective of the other contributes to awareness of illness in schizophrenia. *Schizophrenia Bulletin*, *35*, 1003–1011.

Last, C. G., & Francis, G. (1988). School phobia. In B. B. Lahey & A. E. Kazdin (Eds.), *Advances in clinical child psychology* (Vol. 11, pp. 193–222). New York, NY: Plen.

Laurema, H. (1993). Nocturnal limb movements in conversion paralysis. *Journal of Nervous and Mental Disease*, *181*, 707–708.

Lautch, H. (1971). Dental phobia. *British Journal of Psychiatry*, *119*, 151–158.

Lavigne, K. M., & Woodward, T. S. (2018). Hallucination and speech-specific hypercoupling in frontotemporal auditory and language networks in schizophrenia using combined task-based fMRI data: An fBIRN study. *Human Brain Mapping*, *39*, 1582–1595.

Lazarus, A. A. (1989). Why I am an eclectic (not an integrationist). *British Journal of Guidance and Counselling*, *17*, 248–258.

Lazarus, A. A. (1995). Different types of eclecticism and integration: Let's be aware of the dangers. *Journal of Psychotherapy Integration*, *5*, 27–39.

Lazarus, A. A. (2008). Technical eclecticism and multimodal therapy. In J. L. Lebow (Ed.), *Twenty-first century psychotherapies: Contemporary approaches to theory and practice* (pp. 424–452). Hoboken, NJ: John Wiley & Sons.

Leary, P. M. (2003). Conversion disorder in childhood — diagnosed too late, investigated too much? *Journal of the Royal Society of Medicine*, *96*, 436–438.

Leenaars, A. A., & Lester, D. (1996). Gender and impact of gun control in suicide and homicide. *Archives of Suicide Research*, *2*, 223–234.

Leeper, A. M., Carwile, S., & Huber, R. J. (2002). An Adlerian analysis of the unabomber. *The Journal of Individual Psychology, 58*, 169–176.

Lehman, A. F., Kreyenbuhl, J., Buchanan, R. W., Dickerson, F. B., Dixon, L. B., Goldberg, R., & Green-Paden, L. D. (2004). The schizophrenia patient outcomes research team (PORT): Updated treatment recommendations 2003. *Schizophrenia Bulletin, 30*, 193–217.

Lehman, A. F., Lieberman, J. A., Dixon, L. B., McGlashan, T. M., Miller, A. L., Perkins, D. O., & Kreyenbuhl, J. (2004). *Practice guideline for the treatments of patients with schizophrenia* (2nd ed.). American Psychiatric Association.

Lehman, A. F., Steinwachs, D. M., & the Survey Co-Investigators of the PORT Project. (1998). Pattern of usual care for schizophrenia: Initial results from the schizophrenia patient outcomes research team (PORT) client survey. *Schizophrenia Bulletin, 24*, 11–20.

Leon, G. R. (1990). *Case histories of psychopathology* (4th ed., pp. 319–335). Needham Heights, MA: Allyn & Bacon.

Leonard, W. E. (1927). *The locomotive god*. New York, NY: Appleton-Century.

Lepola, U., Leinonen, E., & Koponen, H. (1996). Citalopram in the treatment of early-onset panic disorder and school phobia. *Pharmacopsychiatry, 29*, 30–32.

Lesser, I. M., Poland, R. E., Holcant, C., & Rose, D. E. (1985). Electroencephalographic study of nighttime panic attacks. *Journal of Nervous and Mental Disease, 173*, 744–746.

Lester, D. (1983). *Why people kill themselves* (2nd ed.). Springfield, IL: Thomas.

Lester, D. (1988a). Rational choice theory and suicide. *Activitas Nervosa Superior, 30*, 309–312.

Lester, D. (1988b). Why do people choose particular methods for suicide? *Activitas Nervosa Superior, 30*, 312–314.

Lester, D. (1993). Firearm availability and accidental deaths from firearms. *Journal of Safety Research, 24*, 167–169

Lester, D. (1997). Communitarianism and suicide prevention: Proposals for the year 2000. *Crisis: The Journal of Crisis Intervention and Suicide Prevention, 18*, 118–123.

Lester, D., & Yang, B. (1996). An approach for examining the rationality of suicide. *Psychological Reports*, *79*, 405–406.

Leucht, S., Cipriani, A., Spineli, L., Mavridis, D., Orey, D., Richter, F., … Davis, J. M. (2013). Comparative efficacy and tolerability of 15 antipsychotic drugs in schizophrenia: A multiple treatments meta-analysis. *The Lancet*, *382*, 951–962.

Levenstein, S., Smith, M. W., & Kaplan, G. A. (2001). Psychosocial predictors of hypertension in men and women. *Archives of Internal Medicine*, *161*, 1341.

Levitt, J. J., Shenton, M. E., McCarley, R. W., Faux, S. F., & Ludwig, A. S. (1994). Premorbid adjustment in schizophrenia: Implications for psychosocial and ventricular pathology. *Schizophrenia Research*, *12*, 159–168.

Levy, R. S., & Jankovic, J. J. (1983). Placebo-induced conversion reaction: A neurobehavioral and EEG study of hysterical aphasia, seizure and coma. *Journal of Abnormal Psychology*, *92*, 243–249.

Lewin, I. (1982). Driver training: A perceptual — motor skill approach. *Ergonomics*, *25*, 917–924.

Lewine, R. J., Watt, N. F., & Fryer, J. H. (1978). A study of childhood social competence, adult premorbid competence, and psychiatric outcome in three schizophrenic subtypes. *Journal of Abnormal Psychology*, *87*, 294–302.

Lewis, H. B. (1981). *Freud and modern psychology* (Vol. 1). New York, NY: Plenum.

Ley, R. (1988). Panic attacks during relaxation and relaxation-induced anxiety: A hyperventilation interpretation. *Journal of Behavior Therapy and Experimental Psychiatry*, *19*, 253–259.

Ley, R. (1989). Dyspneic-fear and catastrophic cognitions in hyperventilatory panic attacks. *Behaviour Research and Therapy*, *27*, 549–554.

Lien, Y.-J., Chang, H.-A., Kao, Y.-C., Tzeng, N.-S., Lu, C.-W., & Loh, C.-H. (2018). The impact of cognitive insight, self-stigma, and medication compliance on the quality of life in patients with schizophrenia. *European Archives of Psychiatry and Clinical Neuroscience*, *268*, 27–38.

Lilienfeld, S. O., Kirsch, I., Sarbin, T. R., Lynn, S. J., Chaves, J. F., Ganaway, G. K., & Powell, R. A. (1999). Dissociative identity disorder and the sociocognitive model: Recalling the lessons of the past. *Psychological Bulletin*, *125*, 507–523.

Lindsay, D. S., & Read, J. D. (1994). Psychotherapy and memories of childhood sexual abuse: A cognitive perspective. *Applied Cognitive Psychology*, *8*, 281–338.

Lochner, C., du Toit, P. L., Zungu-Dirwayi, N., Marais, A., van Kradenburg, J., Seedats, S., Niehaus, D. H., Stein, D. J. (2002). Chidhood trauma in obsessive-compulsive disorder, trichotillomania, and controls. *Anxiety & Depression*, *15*, 66–68.

Loewenstein, R. J. (1991). Rational psychopharmacology in the treatment of multiple personality disorder. *Psychiatric Clinics of North America*, *14*, 721–740.

Loftus, E. F. (1993). The reality of repressed memories. *American Psychologist*, *48*, 518–537.

Loftus, E. F., & Hoffman, H. G. (1989). Misinformation and memory: The creation of new memories. *Journal of Experimental Psychology: General*, *118*, 100–104.

Loftus, E. F., & Klinger, M. R. (1992). Is the unconscious smart or dumb? *American Psychologist*, *47*, 761–765.

Luborsky, L., Rosenthal, R., Diguer, L., Andrusyna, T. P., Berman, J. S., Levitt, J. T., … Krause, E. D. (2002). The dodo verdict is alive and well — mostly. *Clinical Psychology: Science and Practice*, *9*, 2–12.

Lucas, A. R., Beard, C. M., O'Fallon, W. M., & Kurland, L. T. (1991). 50-year trends in the incidence of anorexia nervosa in Rochester, Minn.: A population-based study. *American Journal of Psychiatry*, *148*, 917–922.

Lukaszewski, A. W., & Roney, J. R. (2013). The origins of extraversion: Joint effects of facultative calibration and genetic polymorphism. *Personality and Social Psychology Bulletin*, *37*, 409–421.

Lukoff, D., Snyder, K., Ventura, J., & Nuechterlein, K. H. (1984). Life events, familial stress, and coping in the developmental course of schizophrenia. *Schizophrenia Bulletin*, *10*, 258–292.

Lunt, L., Brmham, J., Morris, R. G., Bullock, P. R., Selway., R. P., Xenitidis, K., & David, A. S. (2012). Prefrontal cortex dysfunction and jumping to conclusions: Bias or deficit? *Journal of Neuropsychology*, *6*, 65–78.

Lynch, D., Laws, K. R., & McKenna, P. J. (2010). Cognitive behavioral therapy for major psychiatric disorder: Does it really work? A meta-analytical review of well-controlled trials. *Psychological Medicine, 40*, 9–24.

Lynn, S. J., Kirsch, I., & Hallquist, M. N. (2008). Social cognitive theories of hypnosis. In M. R. Nash & A. J. Barnier (Eds.), *The Oxford handbook of hypnosis* (pp. 111–139). Oxford, England: University Press.

Lynn, S. J., Lock, T., Loftus, E. F., Krackow, E., & Lilienfeld, S. O. (2003). The remembrance of things past: Problematic memory recovery techniques in psychotherapy. In S. O. Lilienfeld & S. J. Lynn (Eds.), *Science and pseudoscience in clinical psychology*. New York, NY: Guilford Press.

Lysaker, P. H., Buck, K. D., Salvatore, G., Popolo, R., & Dimaggio, G. (2009). Lack of awareness of illness in schizophrenia: Conceptualizations, correlates and treatment approaches. *Expert Review of Neurotherapeutics, 9*, 1035–1043.

Lysaker, P. H., Roe, D., & Yanos, P. T. (2007). Toward understanding the insight paradox: Internalized stigma moderates the association between insight and social functioning, hope, and self-esteem among people with schizophrenia spectrum disorders. *Schizophrenia Bulletin, 33*, 192–199.

Lysiak, M. (2013). *Newtown: An American tragedy*. New York, NY: Gallery Books.

Mackler, D. (Director). (2014, April 8). Take these broken wings [Video file]. Retrieved from https://www.youtube.com/watch?v=EP-fKc-TknWU.

Macmillan, M. (2006). Is Erdelyi's swan a goose? *Behavioral and Brain Sciences, 29*, 525–526.

Magid, A. K. (2009). The unabomber revisited: Reexamining the use of mental disorder diagnoses as evidence of the mental condition of criminal defendants. *Indiana Law Journal, 84*, 1–21.

Magid, K. (2009). The complicated affairs of hormones and humans. *Journal of Evolutionary Psychology, 7*, 351–354.

Mai, F. (1995). Psychiatrists' attitudes to multiple personality disorder: A questionnaire study. *Canadian Journal of Psychiatry, 40*, 154–157.

Malamud, W. (1944). The psychoneuroses. In J. M. Hunt (Ed.), *Personality and the behavior disorders: A handbook based on experimental and clinical research*. New York, NY: Ronald.

Mann, J. J. (1987). Psychobiologic predictors of suicide. *Journal of Clinical Psychiatry, 48*, 39–43.

Mantell, D. M. (1988). Clarifying erroneous child sexual abuse allegations. *American Journal of Orthopsychiatry, 58*, 618–621.

March, J. G. (1978). Bounded rationality, ambiguity, and the engineering of choice. *Bell Journal of Economics, 9*, 587–608.

Marcotte, E. R., Pearson, D. M., & Srivastava, L. K. (2001). Animal models of schizophrenia: A critical review. *Journal of Psychiatry & Neuroscience, 26*, 395–410.

Marcus-Newhall, A., Pedersen, W. C., Carlson, M., & Miller, N. (2000). Displaced aggression is known and well: A meta-analytic review. *Journal of Personality and Social Psychology, 78*, 670–689.

Margraf, J., & Ehlers, A. (1991). Recent research on panic disorder: Review of Marburg studies. *German Journal of Psychology, 15*, 302–319.

Marks, I. M. (1987a). *Fears, phobias and rituals: Panic, anxiety, and their disorders*. New York, NY: Oxford University Press.

Marks, I. M., Crowe, M., Drewe, E., Young, T., & Dewhurst,W. G. (1969). Obsessive-compulsive neurosis in identical twins. *British Journal of Psychiatry, 115*, 991–998.

Marks, I. M., & O'Sullivan, G. (1988). Drugs and psychological treatments for agoraphobia/panic and obsessive-compulsive disorders: A review. *British Journal of Psychiatry, 153*, 650–658.

Marmor, J. (1962). Psychoanalytic therapy as an educational process: Common denominators in the therapeutic approaches of different psychoanalytic schools. In J. H. Masserman (Ed.), *Science and psychoanalysis: Psychoanalytic education* (Vol. 5, pp. 286–299). New York, NY: Grune & Stratton.

Marshall, J. C., Halligan, P. W., Fink, G. R., Wade, D. T., & Frackowiak, R. S. (1997). The functional anatomy of a hysterical paralysis. *Cognition, 64*, B1–B8.

Martin, A. K., Dzafic, I., Robinson, G. A., Reutens, D., & Mowry, B. (2016). Mentalizing in schizophrenia: A multivariate functional MRI study. *Neuropsychologia, 93*, 158–166.

Martin, P. D., & Brantley, P. J. (2004). Stress, coping, and social support in health and behavior. In J. M. Raczynski & L. C. Leviton (Eds.), *Handbook of clinical health psychology: Disorders of behavior and health* (Vol. 2, pp. 233–267). Washington, DC: American Psychological Association.

Martinez-Taboas, A. (1996). Repressed memories: Some clinical data contributing toward its elucidation. *American Journal of Psychotherapy, 50*, 217–230.

Mashour, G. A., Walker, E. E., & Martuza, R. L. (2005). Psychosurgery: Past, present, and future. *Brain Research Reviews, 48*, 409–419.

Masi, G., Pfanner, C., & Brovedani, P. (2013). Antipsychotic augmentation of selective serotonin reuptake inhibitors in resistant tic-related obsessive-compulsive disorder in children and adolescents: A naturalistic comparative study. *Journal of Psychiatric Research, 47*, 1007–1012.

Masserman, J. H. (1946). *Principles of dynamic psychiatry*. Philadelphia, PA: W. B. Saunders Company.

Matheson, S. L., Vijayan, H., Dickson, H., Shepherd, A. M., Carr, V. J., & Laurens, K. R. (2013). Systematic meta-analysis of childhood social withdrawal in schizophrenia, and comparison with data from at-risk children aged 9–14 years. *Journal of Psychiatric Research, 47*, 1061–1068.

Mathew, R. J., Wilson, W. H., Blazer, D. G., & George, L. K. (1993). Psychiatric disorders in adult children of alcoholics: Data from the epidemiologic catchment area project. *American Journal of Psychiatry, 150*, 793–800.

Mathews, A. M., Gelder, M. G., & Johnston, D. W. (1981). *Agoraphobia: Nature and treatment*. New York, NY: Tavistock.

Matsunaga, H., Nagata, T., Hayashida, K., Ohya, K., Kiriike, N., & Stein, D. J. (2009). A long-term trial of the effectiveness and safety of atypical antipsychotic agents in augmenting SSRI-refractory obsessive-compulsive disorder. *The Journal of Clinical Psychiatry, 70*, 863–868.

Mavissakalian, M. R., & Guo, S. (2004). Early detection of relapse in panic disorder. *Acta Psychiatrica Scandinavica, 110*, 393–399.

Mavissakalian, M. R., & Perel, J. M. (1999). Long-term maintenance and discontinuation of imipramine therapy in panic disorder with agoraphobia. *Archives of General Psychiatry, 56*, 821–827.

Mavissakalian, M. R., & Perel, J. M. (2002). Duration of imipramine therapy and relapse in panic disorder with agoraphobia. *Journal of Clinical Psychopharmacology*, *22*, 294–299.

Mavissakalian, M. R., & Ryan, M. T. (1998). Rational treatment of panic disorder with antidepressants. *Annals of Clinical Psychiatry*, *10*, 185–195.

McAndrew, J. F. (1989). Obsessive-compulsive disorder: A behavioral case formulation. *Journal of Behavioral and Experimental Psychiatry*, *20*, 311–318.

McClellan, J., & McCurry, C. (1999). Early onset psychotic disorders: Diagnostic stability and clinical characteristics. *European Child and Adolescent Psychiatry*, *8*, 13–19.

McElroy, L. P. (1992). Early indicators of pathological disassociation in sexually abused children. *Child Abuse and Neglect*, *16*, 833–846.

McGhie, A., & Chapman, J. S. (1961). Disorders of attention and perception in early schizophrenia. *British Journal of Medical Psychology*, *34*, 103–116.

McGillivray, J. A., & McCabe, M. P. (2007). Early detection of depression and associated risk factors in adults with mild/moderate intellectual disability. *Research in Developmental Disabilities*, *28*, 59–70.

McGuire, R. J., & Vallance, M. (1964). Aversion therapy by electric shock: A simple treatment. *British Medical Journal*, *1*, 151–153.

McNally, R. J. (1990). Psychological approaches to panic disorders: A review. *Psychological Bulletin*, *108*, 403–419.

McNally, R. J. (1999). Theoretical approaches to the fear of anxiety. In S. Taylor (Ed.), *The LEA series in personality and clinical psychology. Anxiety sensitivity: Theory, research, and treatment of the fear of anxiety* (pp. 3–16). Mahwah, NJ: Lawrence Erlbaum.

McNally, R. J. (2003). *Remembering trauma*. Cambridge, MA: Harvard University Press.

McNally, R. J. (2006). Let Freud rest in peace. *Behavioral and Brain Sciences*, *29*, 526–527.

McNally, R. J., Clancy, S. A., & Barrett, H. M. (2004). Forgetting trauma? In D. Reisberg & P. Hertel (Eds.), *Memory and emotion*. London, England: Oxford University Press.

McNally, R. J., Hornig, C. D., & Donnell, C. D. (1995). Clinical versus nonclinical panic: A test of suffocation false alarm theory. *Behaviour Research and Therapy*, *33*, 127–131.

McNally, R. J., & Steketee, G. S. (1985). The etiology and maintenance of severe animal phobias. *Behaviour Research and Therapy*, *23*, 431–435.

Meadows, L. A., & Kaslow, N. J. (2002). Hopelessness as a mediator of the link between reports of a history of child maltreatment and suicidality in African-American women. *Cognitive Therapy and Research*, *26*, 657–674.

Mehler-Wex, C., Romanos, M., Kirchheiner, J., & Schulze, U. M. E. (2008). Atypical antipsychotics in severe anorexia nervosa in children and adolescents — Review and case reports. *European Eating Disorders Review*, *16*, 100–108.

Melamed, Y., Mester, R., Margolin, J., & Kalian, M. (2003). Involuntary treatment of anorexia nervosa. *International Journal of Law and Psychiatry*, *26*, 617–626.

Melle, I., & Barrett, E. A. (2012). Insight and suicidal behavior in first-episode schizophrenia. *Expert Review of Neurotherapeutics*, *12*, 353–359.

Mellman, T. A., & Uhde, T. W. (1989a). Sleep panic attacks: New clinical findings and theoretical implications. *The American Journal of Psychiatry*, *146*, 1204–1207.

Mellman, T. A., & Uhde, T. W. (1989b). Electroencephalographic sleep in panic disorder: A focus on sleep-related panic attacks. *Archives of General Psychiatry*, *46*, 178–184.

Memon, A., Hope, L., & Bull, R. (2003). Exposure duration: Effects on eyewitness accuracy and confidence. *British Journal of Psychology*, *94*, 339–354.

Mendick, R. (2015). Andreas Lubitz: Inside the mind of a mass killer. *The Telegraph*. Retrieved from https://www.telegraph.co.uk/news/worldnews/europe/germany/11501981/Andreas-Lubitz-inside-the-mind-of-a-mass-killer.html

Menon, R., Barrett, M. E., & Simpson, D. D. (1990). School, peer group, and inhalant use among Mexican American adolescents. *Hispanic Journal of Behavioral Sciences*, *12*, 408–421.

Mensink, G. J., & Raaijmakers, J. G. (1988). A model for interference and forgetting. *Psychological Review*, *94*, 434–455.

Menzies, R. G., & Clarke, J. C. (1993). A comparison of in vivo and vicarious exposure in the treatment of childhood water phobia. *Behaviour Research and Therapy*, *31*, 9–15.

Merckelbach, H., Horselenberg, R., & Schmidt, H. (2002). Modeling the connection between self-reported trauma and dissociation in a student sample. *Personality and Individual Differences, 32*, 695–705.

Merikangas, K. R., & Gelernter, C. S. (1990). Comorbidity for alcoholism and depression. *Psychiatric Clinics of North America, 13*, 613–632.

Merskey, H. (1979). *The analysis of hysteria.* London, England: Bailliere Tindal.

Merskey, H. (1995). *The analysis of hysteria: Understanding conversion and dissociation.* London, England: Gaskell.

Merskey, H., & Buhrich, N. A. (1975). Hysteria and organic brain disease. *British Journal of Medical Psychology, 48*, 359–366.

Meyer, R. M., & Weaver, C. M. (2013). *Case studies in abnormal behavior*, New York, NY: Parson.

Mialet, J. P., Pope, H. G., & Yurgelun-Todd, D. (1996). Impaired attention in depressive state: A non-specific deficit? *Psychological Medicine, 26*, 1009–1020.

Michael, T., Blechert, J., Vriends, N., Margraf, J., & Wilhelm, F. H. (2007). Fear conditioning in panic disorder: Enhanced resistance to extinction. *Journal of Abnormal Psychology, 116*, 612–617.

Michelson, L., June, K., Vives, A., Testa, S., & Marchione, N. (1998). The role of trauma and dissociation in cognitive-behavioral psychotherapy outcome and maintenance for panic disorder with agoraphobia. *Behaviour and Research Therapy, 36*, 1011–1050.

Mikkelsen, R. L., Middelboe, T., Pisinger, C., & Stage, K. B. (2004). Anxiety and depression in patients with chronic obstructive pulmonary disease (COPD): A review. *Nordic Journal of Psychiatry, 58*, 65–70.

Milgrom, P., Mancl, L., King, B., & Weinstein, P. (1995). Origins of childhood dental fear. *Behaviour Research and Therapy, 33*, 313–319.

Miller, B. G. (2006). Who are Indigenes? A comparative study of Canadian and American practices. *American Behavioral Scientist, 50*, 462–477.

Miller, C. R., & Forbes, J. F. (1990). Camptocormia. *Military Medicine, 155*, 561–565.

Miller, D. D. (2000). The diagnosis and treatment of Dissociative Identity Disorder in children: A critical review. *Dissertation Abstracts International: Section B: The Sciences and Engineering, 60*, 5229.

Miller, D. G. (1983). Hostile emotion and obsessional neurosis. *Psychological Medicine, 13*, 813–819.

Miller, E. (1999). Conversion hysteria: Is it a viable concept? In P. W. Halligan & A. S. David (Eds.), *Conversion hysteria: Towards a cognitive neuropsychological account*. Hove: Psychology Press.

Millon, T. (1983). The *DSM-III*: An insider's perspective. *American Psychologist, 38*, 804–814.

Millon, T. (1986). On the past and future of the *DSM-III*: Personal recollections and projections. In T. Millon & G. L. Klerman (Eds.), *Contemporary directions in psychopathology: Toward the DSM-IV.* New York, NY: Guilford.

Milrod, B., Leon, A. C., Busch, F., Rudden, M., Schwalberg, M., Clarkin, J., … Shear, M. K. (2007). A randomized controlled clinical trial of psychoanalytic psychotherapy for panic disorder. *American Journal of Psychiatry, 164*, 265–272.

Milrod, B., Leon, A. C., & Shear, M. K. (2004). Can interpersonal loss precipitate panic disorder? *American Journal of Psychiatry, 161*, 758–759.

Mineka, S., & Cook, M. (1986). Immunization against the observational conditioning of snake fear in rhesus monkeys. *Journal of Abnormal Psychology, 95*, 307–318.

Mineka, S., & Kihlstrom, J. F. (1978). Unpredictable and uncontrollable events: A new perspective on experimental neurosis. *Journal of Abnormal Psychology, 87*, 256–271.

Mineka, S., & Oehlberg, K. (2008). The relevance of recent developments in classical conditioning to understanding the etiology and maintenance of anxiety disorders. *Acta Psychologica, 127*, 567–580.

Mintz, S., & Alpert, M. (1972). Imagery vividness, reality testing, and schizophrenic hallucinations. *Journal of Abnormal Psychology, 79*, 310–316.

Mirsky, A. F., Silberman, E. K., Latz, A., & Nagler, S. (1985). Adult outcomes of high-risk children: Differential effects of town and kibbutz rearing. *Schizophrenia Bulletin, 11*, 150–154.

Mischel, W., & Mischel, F. (1958). Psychological aspects of spirit possession. *American Anthropologist, 60*, 249–260.

Mistry, S., Harrison, J. R., Smith, D. J., Escott-Price, V., & Zammit, S. (2018). The use of polygenic risk scores to identify phenotypes associated with genetic risk of bipolar disorder and depression: A systematic review. *Journal of Affective Disorders, 234*, 148–155.

Mitchell, J. E., & Eckert, E. D. (1987). Scope and significance of eating disorders. Special issue: Eating disorders. *Journal of Consulting and Clinical Psychology, 55*, 628–634.

Mittal, K., Gonçalves, V. F., Harripaul, R., Cuperfain, A. B., Rollins, B., Tiwari, A. K., … Kennedy, J. L. (2017). A comprehensive analysis of mitochondrial genes variants and their association with antipsychotic-induced weight gain. *Schizophrenia Research, 187*, 67–73.

Mitterauer, B. (1990). A contribution to the discussion of the role of the genetic factor in suicide, based on five studies in an epidemiologically defined area (Province of Salzburg, Austria). *Comprehensive Psychiatry, 31*, 557–565.

Miyamoto, S., Miyake, N., Jarskog, L. F., Fleischhacker, W. W., & Lieberman, J. A. (2012). Pharmacological treatment of schizophrenia: A critical review of the pharmacology and clinical effects of current and future therapeutic agents. *Molecular Psychiatry, 17*, 1206–1227.

Mizes, J. S. (1985). The use of contingent reinforcement in the treatment of a conversion disorder: A multiple baseline study. *Journal of Behavior Therapy and Experimental Psychiatry, 16*, 341–345.

Moller, H. J. (1995). The psychopathology of schizophrenia: An integrated view on positive symptoms and negative symptoms. *International Clinical Psychopharmacology, 10*, 57–64.

Moncrieff, J. (2013). Antipsychotics and brain shirinkage. Mad in America. https://www.madinamerica.com/2013/06/antipsychotics-and-brain-shrinkage-an-update

Motl, T. C., Krieshok, T. S., & Multon, K. D. (2018). The effect of rational and intuitive decision-making strategies on interest appraisals. *Journal of Career Assessment, 26*, 616–630.

Moncrieff, J. (2014). A critique of genetic research on schizophrenia-expensive castles in the air. Retrieved from https://joannamoncrieff.com/.../a-critique-of-genetic-research-on-schizophrenia-expen

Money, C., Davies, H., & Tchanturia, K. (2011). A case study introducing cognitive remediation and emotion skills training for anorexia nervosa inpatient care. *Clinical Case Studies*, *10*, 110–121.

Mongan, D., Ramesar, M., Föcking, M., Cannon, M., & Cotter, D. (2019). Role of inflammation in the pathogenesis of schizophrenia: A review of the evidence, proposed mechanisms and implications for treatment. Early Intervention in Psychiatry. *Advance Online Publication*.

Mooney, G., & Gurrister, T. (2004). Behavioral treatment of psychogenic deafness: A case report. *Rehabilitation Psychology*, *49*, 268–271.

Moore, R., Brødsgaard, I., & Birn, H. (1991). Manifestations, acquisition and diagnostic categories of dental fear in a self-referred population. *Behaviour Research and Therapy*, *29*, 51–60.

Moore, W. E., & Stevenson, J. R. (1991). Understanding trust in the performance of complex automatic sport skills. *The Sport Psychologist*, *5*, 281–289.

Morgan, V. A., Croft, M. L., Valuri, G. M., Zubrick, S. R., Bower, C., McNeil, T. F., & Jablensky, A. V. (2012). Intellectual disability and other neuropsychiatric outcomes in high-risk children of mothers with schizophrenia, bipolar disorder and unipolar major depression. *The British Journal of Psychiatry*, *200*, 282–289.

Morgan, V. A., Leonard, H., Bourke, J., & Jablensky, A. (2008). Intellectual disability co-occurring with schizophrenia and other psychiatric illness: Population-based study. *British Journal of Psychiatry*, *193*, 364–372.

Moritz, S., Vitzthum, F., Randjbar, S., Veckernstedt, R., & Woodward, T. (2010). Detecting and defusing cognitive traps: Metacognitive intervention in schizophrenia. *Current Opinion in Psychiatry*, *23*, 561–569.

Moritz, S., & Woodward, T. S. (2007). Metacognitive training in schizophrenia: From basic research to knowledge translation and intervention. *Current Opinion in Psychiatry*, *20*, 619–625.

Morris, P. (1981). The cognitive psychology of self-reports. In C. Antaki (Ed.), *The psychology of ordinary explanations of social behavior* (pp. 183–203). London, England: Academic Press.

Morrison, A. K. (2009). Cognitive behavior therapy for people with schizophrenia. *Psychiatry*, *6*, 32–39.

Morrison, A. P., & Baker, C. A. (2000). Intrusive thoughts and auditory hallucinations: A comparative study of intrusions in psychosis. *Behaviour Research and Therapy*, *38*, 1097–1106.

Moskowitz, A. K. (2004a). Dissociative pathways to homicide: Clinical and forensic implications. *Journal of Trauma and Dissociation*, *5*, 5–32.

Moskowitz, A. K. (2004b). Dissociation and violence: A review of the literature. *Trauma, Violence and Abuse*, *5*, 21–46.

Mucha, T. F., & Reinhardt, R. F. (1970). Conversion reactions in student aviators. *American Journal of Psychiatry*, *127*, 493–497.

Mueser, K. T., & Berenbaum, H. (1990). Psychodynamic treatment of schizophrenia: Is there a future? *Psychological Medicine*, *20*, 253–262.

Munk-Jorgensen, P., & Mortensen, P. B. (1992). Social outcome in schizophrenia: A 13-year follow-up. *Social Psychiatry and Psychiatric Epidemiology*, *27*, 129–134.

Murray, S., Touyz, S., & Beumont, P. (1990). Knowledge about eating disorders in the community. *International Journal of Eating Disorders*, *9*, 87–93.

Murri, M. B., Amore, M., Calcagno, P. O., Respino, M., Marozzi, V., Masotti, M., … Maj, M. (2016). The "insight paradox" in schizophrenia: Magnitude, moderators and mediators of the association between insight and depression. *Schizophrenia Bulletin*, *42*, 1225–1233.

Mussen, P. H., Conger, J. J., Kagan, J., & Huston, A. C. (1984). *Child development and personality* (6th ed.). New York, NY: Harper & Row.

Nagel, K. L., & Jones, K. H. (1992). Predisposition factors in anorexia nervosa. *Adolescence*, *27*, 381–386.

Nagler, S., & Glueck, Z. (1985). The clinical interview. *Schizophrenia Bulletin*, *11*, 38–47.

Nagler, S., & Mirsky, A. F. (1985). Introduction: The Israeli high-risk study. *Schizophrenia Bulletin*, *11*, 19–29.

Nakic, M., & Thomas, P. (2012). Dissociative identity disorder in the courtroom. *Journal of the American Academy of Psychiatry and the Law*, *40*, 146–148.

Nandi, D. N., Banerjee, G., Bera, S., Nandi, S., & Nandi, P. (1985). Contagious hysteria in a West Bengal Village. *American Journal of Psychotherapy*, *39*, 247–252.

Nasar, S. (1998). *A beautiful mind.* New York, NY: Simon & Schuster.

Nascimento, I., Nardi, A. E., Valença, A. M., Lopes, F. L., Mezzasalma, M. A., Nascentes, R., & Zin, W. A. (2002). Psychiatric disorders in asthmatic outpatients. *Psychiatry Research, 110*, 73–80.

Nash, J. F., Jr. (1994). Autobiography essay. *Les Prix Nobel*, 275–279.

National Institute for Clinical Excellence (2002). London, England: The Stationery Office.

National Institute of Health and Clinical Excellence (2009). *Schizophrenia: Core interventions in the treatment and management of schizophrenia in adults in primary and secondary care.* Clinical Guideline 82. National Institute for Health and Clinical Excellence, London, England.

Neale, J. M., Oltmanns, T. F., & Davison, G. C. (1982). *Case studies in abnormal psychology.* New York, NY: Wiley.

Neelam, K., Garg, D., & Marshall, M. (2011). A systematic review and meta-analysis of neurological soft signs in relatives of people with schizophrenia. *BMC Psychiatry, 11*, Article ID 139.

Newkth, S., & Rachman, S. (2001). The concealment of obsessions. *Behaviour Research and Therapy, 39*, 457–464.

Ng, R. M., Pearson, V., & Chen, E. Y. (2008). What does recovery from schizophrenia mean? Perceptions of psychiatrists. *International Journal of Culture and Mental Health, 1*, 73–84.

Nicol, C. F. (1969). Masks of hysteria: Medical and neurologic. *New York State Journal of Medicine, 69*, 1883–1887.

Nisbett, R. E., & Wilson, T. D. (1977). Telling more than we can know: Verbal reports on mental processes. *Psychological Review, 84*, 231–259.

North, C. S., Ryall, J. M., Ricci, D. A., Wetzel, R. D. (1993). *Multiple personalities, multiple personality disorder: Psychiatric classification and media influence.* New York, NY: Oxford University Press.

Novick, D., Haro, J. M., Suarez, D., Vieta, E., & Naber, D. (2009). Recovery in the outpatient setting: 36-month results from the schizophrenia outpatients' health outcomes (SOHO) study. *Schizophrenia Research, 108*, 223–230.

Noyes, R., Watson, D. B., Carney, C. P., Letuchy, E. M., Peloso, P. M., Black, D. W., & Doebbeling, B. N. (2004). Risk factors for hypochondriacal concerns in a sample of military veterans. *Journal of Psychosomatic Research, 57*, 529–539.

Nuechterlein, K. H., Green, M. F., Calkins, M. E., Greenwood, T. A., Gur, R. E., Gur, R. C., … Braff, D. L. (2015). Attention/vigilance in schizophrenia: Performance results from a large multi-site study of the Consortium on the Genetics of Schizophrenia (COGS). *Schizophrenia Research, 163*, 38–46.

Nuechterlein, K. H., Subotnik, K. L., Ventura, J., Green, M. F., Gretchen-Doorly, D., & Asarnow, R. F. (2012). The puzzle of schizophrenia: Tracking the core role of cognitive deficits. *Development and Psychopathology, 24*, 529–536.

Nurnberger, J. I., & Hingtgen, J. N. (1973). Is symptom substitution an important issue in behavior therapy? *Biological Psychiatry, 7*, 221–236.

Nutt, D., & Lawson, C. (1992). Panic attacks: A neurochemical overview of models and mechanisms. *British Journal of Psychiatry, 160*, 165–178.

O'Brien, G., & Jureidini, J. (2002). Dispensing with the dynamic unconscious. *Philosophy, Psychiatry, & Psychology, 9*, 141–153.

O'Brien, J. T., Sahakian, B. J., & Checkley, S. A. (1993). Cognitive impairments in patients with seasonal affective disorder. *British Journal of Psychiatry, 163*, 338–343.

Ochoa, S., Usall, J., Cobo, J., Labad, X., & Kulkarni, J. (2012). Gender differences in schizophrenia and first-episode psychosis: A comprehensive literature review. *Schizophrenia Research and Treatment, 2012*, 1–9.

O'Conner, K. (2005). Overcoming treatment resistance in obsessive-compulsive disorder. *Acta Psychiatrica Scanidavica, 111*, 257–260.

Okamoto, A., Yamashita, T., Nagoshi, Y., Masui, Y., Wada, Y., Kashima, A., … Fukui, K. (2002). A behavior therapy program combined with liquid nutrition designed for anorexia nervosa. *Psychiatry and Clinical Neurosciences, 56*, 515–520.

O'Kearney, R. (1993). Additional considerations in cognitive-behavioral treatment of obsessional ruminations: A case study. *Journal of Behavior Therapy and Experimental Psychiatry, 24*, 357–365.

Okon, D. M., Greene, A. L., & Smith, J. E. (2003). Family interactions predict intraindividual symptom variation for adolescents with bulimia. *International Journal of Eating Disorders*, *34*, 450–457.

Olfson, M., Uttaro, T., Carson, W. H., & Tafesse, E. (2005). Male sexual dysfunction and quality of life in schizophrenia. *The Journal of Clinical Psychiatry*, *66*, 331–338.

Olin, S. C. S., & Mednick, S. (1996). Risk factors of psychosis: Identifying vulnerable populations premorbidly. *Schizophrenia Bulletin*, *22*, 223–240.

Olin, S. C. S., Mednick, S. A., Cannon, T., Jacobsen, B., Parnas, J., Schulsinger, F., & Schulsinger, H. (1998). School teacher ratings predictive of psychiatric outcome 25 years later. *British Journal of Psychiatry*, *172*, 7–13.

Oliosi, M., & Dalle Grave, R. (2003). A comparison of clinical and psychological features in subgroups of patients with anorexia nervosa. *European Eating Disorders Review*, *11*, 306–314.

Ollendick, T. H. (1995). Cognitive behavioral treatment of panic disorder with agoraphobia in adolescents: A multiple baseline design analysis. *Behavior Therapy*, *26*, 517–531.

Oner, O., & Munir, K. (2005). Attentional and neurocognitive characteristics of high-risk offspring of parents with schizophrenia compared with *DSM-IV* attention deficit hyperactivity disorder children. *Schizophrenia Research*, *76*, 293–299.

Ong, T. (1989). Peers as perceived by drug abusers in their drug-seeking behaviour. *British Journal of Addiction*, *84*, 631–637.

O'Sullivan, G., & Marks, I. (1991). Follow-up studies of behavioral treatment of phobic and obsessive compulsive neuroses. *Psychiatric Annals*, *21*, 368–373.

Ozan, E., Deveci, E., Oral, M., Karahan, U., Oral, E., Aydın, N., & Kırpınar, İ. (2010). Neurocognitive functioning in a group of offspring genetically at high-risk for schizophrenia in Eastern Turkey. *Brain Research Bulletin*, *82*, 218–223.

Park, L. T., Jefferson, J. W., & Greist, J. H. (1997). Obsessive-compulsive disorder: Treatment options. *CNS Drugs*, *7*, 187–202.

Parnas, J., & Jorgensen, A. (1989). Pre-morbid psychopathology in schizophrenia spectrum. *British Journal of Psychiatry*, *155*, 623–627.

Parnas, J., Schulsinger, F., Schulsinger, H., Mednick, S., & Teasdale, T. (1982). Behavioral precursors of schizophrenia spectrum: A prospective study. *Archives of General Psychiatry, 39*, 658–664.

Pate, J. E., Pumariega, A. J., Hester, C., & Garner, D. M. (1992). Cross-cultural patterns in eating disorders: A review. *Journal of the American Academy of Child and Adolescent Psychiatry, 31*, 802–809.

Pato, M. T., Murphy, D. L., & DeVane, C. L. (1991). Sustained plasma concentrations of fluoxetine and/or norfluoxetine four and eight weeks after fluoxetine discontinuation. *Journal of Clinical Psychopharmacology, 11*, 224–225.

Pattison, E. M., & Wintrob, R. M. (1981). Possession and exorcism in contemporary America. *Journal of Operational Psychiatry, 12*, 13–20.

Patton, G. C. (1992). Eating disorders: Antecedents, evaluation and course. *Annals of Medicine, 24*, 281–28

Patton, G. C., Riecher-Rössler, A., & Häfner, H. (1994). Gender differences in schizophrenia: Do computer tomography findings provide an explanation? *New Trends in Experimental and Clinical Psychiatry, 10*, 121–126.

Pauli, P., Marquardt, C., Hartl, L., Nutzinger, D. O., & Strian, F. (1991). Cardiovascular aspects of cardiac phobia: A field approach. *Psychotherapie Psychosomatik Medizinische Psychologie, 41*, 429–436.

Pearce, S. A., Isherwood, S., Hrouda, D., Richardson, P. H., Erskine, A., & Skinner, J. (1990). Memory and pain: Tests of mood congruity and state dependent learning in experimentally induced and clinical pain. *Pain, 43*, 187–193.

Pfeffer, C. R. (1988). Risk factors associated with youth suicide: A clinical perspective. Suicide. *Psychiatric Annals, 18*, 652–656.

Peluso, M. J., Lewis, S. W., Barnes, T. R. E., & Jones, P. B. (2013). Non-neurological and metabolic side effects in the Cost Utility of the Latest Antipsychotics in Schizophrenia Randomized Controlled Trial (CUtLASS-1). *Schizophrenia Research, 144*, 80–86.

Perna, G., Cocchi, S., Politi, E., & Bellodi, L. (1997). CO_2 challenge in non-clinical subjects. *The American Journal of Psychiatry, 154*, 886–887.

Perr, I. N. (1991). Crime and multiple personality disorder: A case history and discussion. *Bulletin of the American Academy of Psychiatry & the Law, 19*, 203–214.

Peterson, C. B., & Mitchell, J. E. (1999). Psychosocial and pharmacological treatment of eating disorders: A review of research findings. *Journal of Clinical Psychology, 55*, 685–697.

Peterson, J. B., & Djikic, M. (2003). You can neither remember nor forget what you do not understand. *Religion and Public Life, 33*, 85–118.

Phelps, L., Cox, D., & Bajorek, E. (1992). School phobia and separation anxiety: Diagnostic and treatment comparisons. *Psychology in the Schools, 29*, 384–394.

Philip, N. S., Carpenter, L., Tyrka, A. R., Whiteley, L., & Price, L. (2009). Varenicline augmentation in depressed smokers: An 8-week, open-label study. *Journal of Clinical Psychiatry, 70*, 1026–1031.

Phillips, L. J., Francey, S. M., Edwards, J., & McMurray, N. (2007). Strategies used by psychotic individuals to cope with life stress and symptoms of illness: A systematic review. *Anxiety, Stress & Coping: An International Journal, 22*, 371–410.

Piacentini, J., & Graae, F. (1997). Childhood OCD. In E. Hollander & D. J. Stein (Eds.), *Obsessive-compulsive disorders: Diagnosis, etiology and treatment.* New York, NY: Marcel Dekker.

Piccinelli, M., Pini, S., Bellantuono, C., & Wilkinson, G. (1995). Efficacy of drug treatment in obsessive-compulsive disorder: A meta-analytic review. *The British Journal of Psychiatry, 166*, 424–443.

Pies, R. (2011). Psychiatry's new-mind and the legend of the "chemical imbalance". *Psychiatric Times*, 11.

Pike, K. M., & Rodin, J. (1991). Mothers, daughters, and disordered eating. *Journal of Abnormal Psychology, 100*, 198–204.

Pilecki, B. C., Clegg, J. W., & McKay, D. (2011). The influence of corporate and political interests on models of illness in the evolution of the *DSM. European Psychiatry, 26*, 194–200.

Piper, A. (1994). Multiple personality disorder. *British Journal of Psychiatry, 164*, 600–612.

Piper, A., Lillevik, L., & Kritzer, R. (2008). What's wrong with believing in repression? A review for legal professionals. *Psychology, Public Policy, and Law, 14*, 223–242.

Piper, A., Pope, H. G., & Borowiecki, J. J. (2000). Custer's last stand: Brown, Scheflin and Whitfield's latest attempt to salvage "dissociative amnesia." *Journal of Psychiatry and Law, 28*, 149–213.

Pisano, S., Catone, G., Pascotto, A., & Gritti, A. (2014). Second generation antipsychotics in adolescent anorexia nervosa: A new hypothesis of eligibility criteria. *Journal of Child and Adolescent Psychopharmacology, 24*, 293–295.

Polivy, J., & Herman, C. P. (1987). Diagnosis and treatment of normal eating. *Journal of Consulting and Clinical Psychology, 55*, 635–644.

Polivy, J., & Herman, C. P. (2002). Causes of eating disorders. *Annual Review of Psychology, 53*, 187–213.

Pollak, J. M. (1979). Obsessive-compulsive personality: A review. *Psychological Bulletin, 86*, 225–241.

Pope, H. G., Champoux, R. F., & Hudson, J. I. (1987). Eating disorder and socioeconomic class: Anorexia nervosa and bulimia in nine communities. *Journal of Nervous and Mental Disease, 175*, 620–623.

Pope, H. G., Hudson, J. I., & Yurgelun-Todd, D. (1984). Anorexia nervosa and bulimia among 300 suburban women shoppers. *American Journal of Psychiatry, 141*, 292–294.

Popper, K. R. (1959). *The logic of scientific discovery*. Oxford, England: Basic Books.

Porzelius, L. K., Berel, S., & Howard, C. (1999). Cognitive behavior therapy. In M. Hersen & A. S. Bellack (Eds.), *Handbook of comparative interventions for adult disorders* (pp. 491–512). Hoboken, NJ: John Wiley & Sons.

Power, M. J., & Brewin, C. R. (1997). *The transformation of meaning in psychological therapies: Integrating theory and practice*. Chichester, England: Wiley.

Perdices, M., Dunbar, N., Grunseit, A., Hall, W., & Cooper, D. A. (1992). Anxiety, depression and HIV related symptomatology across the spectrum of HIV disease. *Australian and New Zealand Journal of Psychiatry, 26*, 560–566.

Premkumar, P., Bream, D., Sapara, A., Fannon, D., Anilkumar, A. P., Kuipers, E., & Kumari, V. (2018). Pituitary volume reduction in schizophrenia following cognitive behavioral therapy. *Schizophrenia Research, 192*, 416–422.

Prenoveau, J. M., Forsyth, J. P., Kelly, M. M., & Barrios, V. (2006). Repeated exposure to 20% CO_2 challenge and risk for developing panic attacks: A controlled 6- and 12-month follow-up in a nonclinical sample. *Journal of Anxiety Disorders*, *20*, 1158–1167.

Pretz, J. (2008). Intuition versus analysis: Strategy and experience in complex everyday problem solving. *Memory & Cognition*, *36*, 554–566.

Proctor, R. W., & Capaldi, E. J. (2001). Empirical evaluation and justification of methodologies in psychological science. *Psychological Bulletin*, *127*, 759–772.

Pruitt, R. D. (1974). Death as an expression of functional disease. *Mayo Clinic Proceedings*, *49*, 627–635.

Prüter, C., Kunert, H. J., & Hoff, P. (2001). ICD-10 mild cognitive disorder following meningitis due to neurosarcoidosis. *Psychopathology*, *34*, 326–327.

Pryor., T. L., Johnson, T., Wiedrman, M. W., & Boswell, D. L. (1995). The clinical significance of symptom denial among women with anorexia nervosa: Another disposable myth? *Eating Disorders*, *3*, 293–303.

Pu, T., Mohamed, E., Imam, K., & El-Roey, A. M. (1986). One hundred cases of hysteria in eastern Libya: A socio-demographic study. *British Journal of Psychiatry*, *148*, 606–609.

Putnam, F. W., & Loewenstein, R. J. (1993). Treatment of multiple personality disorder: A survey of current practices. *American Journal of Psychiatry*, *150*, 1048–1052.

Quick, J. D., Horn, R. S., & Quick, J. C. (1986). Health consequences of stress. *Journal of Organizational Behavior Management*, *8*, 19–36.

Rabe-Jablonska, J. (2003). Anorexia nervosa in adult women. *Psychiatria Polska*, *37*, 29–37.

Rachman, S. (1976). The modification of obsessions: A new formulation. *Behaviour Research and Therapy*, *14*, 437–443.

Rachman, S., Lopatka, C., & Levitt, K. (1988). Experimental analyses of panic: II. Panic patients. *Behaviour Research and Therapy*, *26*, 33–40.

Rachman, S. J. (1990). *Fear and courage* (2nd ed.). New York, NY: Freeman.

Rachman, S. J., & De Silva, P. (1978). Abnormal and normal obsessions. *Behaviour Research and Therapy*, *16*, 233–248.

Rachman, S. J., & Hodgson, R. J. (1980). *Obsessions and compulsions*. Englewood Cliffs, NJ: Prentice Hall.

Rachman, S. J., Levitt, K. C., & Lopatka, C. (1987). Panic: The links between cognitions and bodily symptoms: I. *Behaviour Research and Therapy*, *25*, 411–423.

Rachman, S. J., & Seligman, M. E. P. (1976). Unprepared phobias: "Be prepared." *Behaviour Research and Therapy*, *14*, 333–338.

Ramírez, N., Arranz, B., Sánchez, J. M., Centeno, M., & San, L. (2006). Depression in schizophrenia, can it be treated? A review of the evidence. *Current Psychiatry Reviews*, *2*, 371–379.

Ranganathan, S. (2013). This temple is our natal home!: Women's experiences of marriage and possession in Maharashtra. *Psychological Studies*, *58*, 437–445.

Rapee, R. M. (1995). Psychological factors influencing the affective response to biological challenge procedures in panic disorder. *Journal of Anxiety Disorders*, *9*, 59–74.

Raphael, F. J., Rani, S., Bale, R., & Drummond, L. M. (1996). Religion, ethnicity and obsessive-compulsive disorder. *International Journal of Social Psychiatry*, *42*, 38–44.

Rasmussen, S. A., & Eisen, J. L. (1992). The epidemiology and clinical features of obsessive compulsive disorder. *Psychiatric Clinics of North America*, *15*, 743–758.

Rau, R. (1996). Psychophysiological assessment of human reliability in a simulated complex system. *Biological Psychology*, *42*, 287–300.

Ravenscroft, K. (1965). Voodoo possession: A natural experiment in hypnosis. *International Journal of Clinical and Experimental Hypnosis*, *13*, 157–182.

Ravizza, L., Maina, G., Bogetto, F., Albert, U., Barzega, G., & Bellino, S. (1998). Long term treatment of obsessive compulsive disorder. *CNS Drugs*, *10*, 247–255.

Ray, W., Chung, C., Murray, K., Hall, K., & Stein, M. (2009). Atypical antipsychotic drugs and the risk of sudden cardiac death. *The New England Journal of Medicine*, *360*, 225–235.

Razali, S. M. (1999). Conversion disorder: A case report of treatment with the Main Puteri, a Malay shamanistic healing ceremony. *European Psychiatry*, *14*, 470–472.

Read, J. (1997). Child abuse and psychosis: A literature review and implications for professional practice. *Professional Psychology: Research and Practice*, *28*, 448–456.

Read, J., Agar, K., Barker-Collo, S., Davies, E., & Moskowitz, A. (2001). Assessing suicidality in adults: Integrating childhood trauma as a risk factor. *Professional Psychology: Research and Practice*, *32*, 367–372.

Read, J. D., & Lindsay, D. S. (1994). Moving toward a middle ground on the "false memory debate": Reply to commentaries on Lindsay and Read. *Applied Cognitive Psychology*, *8*, 407–435.

Reich, W. (1982). Psychiatry's second coming. *Psychiatry*, *45*, 189–196.

Reichenberg, A., & Harvey, P. D. (2007). Neuropsychological impairments in schizophrenia: Integration of performance-based and brain imaging findings. *Psychological Bulletin*, *133*, 833–858.

Reinders, A. S., Nijenhuis, E. R., Quak, J., Korf, J., Haaksma, J., Paans, A. M., … Boer, J. A. (2006). Psychobiological characteristics of dissociative identity disorder: A symptom provocation study. *Biological Psychiatry*, *60*, 730–740.

Reutfors, J., Clapham, E., Bahmanyar, S., Brandt, L., Jönsson, E. G., Ekbom, A., . . . Ösby, U. (2016). Suicide risk and antipsychotic side effects in schizophrenia: Nested case–control study. *Human Psychopharmacology: Clinical and Experimental*, *31*, 341–345.

Reisner, A. D. (2005). The common factors, empirically validated treatments, and recovery models of therapeutic change. *Psychological Record*, *55*, 377–399.

Reynolds, E. H. (2018). Hysteria in ancient civilisations: A neurological review: Possible significance for the modern disorder. *Journal of the Neurological Sciences*, *388*, 208–213.

Rich, C. L., Warstadt, G. M., Nemiroff, R. A., Fowler, R. C., & Young, D. (1991). Suicide, stressors, and the life cycle. *American Journal of Psychiatry*, *148*, 524–527.

Richards, J. C., Klein, B., & Austin, D. W. (2006). Internet cognitive behavioral therapy for panic disorder: Does the inclusion of stress management information improve end-state functioning? *Clinical Psychologist*, *10*, 2–15.

Richardson, M., Isbister, G., & Nicholson, B. (2018). A novel treatment protocol (Nocebo Hypothesis Cognitive Behavioural Therapy; NH-CBT) for Functional Neurological Symptom Disorder/Conversion Disorder: A retrospective consecutive case series. *Behavioural and Cognitive Psychotherapy*, *46*, 497–503.

Richter, C. P. (1957). On the phenomenon of sudden death in animals and man. *Psychosomatic Medicine*, *19*, 191–198.

Rieber, R. W. (1999). Hypnosis, false memory and multiple personality: A trinity of affinity. *History of Psychiatry*, *10*, 3–11.

Rief, W., & Hermanutz, M. (1996). Responses to activation and rest in patients with panic disorder and major depression. *British Journal of Clinical Psychology*, *35*, 605–616.

Rimm, D. C., & Somervill, J. W. (1977). *Abnormal psychology*. New York, NY: Academic Press.

Rind, B., Tromovitch, P., & Bauserman, R. (1998). A meta-analytic examination of assumed properties of child sexual abuse using college samples. *Psychological Bulletin*, *124*, 22–53.

Riplee (2012). *Overcoming paranoid schizophrenia: The inspiring cases of John Forbers Nash, Jr.*

Robbins, C. A. (1989). Sex differences in psychosocial consequences of alcohol and drug abuse. *Journal of Health and Social Behavior*, *30*, 117–130.

Robbins, M. (2002). "Psychoanalysis and schizophrenia: A cautionary tale": Comment. *Journal of the American Psychoanalytic Association*, *50*, 310–314.

Roberson-Nay, R., McClure, E. B., Monk, C. S., Nelson, E. E., Guyer, A. E., Fromm, S. J., … Pine, D. S. (2006). Increased amygdala activity during successful memory encoding in adolescent major depressive disorder: An fMRI study. *Biological Psychiatry*, *60*, 966–973.

Roberts, G. (1991). Delusional belief systems and meaning in life: A preferred reality? *The British Journal of Psychiatry*, *159*, 19–28.

Rodger, E. (2014). *My twisted world: The story of Elliot Rodger*. Retrieved from https://www.documentcloud.org/documents/1173808-elliot-rodger-manifesto.html

Roelofs, K., Keijsers, G. P. J., Hoogduin, C. A. L., Näring, G. W. B., & Moene, F. C. (2002). Childhood abuse in patients with conversion disorder. *The American Journal of Psychiatry*, *159*, 1908–1913.

Rofé, Y. (1989). *Repression and fear: A new approach to resolve the crisis in psychopathology*. New York, NY: Hemisphere.

Rofé, Y. (2000). *The rationality of psychological disorders: Psychobizarreness theory*. New York, NY: Kluwer Academic.

Rofé, Y. (2008). Does repression exist? Memory, pathogenic, unconscious, and clinical evidence. *Review of General Psychology*, *12*, 63–85.

Rofé, Y. (2010). The rational-choice theory of neurosis: Unawareness and an integrative therapeutic approach. *Journal of Psychotherapy Integration*, *20*, 152–202.

Rofé, Y. (2016). Which diagnostic approach is more valid? The *DSM* or the rational choice theory of neurosis. *International Journal of Psychological Studies*, *8*, 98–110.

Rofé, Y., & Rofé, Y. (2013). Conversion disorder: A review through the prism of the rational-choice theory of neurosis. *Europe's Journal of Psychology*, *9*, 832–868.

Rofé, Y., & Rofé, Y. (2015). Fear and phobia: A critical review and the rational-choice theory of neurosis. *International Journal of Psychological Studies*, *7*, 37–73.

Roghanizad, M. M., & Neufeld, D. J. (2015). Intuition, risk, and the formation of online trust. *Computers in Human Behavior*, *50*, 489–498.

Rolf, J. E. (1972). The social and academic competence of children vulnerable to schizophrenia and other behavior pathologies. *Journal of Abnormal Psychology*, *80*, 225–243.

Rolf, J. E., & Garmezy, N. (1974). The school performance of children vulnerable to behavior pathology. In D. F. Ricks, A. Thomas, & M. Roff (Eds.), *Life history research in psychopathology* (Vol. 3). Minneapolis, MN: University of Minnesota Press.

Romanov, K., Varjonen, J., Kaprio, J., & Koskenvuo, M. (2003). Life events and depressiveness — the effect of adjustment for psychosocial factors, somatic health and genetic liability. *Acta Psychiatrica Scandinavica*, *107*, 25–33.

Rose, E. J., & Ebmeier, K. P. (2006). Pattern of impaired working memory during major depression. *Journal of Affective Disorders*, *90*, 149–161.

Rosen, G. M., & Davison, G. C. (2003). Psychology should list empirically supported principles of change (ESPs) and not credential trademarked therapies or other treatment packages. *Behavior Modification*, *27*, 300–312.

Rosenbaum, J. F., Pollock, R. A., Otto, M. W., & Pollack, M. H. (1995). Integrated treatment of panic disorder. *Bulletin of the Menninger Clinic*, *59*, A4–A26.

Rotge, J., Lambrecq, V., Marchal, C., Pedespan, J., Burbaud, P., Rougier, A., & Michel, V. (2009). Conversion disorder and coexisting nonepileptic seizures in patients with refractory seizures. *Epilepsy and Behavior, 16*, 350–352.

Rothschild, A. J. (2000). Sexual side effects of antidepressants. *The Journal of Clinical Psychiatry, 61*, 28–36.

Routledge, K. M., Burton, K. L. O., Williams, L. M., Harris, A., Schofield, P. R., Clark, C. R., & Gatt, J. M. (2017). The shared and unique genetic relationship between mental well-being, depression and anxiety symptoms and cognitive function in healthy twins. *Cognition and Emotion, 31*, 1465–1479.

Roy-Byrne, P., Craske, M. G., & Stein, M. B. (2006). Panic disorder. *The Lancet, 368*, 1023–1032.

Roy, A., Segal, N. L., Centerwall, B. S., & Robinette, C. D. (1991). Suicide in twins. *Archives of General Psychiary, 48*, 29–32.

Rudd, M. D. (1990). An integrative model of suicidal ideational. *Suicide and Life Threatening Behavior, 20*, 16–30.

Rund, B. R. (1994). Cognitive dysfunctions and psychosocial treatment of research of schizophrenia: Future and past perspective. *Acta Psychiatrica Scandinavica, 90*, 9–16.

Sackeim, H. A., & Gur, R. C. (1978). Lateral asymmetry in intensity of emotional expression. *Neuropsychologia, 16*, 473–481.

Sackeim, H. A., Nordlie, J. W., & Gur, C. R. (1979). A model of hysterical and hypnotic blindness: Cognition, motivation and awareness. *Journal of Abnormal Psychology, 88*, 474–489.

Sadler-Smith, E. (2008). *Inside intuition*. New York, NY: Routledge.

Sahm, M., & von Weizsäcker, R. K. (2016). Reason, intuition, and time. *Managerial & Decision Economics, 37*, 195–207.

Sakamoto, K., & Crowley, J. J. (2018). A comprehensive review of the genetic and biological evidence supports a role for MicroRNA-137 in the etiology of schizophrenia. *American Journal of Medical Genetics Part B: Neuropsychiatric Genetics, 177*, 242–256.

Sakes, E. R. (2007). *The center cannot hold: My journey through madness*. New Yourk: Hyperion.

Saks, E. R., & Behnke, S. H. (1997). *Jekyll on trial: Multiple personality disorder and criminal law*. New York, NY, US: New York University Press.

Salkovskis, P. M., & Clark, D. M. (1986). Cognitive and physiological processes in the maintenance and treatment of panic attacks. In Hand, I. & Wittchen, U. H. (Eds.), *Panic and phobias*, New York, NY: Springer.

Salkovskis, P. M., & Clark, D. M. (1991). Cognitive therapy for panic attacks. *Journal of Cognitive Psychotherapy, 5*, 215–226.

Salkovskis, P. M., Clark, D. M., & Hackmann, A. (1991). Treatment of panic attacks using cognitive therapy without exposure or breathing retraining. *Behaviour Research and Therapy, 29*, 161–166.

Salkovskis, P. M., & Warwick, H. M. C. (1986). Morbid preoccupations, health anxiety and reassurance: A cognitive-behavioral approach to hypochondriasis. *Behaviour Research and Therapy, 24*, 597–602.

Salkovskis, P. M., Warwick, H. M. C., Clark, D. M., & Wessels, D. J. (1986). A demonstration of acute hyperventilation during naturally occurring panic attacks. *Behaviour Research and Therapy, 24*, 91–94.

Salkovskis, P. M., & Westbrook, D. (1989). Behavior therapy and obsessional ruminations: Can failure be turned into success? *Behaviour Research and Therapy, 27*, 149–160.

Sally, C. J. (1998, September 11). Psychiatric competence of Dr. Sally C, Johnson.

Salokangas, R. K., & Stengård, E. (1990). Gender and short-term outcome in schizophrenia. *Schizophrenia Research, 3*, 333–345.

Sampson, H. (1992). The role of "real" experience in psychopathology and treatment. *Psychoanalytic Dialogues, 2*, 509–528.

Samuels, J., Bienvenu, O. J., III., Riddle, M. A., Cullen, B. A. M., Grados, M. A., Liang, K. Y., … Nestadt, G. (2002). Hoarding in obsessive compulsive disorder: Results from a case-control study. *Behaviour Research and Therapy, 40*, 517–528.

Sanborn, C. J. (1990). Gender socialization and suicide: American Association of Suicidology presidential address, 1989. *Suicide and Life-Threatening Behavior, 20*, 148–155.

Sanderson, W. C., & Beck, A. T. (1989). Classical conditioning. Model of panic disorder: Response to Wolpe and Rowan. *Behaviour Research and Therapy, 27*, 581–582.

Sar, V., Alioglu, F., & Akyuz, G. (2014). Experiences of possession and paranormal phenomena among women in the general population: Are they related to traumatic stress and dissociation? *Journal of Trauma & Dissociation, 15*, 303–318.

Şar, V., Dorahy, M. J., & Krüger, C. (2017). Revisiting the etiological aspects of dissociative identity disorder: A biopsychosocial perspective. *Psychology Research and Behavior Management, 10*, 137–146.

Sar, V., Unal, S. N., & Ozturk, E. (2007). Frontal and occipital perfusion changes in dissociative identity disorder. *Psychiatry Research: Neuroimaging, 156*, 217–223.

Sarin, F., & Wallin, L. (2014). Cognitive model and cognitive behavior therapy for schizophrenia: An overview. *Nordic Journal of Psychiatry, 68*, 145–163.

Sarin, F., Wallin, L., & Widerlöv, B. (2011). Cognitive behavior therapy for schizophrenia: A meta-analytical review of randomized controlled trials. *Nordic Journal of Psychiatry, 65*, 162–174.

Sarma, S. J., & Garfield, D. A. S. (2001). The rationality of psychological disorders: Psychobizarreness theory. *Psychiatric Services, 52*, 1264–1265.

Sarmány-Schuller, I. (2010). Decision making under time pressure in regard to preferred cognitive style (analytical-intuitive and study orientation). *Studia Psychologica, 52*, 285–289.

Sasson, Y., Dekel, S., Nacasch, N., Chopra, M., Zinger, Y., Amital, D., & Zohar, J. (2005). Posttraumatic obsessive-compulsive disorder: A case series. *Psychiatry Research, 135*, 145–152.

Savoy, R. L., Frederick, B. B., Keuroghlian, A. S., & Wolk, P. C. (2012). Voluntary switching between identities in dissociative identity disorder: A functional MRI case study. *Cognitive Neuroscience, 3*, 112–119.

Sawer, P. (2015a, May 6). Andreas Lubitz: Everything we know about Germanwings plane crash co-pilot. *The Telegraph.*

Sawer, P. (2015b, March 27). Germanwings: Andreas Lubitz breakdown six years ago offers clue. *The Sydney Morning Herald.*

Sayegh, L., Anthony, W. P., & Perrewe, P. L. (2004). Managerial decision-making under crisis: The role of emotion in an intuitive decision process. *Human Resource Management Review, 14*, 179–199.

Schaeffer, M. H. (1989). Environmental stress and individual decision-making: Implications for the patient. *Patient Education and Counseling, 13*, 221–235.

Schiffman, J., Maeda, J. A., Hayashi, K., Michelsen, N., Sorensen, H. J., Ekstrom, M., … Mednick, S. A. (2006). Premorbid childhood ocular alignment abnormalities and adult schizophrenia-spectrum disorder. *Schizophrenia Research, 81*, 253–260.

Schinke, S. P., Moncher, M. S., Palleja, J., Zayas, L. H., & Schilling, R. F. (1988). Hispanic youth, substance abuse, and stress: Implications for preventation research. *International Journal of the Addictions, 23*, 809–826.

Schredl, M., Kronenberg, G., Nonnell, P., & Heuser, I. (2001). Dream recall, nightmare frequency, and nocturnal panic attacks in patients with panic disorder. *Journal of Nervous and Mental Disease, 189*, 559–562.

Schruers, K., Koning, K., Luermans, J., Haack, M. J., & Griez, E. (2005). Obsessive-compulsive disorder: A critical review of therapeutic perspectives. *Acta Psychiatrica Scandinavica, 111*, 261–271.

Schulsinger, H. (1976). A ten-year follow-up of children of schizophrenic mothers: Clinical assessment. *Acta Psychiatrica Scandinavica, 53*, 371–386.

Schwartz, S. (2000). *Abnormal psychology*. Mountain View, CA: Mayfield.

Scigliano, G., & Ronchetti, G. (2013). Antipsychotic-induced metabolic and cardiovascular side effects in schizophrenia: A novel mechanistic hypothesis. *CNS Drugs, 27*, 249–257.

Scocco, P., Barbieri, I., & Frank, E. (2007). Interpersonal problem areas and onset of panic disorder. *Psychopathology, 40*, 8–13.

Searle, J. (1992). *The rediscovery of the mind*. Cambridge, MA: MIT Press.

Seligman, M. E. P. (1974). Depression and learned helplessness. In R. J. Friedman & M. M. Katz (Eds.), *The psychology of depression: Contemporary theory and research*. Washington, DC: Winston.

Seligman, M. E. P. (1975). *A series of books in psychology. Helplessness: On depression, development, and death*. New York, NY: W H Freeman/Times Books/Henry Holt.

Seligman, M. E. P. (1988). Competing theories of panic. In S. Rachman & J. D. Maser (Eds.), *Panic: Psychological perspectives*. Hillsdale, NJ: Erlbaum.

Seltzer, A. (1983). Psychodynamics of spirit possession among the Inuit. *Canadian Journal of Psychiatry, 28*, 52–56.

Sergi, M. J., Green, M. F., Widmark, C., Reist, C., Erhart, S., Braff, D. L., … Mintz, J. (2007). Cognition and neurocognition: Effects of risperidone, olanzapine, and haloperidol. *The American Journal of Psychiatry, 164*, 1585–1594.

Shane, M. S., & Peterson, J. B. (2004). Self-induced memory distortions and allocations of processing resources at encoding and retrieval. *Cognition and Emotion, 18*, 533–558.

Shankar, R., Kamath, S., & Joseph, A. A. (1995). Gender differences in disability: A comparison of married patients with schizophrenia. *Schizophrenia Research, 16*, 17–23.

Shavitt, R. G., Gentil, V., & Mandetta, R. (1992). The association of panic/agoraphobia and asthma: Contributing factors and clinical implications. *General Hospital Psychiatry, 14*, 420–423.

Shenton, M. E., Dickey, C. C., Frumin, M., & Mccarley, R. W. (2001). A review of MRI findings in schizophrenia. *Schizophrenia Research, 49*, 1–52.

Sherman, M. (1938). *Mental conflicts and personality*. New York, NY: Longmans, Green.

Shevrin, H., & Dickman, S. (1980). The psychology of unconscious: A necessary assumption for all psychological theory? *American Psychologist, 35*, 421–434.

Shilkret, C. J. (2002). The role of unconscious pathogenic beliefs in agoraphobia. *Psychotherapy: Theory, Research, Practice, Training, 39*, 368–375.

Shisslak, C. M., Crago, M., Neal, M. E., & Swain, B. (1987). Primary prevention of eating disorders. *Journal of Consulting and Clinical Psychology, 55*, 660–667.

Shiv, B., & Fedorikhin, A. (1999). Heart and mind in conflict: The interplay of affect and cognition in consumer decision making. *Journal of Consumer Research, 26*, 278–292.

Shiv, B., & Fedorikhin, A. (2002). Spontaneous versus controlled influences of stimulus-based effect of choice behavior. *Organizational Behavior and Human Decision Processes, 87*, 342–370.

Siebert, A. (1999). Brain disease hypothesis for schizophrenia disconfirmed by all evidence. *Ethical Human Sciences & Services, 1*, 179–189.

Siebert, A. (2000). How non-diagnostic listening led to a rapid recovery from paranoid schizophrenia: What is wrong with psychiatry? *Journal of Humanistic Psychology*, *40*, 34–58.

Siegel, M., & Barthel, R. P. (1986). Conversion disorders on a child psychiatry consultation service. *Psychosomatics*, *27*, 201–204.

Silver, A. L. (2008). Karon's case of Mr. X and the "International society for the psychological treatments of schizophrenia and other psychoses" (ISPS). *Pragmatic Case Studies in Psychotherapy*, *4*, 44–54.

Simon, H. A. (1955). A behavioral model of rational choice. *Quarterly Journal of Economics*, *69*, 99–118.

Simon, H. A. (1956). Rational choice and the structure of the environment. *Psychological Review*, *63*, 129–138.

Simon, H. A. (1978). Rationality as process and as product of thought. *American Economic Association*, *68*, 1–16.

Sinclair, M., Ashkanasy, N., & Chattopadhyay, P. (2010). Affective antecedents of intuitive decision making. *Journal of Management & Organization*, *16*, 382–398.

Siris, S. G., Rifkin, A., Reardon, G. T., Endicott, J., Pereira, D. H., Hayes, R., & Casey, E. (1984). Course-related depressive syndromes in schizophrenia. *American Journal of Psychiatry*, *141*, 1254–1257.

Škodlar, B., Henriksen, M. G. (2019). Toward a phenomenological psychotherapy for schizophrenia. *Psychotherapy Online*.

Škodlar, B., Henriksen, M. G., Sass, L. A., Nelson, B., & Parnas, J. (2013). Cognitive-behavioral therapy for schizophrenia: A critical evaluation of its theoretical framework from a clinical-phenomenological perspective. *Psychopathology*, *46*, 249–265.

Skrabanek, P. (1984). Biochemistry of schizophrenia: A pseudoscientific model. *Integrative Psychiatry*, *2*, 224–228.

Skrzypek, S., Wehmeier, P. M., & Remschmidt, H. (2001). Body image assessment using body size estimation in recent studies on anorexia nervosa. A brief review. *European Child & Adolescent Psychiatry*, *10*, 215–221.

Sober, E. (1981). The principle of parsimony. *The British Journal for the Philosophy of Science*, *32*, 145–156.

Sohlberg, S. C., & Yaniv, S. (1985). Social adjustment and cognitive performance of high-risk children. *Schizophrenia Bulletin, 11*, 61–65.

Spanos, N. P. (1994). Multiple identity enactments and multiple personality disorder: A sociocognitive perspective. *Psychological Bulletin, 116*, 143–165.

Spanos, N. P. (1996). *Multiple identities and false memories: A sociocognitive perspective.* Washington, DC: American Psychological Association.

Spanos, N. P., & Burgess, C. (1994). Hypnosis and multiple personality disorder: A sociocognitive perspective. In S. J. Steven & J. W. Rhue (Eds.), *Dissociation: Clinical and theoretical perspectives*. New York, NY: Guilford Press.

Spanos, N. P., Weekes, J. R., & Bertrand, L. D. (1985). Multiple personality: A social psychological perspective. *Journal of Abnormal Psychology, 94*, 362–376.

Spanos, N. P., Weekes, J. R., Menary, E., & Bertrand, L. D. (1986). Hypnotic interview and age regression procedures in the elicitation of multiple personality symptoms: A simulation study. *Psychiatry: Journal for the Study of Interpersonal Processes, 49*, 298–311.

Spence, S. A. (1999). Hysterical paralyses as disorders of action. In P. W. Halligan & A. S. David (Eds.), *Conversion hysteria: Towards a cognitive Neurolpsychological Account.*

Spence, S. H., & McCathie, H. (1993). The stability of fears in children: A two-year prospective study: A research note. *Child Psychology & Psychiatry & Allied Disciplines, 34*, 579–585.

Spettigue, W., & Henderson, K. A. (2004). Eating disorders and the role of the media. *Canadian Child and Adolescent Psychiatry Review, 13*, 16–19.

Spierings, C., Poels, P. J. E., Sijben, N., Gabreëls, F. J. M., & Renier, W. O. (1990). Conversion disorders in childhood: A retrospective follow-up study of 84 inpatients. *Developmental Medicine and Child Neurology, 32*, 865–871.

Spitzer, R. L., Skodol, A. E., Gibbon, M., & Williams, J. B. W. (1983). *Psychopathology: A case book.* New York, NY: McGraw-Hill.

Spring, B., & Coons, H. (1982). Stress as a precursor of schizophrenia. In R. W. J. Neufeld (Ed.), *Psychological stress and psychopathology*. New York, NY: McGraw-Hill.

Stack, S. (1988). Suicide: Media impacts in war and peace, 1910–1920. *Suicide and Life Threatening Behavior, 18*, 342–357.

Stack, S. (1993). The media and suicide: A nonaddictive model, 1968–1980. *Suicide and Life Threatening Behavior, 23*, 63–66.

Stanley, M. A., & Turner, S. M. (1995). Current status of pharmacological and behavioral treatment of obsessive-compulsive disorder. *Behavior Therapy, 26*, 163–186.

Stein, D. J., & Hollander, E. (1993). Impulsive aggression and obsessive-compulsive disorder. *Psychiatric Annals, 23*, 389–395.

Stein, D. J., Hollander, E., DeCaria, C. M., Trungold, S. (1991). OCD: A disorder with anxiety, aggression, impulsivity, and depressed mood. *Psychiatry Research, 36*, 237–239.

Steinberg, J. L., Garver, D. L., Moeller, F. G., Raese, J. D., Orsulak, P. J. (1993). Serum homovanillic acid levels in schizophrenic patients and normal control subjects. *Psychiatry Research, 48*, 93–106.

Steketee, G., Quay, S., & White, K. (1991). Religion and guilt in OCD patients. *Journal of Anxiety Disorders, 5*, 359–367.

Stevens, H. (1969). Conversion hysteria — revisited by the pediatric neurologist. *Clinical Proceedings of Children Hospital, 25*, 27–32.

Stice, E. (1994). Review of the evidence for a sociocultural model of bulimia nervosa and an exploration of the mechanisms of action. *Clinical Psychology Review, 14*, 633–661.

Stone, J., LaFrance, W. C., Jr., Brown, R., Spiegel, D., Levenson, J. L., & Sharpe, M. (2011). Conversion disorder: Current problems and potential solutions for *DSM-5*. *Journal of Psychosomatic Research, 71*, 369–376.

Stone, J., LaFrance, W. C., Jr., Levenson, J. L., & Sharpe, M. (2010). Issues for *DSM-5*: Conversion disorder. *The American Journal of Psychiatry, 167*, 626–627.

Stone, J., & Sharpe, M. (2006). Functional symptoms in neurology: Case studies. *Neurologic Clinics, 24*, 385–403.

Stone, J., Warlow, C., Sharpe, M. (2012). Functional weakness: Clues to mechanism from the nature of onset. *Journal of Neurology, Neurosurgery & Psychiatry, 83*, 67–69.

Striegel-Moore, R. H., Silberstein, L. R., & Rodin, J. (1986). Toward an understanding of risk factors for bulimia. *American Psychologist, 41*, 246–263.

Subotnik, K. L., Ventura, J., Gretchen-Doorly, C., Hellemann, G. S., Agee, E. R., Casaus, L. R., … Nuechterlein, K. H. (2014). The impact of second-generation antipsychotic adherence on positive and negative symptoms in recent-onset schizophrenia. *Schizophrenia Research, 159,* 95–100.

Sunday, S. R., Halmi, K. A., & Einhorn, A. (1995). The Yale-Brown-Cornell eating disorder scale: A new scale to assess eating disorders symptomatology. *International Journal of Eating Disorders, 18,* 237–245.

Suokas, J. T., Suvisaari, J. M., Haukka, J., Korhonen, P., & Tiihonen, J. (2013). Description of long-term polypharmacy among schizophrenia outpatients. *Social Psychiatry and Psychiatric Epidemiol, 48,* 631–638.

Szałek, P. (2015). Phenomenological and Psychodynamic understanding of schizophrenia (Silvano Arieti, Eugène Minkowski). *Polish Psychological Bulletin, 46,* 112–121.

Tai, S., & Turkington, D. (2009). The evolution of cognitive behavior therapy for schizophrenia current practice and recent developments. *Schizophrenia Bulletin, 35,* 865–873.

Tandon, R., Keshavan, M., & Nasrallah, H. A. (2008). Schizophrenia, "just the facts": What we know in 2008. Epidemiology and etiology. *Schizophrenia Research, 102,* 1–18.

Tarter, R. E., & Edwards, K. L. (1987). Vulnerability to alcohol and drug abuse: A behavior-genetic view. *Journal of Drug Issues, 17,* 67–81.

Taylor, S. (2000). *Understanding and treating panic disorder: Cognitive-behavioral approaches.* West Sussex, England: Wiley.

Taylor, S. (2002). Cognition in obsessive compulsive disorder: An overview. In R. O. Frost & G. Steketee (Eds.), *Cognitive approaches to obsessions and compulsions: Theory, assessment, and treatment* (pp. 1–12). Oxford, England: Pergamon Press.

Taylor, W. S., & Culler, E. (1929). The problem of the locomotive god. *Journal of Abnormal and Social Psychology, 24,* 342–399.

Taylor, W. S., & Culler, E. (1931). Note on "The problem of the Locomotive-God." *The Journal of Abnormal and Social Psychology, 26,* 340–341.

Teague, G. B., Drake, R. E., & Bartels, S. J. (1989). Stress and schizophrenia: A review of research models and findings. *Stress Medicine, 5,* 153–165.

Tearnan, B. H., Telch, M. J., & Keefe, P. (1984). Etiology and onset of agoraphobia: A critical review. *Comprehensive Psychiatry, 25*, 51–62.

Teasell, R. W., & Shapiro, A. P. (1994). Strategic-behavioral intervention in the treatment of chronic nonorganic motor disorders. *American Journal of Physical Medicine and Rehabilitation, 73*, 44–50.

Telch, M. J. (1988). Combined pharmacological and psychological treatment. In C. G. Last & M. Hersen (Eds.), *Pergamon general psychology series. Handbook of anxiety disorders* (Vol. 151, pp. 507–527). Elmsford, NY: Pergamon Press.

Telch, M. J., Brouillard, M., Telch, C. F., Agras, W. S., & Taylor, C. B. (1989). Role of cognitive appraisal in panic-related avoidance. *Behaviour Research and Therapy, 27*, 373–383.

Temple, N. (2001). Psychodynamic psychotherapy in the treatment of conversion hysteria. In P. W. Halligan, C. Bass, & J. F. Marshall (Eds.), *Contemporary approaches to the study of hysteria* (pp. 283–297). New York, NY: Oxford.

Tennant, C. (2002). Life events, stress and depression: A review of the findings. *Australian and New Zealand Journal of Psychiatry, 36*, 173–182.

Terry, A. V., & Mahadik, S. P. (2007). Time-dependent cognitive deficits associated with first and second generation antipsychotics: Cholinergic dysregulation as a potential mechanism. *The Journal of Pharmacology and Experimental Therapeutics, 320*, 961–968.

Terzian, A. C., Andreoli, S. B., de Oliveira, L., de Jesus, M., & McGrath, J. (2007). A cross-sectional study to investigate current social adjustment of offspring of patients with schizophrenia. *European Archives of Psychiatry and Clinical Neuroscience, 257*, 230–236.

Thapar, A. (2017). Intellectual disability and attention-deficit/hyperactivity disorder: What does the clinical and genetic overlap mean for practice and research? *Journal of the American Academy of Child & Adolescent Psychiatry, 56*, 105–106.

Thara, R., & Joseph, A. A. (1995). Gender differences in symptoms and course of schizophrenia. *Indian Journal of Psychiatry, 37*, 124–128.

Thara, R., & Kamath, S. (2015). Women and schizophrenia. *Indian Journal of Psychiatry, 57*, S245–S251.

Thara, R., & Rajkumar, S. (1992). Gender differences in schizophrenia: Results of a follow-up study from India. *Schizophrenia Research, 7*, 65–70.

The Irish Times (2015, March 28). Lubitz's ex-girlfriend says he "planned to be remembered". Retrieved from https://www.irishtimes.com/news/world/europe/lubitz-s-ex-girlfriend-says-he-planned-to-be-remembered-1.2157389

Thorpe, G. L., & Burns, L. E. (1983). *The agoraphobic syndrome: Behavioral approaches to evaluation and treatment*. New York: Wiley.

Thorpe, J. G., Schmidt, E., Brown, P. T., & Castell, D. (1964). Aversion-relief therapy: A new method for general application. *Behavior Research and Therapy, 2*, 71–82.

Tienari, P., Wynne, L. C., Moring, J., Wahlberg, K. E., Sorri, A., Naarala, M., & Lahti, I. (1993). Genetic vulnerability or family environment? Implications from the Finnish adoptive family study of schizophrenia. *Psychiatria Fennica, 24*, 23–41.

Tiihonen, J., Mittendorfer-Rutz, E., Torniainen, M., Alexanderson, K., & Tanskanen, A. (2016). Mortality and cumulative exposure to antipsychotics, antidepressants, and benzodiazepines in patients with schizophrenia: An observational follow-up study. *American Journal of Psychiatry, 173*, 600–606.

Tiihonen, J., Suokas, J. T., Suvisaari, J. M., Haukka, J., & Korhonen, P. (2012). Polypharmacy with antipsychotics, antidepressants, or benzodiazepines and mortality in schizophrenia. *JAMA Psychiatry, 69*, 476–483.

Torres, U. S., Portela-Oliveira, E., Borgwardt, S., & Busatto, G. F. (2013). Structural brain changes associated with antipsychotic treatment in schizophrenia as revealed by voxel-based morphometric MRI: An activation likelihood estimation meta-analysis. *BMC Psychiatry, 13*, 1–14.

Toscano, L. (1990). *Triple cross: Israel, the atomic bomb and the man who spilled the secrets*. New York, NY: Birch Lane Press.

Touyz, S. W., Beumont, P. J. V., Glaun, D., Phillips, T., & Cowie, I. (1984). A comparison of lenient and strict operant conditioning programmes in refeeding patients with anorexia nervosa. *British Journal of Psychiatry, 144*, 517–520.

Tremblay, S., Nicholls, A. P., Parmentier, F. B. R., & Jones, D. M. (2005). Visual distraction and visual-spatial memory: A sandwich effect. *Memory, 13*, 357–363.

Tryon, W. (2005). Possible mechanisms for why desensitization and exposure therapy work. *Clinical Psychology Review, 25*, 67–9.

Tryon, W. W. (2008). Whatever happened to symptom substitution? *Clinical Psychology Review, 28*, 963–968.

Tsai, G. E., Condie, D., Wu, M. T., & Chang, I. W. (1999). Functional magnetic resonance imaging of personality switches in a woman with dissociative identity disorder. *Harvard Review of Psychiatry, 7*, 119–122.

Tucher, J., & Long, M. A. D. (1985). A multicomponent behavioral treatment of conversion visual loss. *Behavior Therapist, 8*, 3–4.

Tundo, A., Salvati, L., Busto, G., Di-Spigno, D., & Falcini, R. (2007). Addition of cognitive-behavioral therapy for nonresponders to medication for obsessive-compulsive disorder: A naturalistic study. *Journal of Clinical Psychiatry, 68*, 1552–1556.

Turkington, D., Kingdon, D., & Weiden, P. J. (2006). Cognitive behavior therapy for schizophrenia. *The American Journal of Psychiatry, 163*, 365–373.

Turkington, D., Sensky, T., Scott, J., Barnes, T. R. E., Nur, U., Siddle, R., … Kingdon, D. (2008). A randomized controlled trial of cognitive-behavior therapy for persistent symptoms in schizophrenia: A five-year follow-up. *Schizophrenia Research, 98*, 1–7.

Tyrere, P. (2012). The end of psychopharmacological revolution. *British Journal of Psychiatry, 201*, 168.

Tyron, W. W. (2005). Possible mechanisms for why desensitization and exposure therapy work. *Clinical Psychology Review, 25*, 67–95.

Uchino, B. N., Trettevik, R., Kent de Grey, R. G., Cronan, S., Hogan, J., & Baucom, B. R. W. (2018). Social support, social integration, and inflammatory cytokines: A meta-analysis. *Health Psychology, 37*, 462–471.

Uchinuma, Y., & Sekine, Y. (2000). Dissociative identity disorder (DID) in Japan: A forensic case report and the recent increase in reports of DID. *International Journal of Psychiatry in Clinical Practice, 4*, 155–160.

Uhrlass, D. J., Schofield, C. A., Coles, M. E., & Gibb, B. E. (2009). Self-perceived competence and prospective changes in symptoms of depression and social anxiety. *Journal of Behavior Therapy and Experimental Psychiatry*, *40*, 329–337.

Ullmann, L. P., & Krasner, L. (1975). *A psychological approach to abnormal behavior* (2nd ed.). Englewood Cliffs, NJ: Prentice Hall.

Usall, J., López-Carrilero, R., Iniesta, R., Roca, M., Caballero, M., Rodriguez-Jimenez, R., ... Abordaje Síntomas Negativos Esquizofrenia (ASINE) Group (2014). Double-blind, placebo-controlled study of the efficacy of reboxetine and citalopram as adjuncts to atypical antipsychotics for negative symptoms of schizophrenia. *Journal of Clinical Psychiatry*, *75*, 608–615.

Valença, A. M., Falcào, R., Freire, R. C., Nascimento, I., Nascentes, R., Zin, W. A., & Nardi, A. E. (2006). The relationship between the severity of asthma and comorbidities with anxiety and depressive disorders. *Revista Brasileira de Psiquiatria*, *28*, 206–208.

Valença, A. M., Mendlowicz, M. V, Nascimento, I., & Nardi, A. E. (2011). Filicide, attempted filicide, and psychotic disorders. *Journal of Forensic Sciences*, *56*, 551–554.

Van Balkom, A. J. L. M., Van Oppen, P., Vermeulen, A. W., Van Dyck, R., Nauta, M. C. E., & Vorst, H. C. M. (1994). A meta-analysis on the treatment of obsessive compulsive disorder: A comparison of antidepressants, behavior, and cognitive therapy. *Clinical Psychology Review*, *14*, 359–381.

Van Beilen, M., Vogt, B. A., & Leenders, K. L. (2010). Increased activation in cingulate cortex in conversion disorder: What does it mean? *Journal of the Neurological Sciences*, *289*, 155–158.

Van Pelt, S. J. (1975). The role of hypnotic suggestion in the etiology and treatment of the psychoneurotic. *Journal of the American Institute of Hypnosis*, *16*, 27–33.

Van Putten, T., Crumpton, E., & Yale, C. (1976). Drug refusal in schizophrenia and the wish to be crazy. *Archives of General Psychiatry*, *33*, 1443–1446.

Vandereycken, W. (2006a). Denial of illness in anorexia nervosa — a conceptual review: Part 1 diagnostic significance and assessment. *European Eating Disorder Review*, *14*, 341–351.

Vandereycken, W. (2006b). Denial of illness in anorexia nervosa — a conceptual review: Part 2 different forms and meanings. *European Eating Disorder Review, 14*, 352–368.

Vanunu, M. (1990). Cr. App 172/88 Vanunu v. State of Israel, Pd., *44*(1) 265–304.

Varma, V. K., Bouri, M., & Wig, N. N. (1981). Multiple personality in India: Comparison with hysterical possession state. *American Journal of Psychotherapy, 35*, 113–120.

Vaswani, M., Ramesh, S., Kalra, H., & Sagar, R. (2005). Use of selective serotonin reuptake inhibitors in neuropsychiatric disorders. In Shohov, S. P. (Ed.), *Advances in Psychology Research*. Hauppauge: Nova Science.

Veijola, J., Guo, J. Y., Moilanen, J. S., Jääskeläinen, E., Miettunen, J., Kyllönen, M., … Murray, G. K. (2014). Longitudinal changes in total brain volume in schizophrenia: Relation to symptom severity, cognition, and antipsychotic medication. *PLoS ONE, 9*(7), e101689.

Velligan, D. I., Miller, A. L., Eckert, S. L., Funderburg, L. G., True, J. E., Mahurin, R. K., … Hazelton, B. (1996). The relationship between parental communication deviance and relapse in schizophrenic patients in the 1-year period after hospital discharge. *Journal of Nervous and Mental Disease, 184*, 490–496.

Ventura, J., Subotnik, K. L., Guzik, L. H., Hellemann, G. S., Gitlin, M. J., Wood, R. C., & Nuechterlein, K. H. (2011). Remission and recovery during the first outpatient year of the early course of schizophrenia. *Schizophrenia Research, 132*, 18–23.

Venturello, S., Barzega, G., Maina, G., & Bogetto, F. (2002). Premorbid conditions and precipitating events in early-onset panic disorder. *Comprehensive Psychiatry, 43*, 28–36.

Ver Eecke, W. (2003). The role of psychoanalytic theory and practice in understanding and treating schizophrenia: A rejoinder to the PORT report's condemnation of psychoanalysis. *Journal of the American Academy of Psychoanalysis and Dynamic Psychiatry, 31*, 11–29.

Verburg, K., Griez, E., Meijer, J., & Pols, H. (1995). Respiratory disorders as a possible predisposing factor for panic disorder. *Journal of Affective Disorders, 33*, 129–134.

Vermetten, E., Schmahl, C., Lindner, S., Loewenstein, R. J., & Bremner, J. D. (2006). Hippocampal and amygdalar volumes in dissociative identity disorder. *The American Journal of Psychiatry, 163*, 630–636.

Vernon, J. A., Grudnikoff, E., Seidman, A. J., Frazier, T. W., Sandhya Vemulapalli, M., Pareek, P., … Correll, C. U. (2014). Antidepressants for cognitive impairment in schizophrenia: A systematic review and meta-analysis. *Schizophrenia Research, 159*, 385–394.

Viederman, M. (1995). Metaphor and meaning in conversion disorder: A brief active therapy. *Psychosomatic Medicine, 57*, 403–409.

Vissia, E. M., Giesen, M. E., Chalavi, S., Nijenhuis, E. R. S., Draijer, N., Brand, B. L., & Reinders, A. A. T. S. (2016). Is it trauma– or fantasy-based? Comparing dissociative identity disorder, post-traumatic stress disorder, simulators, and controls. *Acta Psychiatrica Scandinavica, 134*, 111–128.

Vitousek, K. B., & Hollon, S. D. (1990). The investigation of schematic content and processing in eating disorders. *Cognitive Therapy and Research, 14*, 191–214.

Volkmar, F. R., Poll, J., & Lewis, M. (1984). Conversion reactions in childhood and adolescence. *American Academy of Child Psychiatry, 23*, 424–430.

Von Hippel, W., & Trivers, R. (2011). The evolution and psychology of self-deception. *Behavioral and Brain Sciences, 34*, 1–56.

Voon, V. (2006). Treatment of psychogenic movement disorder: Psychotropic medications. In M. Hallet, F. Stanley, J. Jankovic, A. E. Lang., C. R. Cloninger, et al. (Eds.), *Psychogenic movement disorders: Neurology and neuropsychiatry* (pp. 302–310). Philadelphia, PA: Lippincott Williams & Wilkins.

Voon, V., & Lang, A. E. (2005). Antidepressant treatment outcomes of psychogenic movement disorder. *Journal of Clinical Psychiatry, 66*, 1529–1534.

Voss, M., Moore, M., Hauser, M., Gallinat, J., Heinz, A., & Haggard, P. (2010). Altered awareness of action in schizophrenia: A specific deficit in predicting action consequences. *A Journal of Neurology, 133*, 3104–3112.

Wachtel, P. L. (1977). *Psychoanalysis and behavior therapy: Toward an integration*. New York, NY: Basic Books.

Wagstaff, G. F., & Frost, R. (1996). Reversing and breaching posthypnotic amnesia and hypnotically created pseudomemories. *Contemporary Hypnosis*, *13*, 191–197.

Waiess, E. A. (2006). Treatment of dissociative identity disorder: "Tortured child syndrome". *Psychoanalytic Review*, *93*, 477–500.

Wakefield, J. C. (1999). Philosophy of science and the progressiveness of the *DSM's* theory-neutral nosology: Response to Follette and Houts: Part I. *Behaviour Research and Therapy*, *37*, 963–999.

Waldman, A., Loomes, R., Mountford, V. A., & Tchanturia, K. (2013). Attitudinal and perceptual factors in body image distortion: An exploratory study in patients with anorexia nervosa. *Journal of Eating Disorders*, *1*, 17.

Walker, E. F., & Diforio, D. (1997). Schizophrenia: A neural diathesis-stress model. *Psychological Review*, *104*, 667–685.

Wang, H. R., Woo, Y. S., & Bahk, W. (2014). The potential role of atypical antipsychotics in the treatment of panic disorder. *Human Psychopharmacology: Clinical and Experimental*, *29*, 405–413.

Wänke, M., & Friese, M. (2005). The role of experience in consumer decisions: The case of brand loyalty. In T. Betsch & S. Haberstroh (Eds.), *The routines of decision making* (pp. 289–309). London, England: Erlbaum.

Wardle, J., Hayward, P., Higgit, A., Brewin, C. R., & Gray, J. (1997). Causes of agoraphobia: The patient's perspective. *Behavioural and Cognitive Psychotherapy*, *25*, 27–37.

Warelow, P., & Holmes, C. A. (2011). Deconstructing the *DSM-IV*-TR: A critical perspective. *International Journal of Mental Health Nursing*, *20*, 383–391.

Warwick, H. M., & Salkovskis, P. M. (1990). Unwanted erections in obsessive-compulsive disorder. *The British Journal of Psychiatry*, *157*, 919–921.

Watt, N. F. (1978). Patterns of childhood social development in adult schizophrenics. *Archives of General Psychiatry*, *35*, 160–165.

Watt, N. F., Grubb, T. W., & Erlenmeyer-Kimiling, L. (1982). Social, emotional, and intellectual behavior at school among children at high risk for schizophrenia. *Journal of Consulting and Clinical Psychology*, *2*, 171–181.

Watt, N. F., & Lubensky, A. W. (1976). Childhood roots of schizophrenia. *Journal of Consulting and Clinical Psychology*, *44*, 363–375.

Weiden, P. J. (2002). Why did John Nash stop his medication? *Journal of Psychiatric Practice*, *8*, 386–392.

Weinstein, E. A., Eck, R. A., & Lyerly, O. G. (1969). Conversion hysteria in Appalachia. *Psychiatry*, *32*, 334–341.

Weintraub, S., Liebert, D., & Neale, J. M. (1975). Teacher ratings of children vulnerable to psychopathology. *American Journal of Orthopsychiatry*, *45*, 838–845.

Welch, K. A., Lawrie, S. M., Muir, W., & Johnstone, E. C. (2011). Systematic review of the clinical presentation of schizophrenia in intellectual disability. *Journal of Psychopathology and Behavioral Assessment*, *33*, 246–253.

Wentz, E., Gillberg, I. C., Gillberg, C., & Rástam, M. (2005). Fertility and history of sexual abuse at 10-year follow-up of adolescent-onset anorexia nervosa. *International Journal of Eating Disorders*, *37*, 294–298.

Westen, D., & Morrison, K. (2001). A multidimensional meta-analysis of treatments for depression, panic, and generalized anxiety disorder: An empirical examination of the status of empirically supported therapies. *Journal of Consulting and Clinical Psychology*, *69*, 875–899.

Westen, D., Novotny, C. M., & Thompson-Brenner, H. (2004). The empirical status of empirically supported psychotherapies: Assumptions, findings, and reporting in controlled clinical trials. *Psychological Bulletin*, *130*, 631–663.

Westenberg, H. G. M. (1996). Developments in the drug treatment of panic disorder: What is the place of the selective serotonin reuptake inhibitors? *Journal of Affective Disorders*, *40*, 85–93.

Whitaker, R. (2010). *Anatomy of epidemic: Magic, bullets, psychiatric drugs and the astonishing rise of mental illness*. New York: Crown Publishers.

Whitaker, R. (2015). *Anatomy of epidemic: Magic, bullets, psychiatric drugs and the astonishing rise of mental illness*. New York: Broadway Books.

Whitaker, A., Davies, M., Shaffer, D., Johnson, J., Abrams, S., Walsh, B.T., & Kalikow, K. (1989). The struggle to be thin: A survey of anorexic and bulimic symptoms in a non-referred adolescent population. *Psychological Medicine*, *19*, 143–163.

Whitaker, A., Davies, M., Shaffer, D., Johnson, J., Abrams, S., Walsh, B. T., & Kalikow, K. (1989). The struggle to be thin: A survey of anorexic and bulimic symptoms in a non-referred adolescent population. *Psychological Medicine, 19*, 143–163.

White, R. W. (1964). *The abnormal personality* (3rd ed.). New York, NY: Ronald Press.

White, R. W., & Watt, N. F. (1981). *The abnormal personality* (5th ed.). New York, NY: Wiley.

Whitehead, C., Moss, S., Cardno, A., & Lewis, G. (2003). Antidepressants for the treatment of depression in people with schizophrenia: A systematic review. *Psychological Medicine, 33*, 589–599.

Whiteside, S. P., & Abramowitz, J. S. (2005). The expression of anger and its relationship to symptoms and cognitions in obsessive-compulsive disorder. *Depression and Anxiety, 21*, 106–111.

Whitlock, F. A. (1967). The etiology of hysteria. *Acta Psychiatrica Scandinavica, 43*, 144–162.

Whittal, M. L., & Goetsch, V. L. (1995). Physiological, subjective, and behavioral responses to hyperventilation in clinical and infrequent panic. *Behaviour Research and Therapy, 33*, 415–422.

Wijesinghe, C. P., Dissanayake, S. A. W., & Mendis, N. (1976). Possession trance in a semi-urban community in Sri Lanka. *Australian and New Zealand Journal of Psychiatry, 10*, 135–139.

Wilbur, C. B. (1984). Treatment of multiple personality. *Psychiatric Annals, 14*, 27–31.

Willi, J., Giacometti, G., & Limacher, B. (1990). Update on the epidemiology of anorexia nervosa in a defined region of Switzerland. *American Journal of Psychiatry, 147*, 1514–1517.

Williams, K. E., Chambless, D. L., & Ahrens, A. (1997). Are emotions frightening? An extension of the fear of fear construct. *Behaviour Research and Therapy, 35*, 239–248.

Williams, K. L., & Galliher, R. V. (2006). Predicting depression and self-esteem from social connectedness, support, and competence. *Journal of Social and Clinical Psychology, 25*, 855–874.

Williams, P. (2012). *Rethinking madness: Towards a paradigm shift in our understanding and treatment of psychoses*. San Francisco, CA: Sky's Edge Publishing.

Willick, M. S. (2001). Psychoanalysis and schizophrenia: A cautionary tale. *Journal of the American Psychoanalytic Association*, *49*, 27–56.

Willick, M. S. (2002). Martin S. Willick replies. *Journal of the American Psychoanalytic Association*, *50*, 316–319.

Wills, T. A. (1981). Downward comparison principles in social psychology. *Psychological Bulletin*, *90*, 245–271.

Wilson, G. T. (1999). Cognitive behavior therapy for eating disorders: Progress and problems. *Behaviour Research and Therapy*, *37*, S79–S95.

Wilson, T. D., & Dunn, E. W. (2004). Self-knowledge: Its limits, value and potential for improvement. *Annual Review of Psychology*, *55*, 493–518.

Wisner, K. M., Chiappelli, J., Savransky, A., Fisseha, F., Rowland, L. M., Kochunov, P., & Hong, L. E. (2019). Cingulum and abnormal psychological stress response in schizophrenia. *Brain Imaging and Behavior*. Advance Online Publication

Wittchen, H. U, Nocon, A., Beesdo, K., Pine, D. S., Höfler, M., Lieb, R., & Gloster, A. T. (2008). Agoraphobia and panic. *Psychotherapy and Psychosomatics*, *77*, 147–157.

Wittkower, E., Rodger, T. F., Scott, G. I., & Semeonoff, B. (1941). "Night-blindness" — a psychophysiological study. *British Medical Journal*, *2*, 571–575, 607–611.

Witztum, E., Grisaru, N., & Budowski, D. (1996). The "Zar" possession syndrome among Ethiopian immigrants to Israel: Cultural and clinical aspects. *British Journal of Medical Psychology*, *69*, 207–225.

Wolach, I., & Pratt, H. (2001). The mode of short-term memory encoding as indicated by event-related potentials in a memory scanning task with distractions. *Clinical Neurophysiology*, *112*, 186–197.

Wolf, A., Leucht, S., & Pajonk, F. (2017). Do antipsychotics lead to cognitive impairment in dementia? A meta-analysis of randomized placebo-controlled trials. *European Archives of Psychiatry and Clinical Neuroscience*, *267*, 187–198.

Wolfe, B. E. (1995). Dimensions of response to antidepressant agents in bulimia nervosa: A review. *Archives of Psychiatric Nursing*, *9*, 111–121.

Wolitzky, D. L., & Eagle, M. N. (1999). Psychoanalytic approaches. In M. Hersen & A. S. Bellack (Eds.), *Handbook of comparative interventions for adult disorders* (pp. 181–224). Hoboken, NJ: John Wiley.

Wolpe, J. (1981). The dichotomy between classical conditioned and cognitively learned anxiety. *Journal of Behavior Therapy and Experimental Psychiatry, 12*, 35–42.

Wolpe, J., & Rowan, V. C. (1988). Panic disorder: A product of classical conditioning. *Behaviour Research and Therapy, 26*, 441–450.

Wood, A. M., & Joseph, S. (2010). Correspondence. *Psychological Medicine, 40*, 1055–1056.

Woodward, T. S., Munz, M., LeClerc, C., & Lecomte, T. (2009). Change in delusions is associated with change in "jumping to conclusions." *Psychiatry Research, 170*, 124–127.

Woody, J. M. (2003). The unconscious as a hermeneutic myth: A defense of the imagination. In J. Phillips & J. Morley (Eds.), *Imagination and its pathologies*. London, England: MIT Press.

Wykes, T., Steel, C., Everitt, B., & Tarrier, N. (2008). Cognitive behavior therapy for schizophrenia: Effect sizes, clinical models, and methodological rigor. *Schizophrenia Bulletin, 34*, 523–537.

Xiang, Y. T., Weng, Y. Z., Leung, C. M., Tang, W. K., & Ungvari, G. S. (2007). Clinical and social determinants of long-term use of benzodiazepines and its impact on quality of life of Chinese schizophrenia patients. *Pharmacopsychiatry, 40*, 269–274.

Yama, M. F., Tovey, S. L., & Fogas, B. S. (1993). Childhood family environment and sexual abuse as predictors of anxiety and depression in adult women. *American Journal of Orthopsychiatry, 63*, 136–141.

Yellowlees, P. M., & Kalucy, R. S. (1990). Psychobiological aspects of asthma and the consequent research implications. *Chest, 97*, 628–634.

Yogaratnam, J., Biswas, N., Vadivel, R., & Jacob, R. (2013). Metabolic complications of schizophrenia and antipsychotic medications. An updated review. *East Asian Archives of Psychiatry, 23*, 21–28.

Yorker, B. C., Kizer, K. W., Lampe, P., Forrest, A. R. W., Lannan, J. M., & Russell, D. A. (2006). Serial murder by healthcare professionals. *Journal of Forensic Sciences, 51*, 1362–1371.

Young, W. C. (1987). Emergence of a multiple personality in a posttraumatic stress disorder of adulthood. *American Journal of Clinical Hypnosis, 29*, 249–254.

Zaidah, Z. (2007). Case study as a research method. *Journal of Kemanusiaan, 9*, 1–6.

Zaitsoff, S. L., Fehon, D. C., & Grilo, C. M. (2009). Social competence and social-emotional isolation and eating disorder psychopathology in female and male adolescent psychiatric inpatients. *International Journal of Clinical and Health Psychology, 9*, 219–228.

Zandbergen, J., Bright, M., Pols, H., Fernandez, I., de Loof, C., & Griez, E. J. L. (1991). Higher lifetime prevalence of respiratory diseases in panic disorder? *American Journal of Psychiatry, 148*, 1583–1585.

Zaragoza, M. S., & Lane, S. M. (1994). Source misattributions and the suggestibility of eyewitness memory. *Journal of Experimental Psychology: Learning and Cognition, 20*, 934–945.

Ziegler, F. J., Imboden, J. B., & Meyer, E. (1960). Contemporary conversion reactions: A clinical study. *American Journal of Psychiatry, 116*, 901–910.

Zigler, E., & Glick, M. (1984). Paranoid schizophrenia: An unorthodox view. *American Journal of Orthopsychiatry, 54*, 43–70.

Zimmer-Gembeck, M. J., & Mortimer, J. T. (2006). Adolescent work, vocational development, and education. *Review Educational Research, 76*, 537–566.

Zimmerman J., & Grosz, H. J. (1966). Visual performance of a functionally blind person. *Behaviour Research and Therapy, 4*, 119–134.

Zipursky, R. B., Reilly, T. J., & Murray, R. M. (2013). The myth of schizophrenia as a progressive brain disease. *Schizophrenia Bulletin, 39*, 1363–1372.

Zhou, D.-D., Zhou, X.-X., Lv, Z., Chen, X.-R., Wang, W., Wang, G.-M., . . . Kuang, L. (2019). Comparative efficacy and tolerability of antipsychotics as augmentations in adults with treatment-resistant obsessive-compulsive disorder: A network meta-analysis. *Journal of Psychiatric Research, 111*, 51–58.

Zucker, D., Taylor, C. B., Brouillard, M., Ehlers, A., Margraf, J., Telch, M., … Agras, W. S. (1989). Cognitive aspects of panic attacks:

Content, course and relationship to laboratory stressors. *British Journal of Psychiatry*, *155*, 86–91.

Zuk, G. H, & Zuk, C. V. (2000). Negation theory as a cause of delusion: The case of the Unabomber. *Contemporary Family Therapy: An International Journal*, *22*, 329–36.

Index

CPSIA information can be obtained
at www.ICGtesting.com
Printed in the USA
BVHW092357150320
574806BV00002BA/6

9 789811 208881